REAL-LIFE GUIDE *to* DIABETES

Practical Answers to Your Diabetes Problems

HOPE S. WARSHAW MMSc, RD, CDE, BC-ADM
JOY PAPE RN, BSN, CDE, WOCN, CFCN

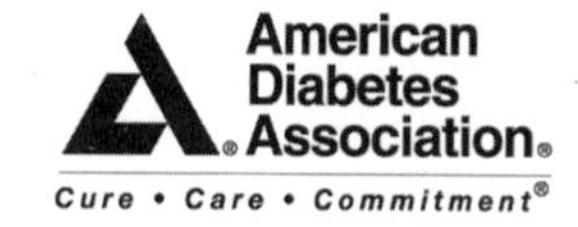

Director, Book Publishing, Robert Anthony; Managing Editor, Book Publishing, Abe Ogden; Editor, Rebekah Renshaw; Production Manager, Melissa Sprott; Composition, pixiedesign, llc; Cover Design, Jody Billert; Printer, R.R. Donnelley.

Printed in the United States of America

1 3 5 7 9 10 8 6 4 2

The suggestions and information contained in this publication are generally consistent with the Clinical Practice Recommendations and other policies of the American Diabetes Association, but they do not represent the policy or position of the Association or any of its boards or committees. Reasonable steps have been taken to ensure the accuracy of the information presented. However, the American Diabetes Association cannot ensure the safety or efficacy of any product or service described in this publication. Individuals are advised to consult a physician or other appropriate health care professional before undertaking any diet or exercise program or taking any medication referred to in this publication. Professionals must use and apply their own professional judgment, experience, and training and should not rely solely on the information contained in this publication before prescribing any diet, exercise, or medication. The American Diabetes Association—its officers, directors, employees, volunteers, and members—assumes no responsibility or liability for personal or other injury, loss, or damage that may result from the suggestions or information in this publication.

∞ The paper in this publication meets the requirements of the ANSI Standard Z39.48-1992 (permanence of paper).

ADA titles may be purchased for business or promotional use or for special sales. To purchase more than 50 copies of this book at a discount, or for custom editions of this book with your logo, contact the American Diabetes Association at the address below, at booksales@diabetes.org, or by calling 703-299-2046.

For all other inquiries, please call 1-800-DIABETES.

American Diabetes Association
1701 North Beauregard Street
Alexandria, Virginia 22311

Library of Congress Cataloging-in-Publication Data

Warshaw, Hope S., 1954-
Real-life guide to diabetes : what you need to know / Hope Warshaw and Joy Pape.
p. cm.
Includes index.
ISBN 978-1-58040-314-6 (alk. paper)
1. Diabetes--Popular works. I. Pape, Joy. II. Title.

RC660.4.W37 2009
616.4'62--dc22

2008049715

Table of Contents

DEDICATION

To you, our readers:

May the knowledge and support you gain from the pages ahead help you and members of your support networks learn how to care for your diabetes; get the encouragement you need from loved ones, other people with diabetes, and your health care providers; and stay healthy today, tomorrow, and for many years to come.

Acknowledgments

No book, and particularly not a book of this breadth and size, comes together without the help of countless dedicated people. *Real-life Guide to Diabetes* is no exception. A few special thanks are in order.

Thanks go to colleagues who took hours to review the contents of this book and provide their thoughtful critique and suggestions to improve the content: Janis Roszler, RD, CDE, LD/N; Barbara J. Anderson, PhD; and Joan Hill, RD, CDE, LD.

Thanks to people with diabetes and their caretakers whom we, as health care providers, have cared for and learned from for more than 60 collective years. It is you who have taught us so much about the need to be realistic and supportive in the care of diabetes. A special thanks to Sara Brodsky Siemen and Janet Musick. Sara is a special woman and friend, who has lived well with diabetes for many years and contributed many of the *If I Only Knew* segments in the book. Janet Musick is another special woman and friend, who lives with type 2 diabetes. Janet helped us make sure we covered the "real" issues in this book.

Thanks to the dedicated book publication staff at ADA. Thanks go to Rob Anthony, Director, Book Publishing for his understanding of the need for this title and his vision to see it to fruition. Thanks to Abe Ogden, Managing Editor, Book Publishing, for his gentle way and careful oversight of this book. A special thanks to Rebekah Renshaw, Development Editor, who edited this book and saw it through the entire production process. Her dedication to crafting this book into its final form was never-ending. Thanks also to pixiedesign, llc, for all the hard work on designing this lovely, easy-to-navigate book.

And thanks to several other dedicated ADA staff members who took time from their busy schedules to review sections of this book, including Shereen Arent, JD; Crystal C. Jackson, ADA Legal Advocacy; M. Sue Kirkman, MD; and Stephanie Dunbar, RD, CDE.

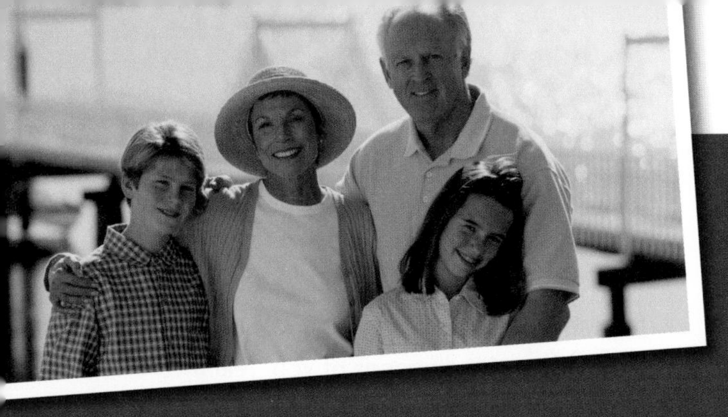

INTRODUCTION

Real-Life Guide to Diabetes

By opening the *Real-Life Guide to Diabetes* you've already taken a positive step to managing your diabetes. Young, old, or middle-aged, it can be a shock to be told you have diabetes. Managing diabetes is a balancing act between doing what needs to be done to care for your diabetes to stay healthy, and doing and accomplishing your tasks and life goals. There will be days when managing diabetes will be more center-stage and others when the commitments you have as an employer, employee, father, mother, wife, husband, student, grandparent, or grandchild won't allow you to complete your diabetes self-care list. As the saying goes, such is life!

Diabetes is a disease that puts you in the driver's seat—steering your daily activities to get and stay healthy. Daily diabetes self-care means you're on the job 24/7, 365 days a year. You'll figure out ways to manage your diabetes along with all the other aspects of your life—work, family, social relationships, religious connections, time constraints, financial concerns, other medical conditions...and more.

Research shows that you will be more successful over the long haul if you slowly, but surely, set and accomplish lifestyle changes, such as eating more vegetables each day or walking at lunch time. Over the last 20 years, new and improved blood glucose–lowering medications and faster and more accurate glucose-monitoring devices have come into the marketplace. And many more are on the way! This means that it's easier than ever to find a diabetes care plan that works for you.

Real-Life Guide to Diabetes is filled with information. Each chapter begins with a list of key points covered (What You'll Learn). Chapter contents provide you with the latest key research studies (Research Briefs), numbers to put content into perspective (By the Numbers), and definitions of common terms (Definitions). The content also dispels common myths (Myths and Facts), provides answers to common questions (Wonder?), offers practical pointers (Tips and Tactics), provides expert insights (Psst!), and even offers caution signs (Red Flag).

Real-Life Guide to Diabetes is divided into three sections:

Section 1: Build Your Strong Foundations

This section provides the initial building blocks to help you form your solid foundations for high-quality diabetes care and long-term health—knowledge and support.

Section 2: Create Your Real-Life Diabetes Plan

This section focuses on the key elements of daily diabetes self-care—choosing healthy foods, becoming physically active, taking blood glucose–lowering medications, and other diabetes-related medications.

Section 3: When Life Happens

This section accepts the realities that life doesn't always go as planned, and diabetes is expensive. Daily life contains ups and downs. You'll learn how to find a balance between caring for your diabetes and doing and accomplishing your day-to-day tasks and lifelong goals.

This book doesn't sugarcoat managing diabetes or provide pie-in-the-sky advice. We acknowledge that diabetes care takes effort, energy, and determination. We encourage you not to beat yourself up if you don't achieve perfection. You are human! We encourage you to balance the demands of your real life with those of diabetes care and to slowly change your lifestyle to live healthier and stay healthy with diabetes.

Don't delay any further. Don't spend time regretting what you've done (or haven't done) or how you've lived in the past. Today is the first day of the rest of your life!

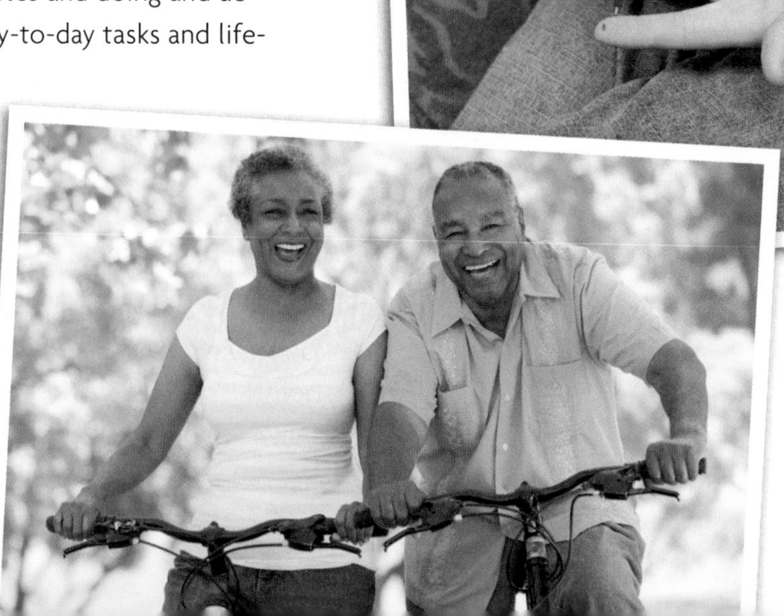

Section 1

Build Your Strong Foundations

Managing your diabetes well day to day and staying healthy over the years require you to build strong foundations of both knowledge and support. Initially you'll want the answers to a few basic questions:

- What type of diabetes do I have?
- What medications do I need to take?
- What should my blood glucose levels be?
- What can I eat?
- What do I need to do to prevent complications?

You'll find the answers to these and many more questions in section 1. You'll also want to know which health care providers care for people with diabetes and where to seek the knowledge and support you need.

The goal of section 1 of the *Real-Life Guide to Diabetes* is to provide the initial building blocks to help you form your solid foundations of both knowledge and support. Here's briefly what the three chapters in this section cover:

Chapter 1

Understanding Diabetes: This chapter helps you learn about diabetes in general and about the various types of diabetes. You'll learn what causes diabetes and how it is diagnosed. You'll learn about why there are currently epidemics of pre-diabetes and type 2 diabetes and about the connection to being overweight.

Chapter 2

Know and Control Your ABCs: Through numerous research studies, it has become well accepted that in order to stay healthy with diabetes, it's critical to get and keep your blood glucose, blood pressure, and blood lipids under good control. This chapter helps you understand the connections between diabetes and heart and blood pressure health, and provides you with the target numbers for control.

Chapter 3

Seek and Find Care and Support: To get to and keep your blood glucose, blood pressure, and blood lipids under control, you'll need to seek and find health care providers with whom you can form a successful and honest partnership. You'll learn how in this chapter. Beyond your health care providers, you'll need support from your loved ones, spiritual leaders, social network, and community. You'll gather tips to build your support networks. Lastly you'll learn how and where to connect with the diabetes community, both locally and globally.

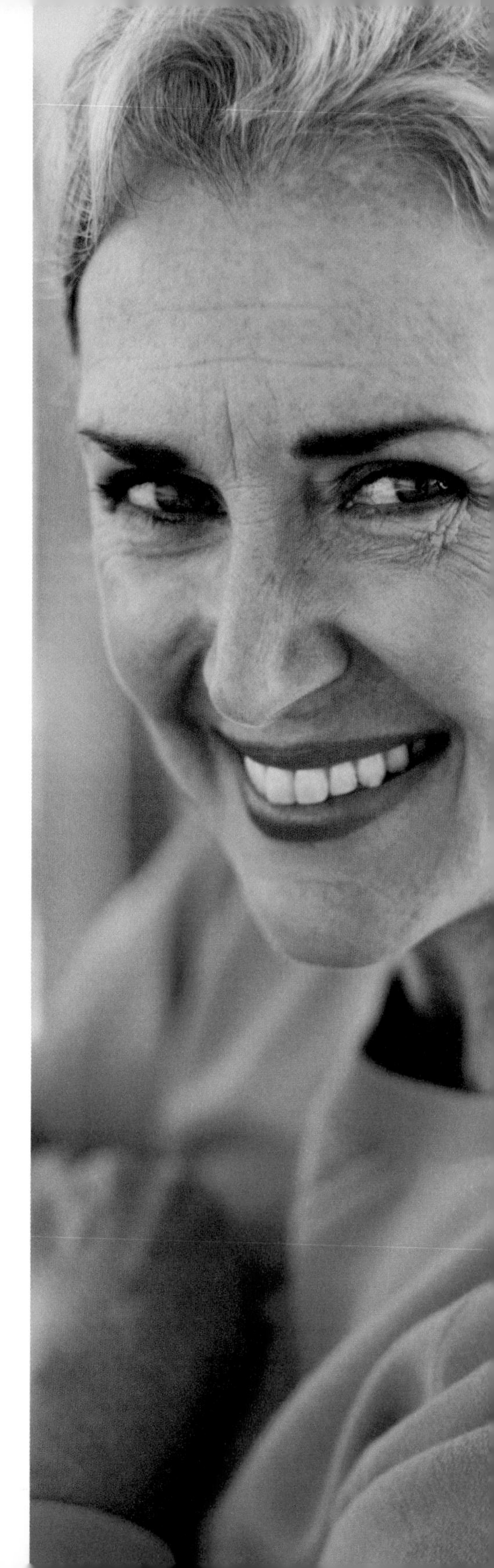

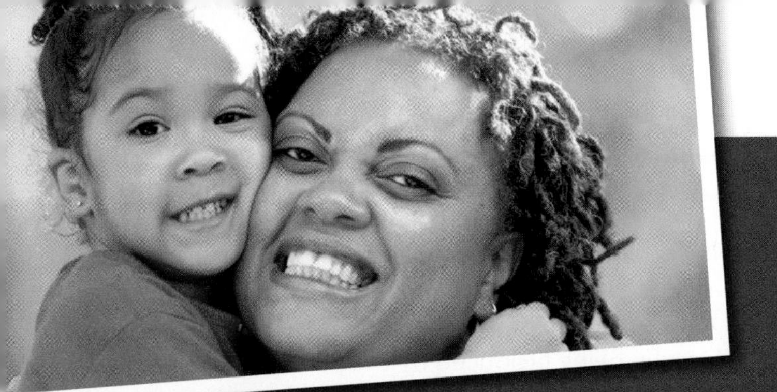

CHAPTER 1

Understanding Diabetes

Young, old, or middle-aged, it can be a shock to be told you have diabetes. You may have several family members with diabetes, may have been warned by your health care provider that you were at risk for diabetes, or may have had diabetes appear out of the blue.

You will have unique thoughts and feelings about being diagnosed with diabetes. You will have unique ways of learning about diabetes and how to manage your diabetes, specifically. A word to the wise—give yourself time and space to allow the diagnosis to sink in, move to accept that you have it, and share the diagnosis with family and friends. You will do all of the above on your own timeline.

You probably have many questions. You may have just walked from your health care provider's office into a bookstore, hopped online, and done a search for diabetes books, or may have been recently hospitalized for surgery or a heart attack and told that your blood glucose was high. Or perhaps you have had diabetes for years and are now ready to plunge into action because you just had a health scare, such as a small stroke or retinal hemorrhage that was related to your years of having diabetes.

What's most important is that you take the diagnosis of pre-diabetes or diabetes seriously and put your diabetes plan into action. The good news is that staying healthy with diabetes for many years is very possible.

What You'll Learn:

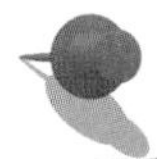

- To define and differentiate the main types of diabetes
- How diabetes is diagnosed
- What causes diabetes
- The connection between being overweight and developing pre- and type 2 diabetes
- How insulin resistance and inflammation trigger pre- and type 2 diabetes
- Essential details about insulin made by the pancreas and insulin taken by injection

Diabetes Defined

Diabetes, officially called diabetes mellitus, dates back to 1500 B.C. Even today, multitudes of scientists around the world are still trying to zero in on why and how diabetes happens… and the reasons appear to be many, and the whys are complex.

Defining diabetes today is becoming more complex. The waters are becoming muddy between type 1 and type 2. Consider these examples: adults, even children, are developing type 2 diabetes at younger ages due, in part, to obesity. Additionally, more adults are developing type 1 diabetes, often referred to as latent auto-immune diabetes in adults (LADA). It is likely that as research continues—particularly the human genome projects—we'll learn that there are actually more discrete types of diabetes.

Bearing this complexity in mind, let's start with a simple definition: Diabetes is a group of diseases that are defined by higher-than-normal blood glucose levels. The major explanation for the high blood glucose levels has to do with either insufficient amounts of insulin being produced by the pancreas and/or the inability to properly use the insulin made by the pancreas due to the phenomenon of insulin resistance.

Unfortunately, the number of people who have and are developing both pre-diabetes and type 2 diabetes is growing in epidemic proportions. It is clear that the escalation of these diseases in the U.S. and around the world closely follows the dramatic rise in obesity. Obesity is directly related to the modern way of life—unhealthy eating habits and food choices, large food portions, and too little physical activity. Today, 240 million people worldwide have diabetes, and 400 million are expected to have diabetes by 2025. If there is strength in numbers, clearly you are not alone [also check out *By the Numbers: The World View and The U.S. View*, pages 6 and 7].

By the Numbers

The World View

People diagnosed with diabetes:

- More than 240 million worldwide
  - 90–95% with type 2 diabetes
  - 7.3% of adults 20–79 years old (average around the world)
  - 9.2% of adults 20–79 years old in North America
  - Slightly more women than men

2025: Estimate 400 million

Source: International Diabetes Federation (www.idf.org)

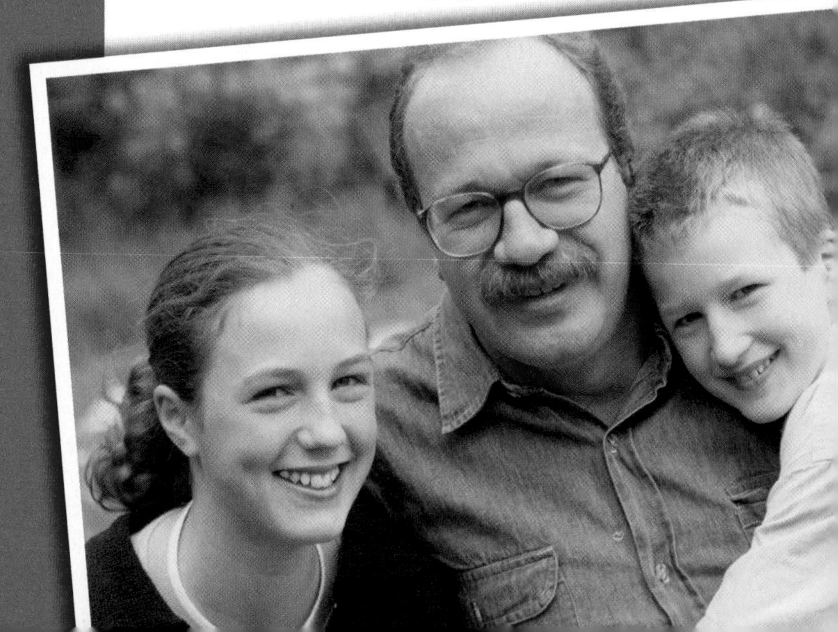

DEFINITIONS:

diabetes mellitus: a condition characterized by blood glucose levels that are higher than normal (also called hyperglycemia) due to either insufficient amounts of insulin being produced by the pancreas and/or the inability to properly use the insulin made by the pancreas due to the phenomenon of insulin resistance. This results in the body's inability to use blood glucose for energy.

pancreas: a vital organ that is a comma-shaped gland located just behind the stomach that has several essential functions. It produces digestive enzymes to break food into digestible parts and hormones, such as insulin, glucagon, and amylin that help regulate blood glucose levels.

insulin resistance: a condition characterized by the body's inability to respond to and use the insulin that it produces in the pancreas, meaning that insulin cannot function properly and over time results in the need for higher and higher amounts of insulin to control blood glucose.

By the Numbers

The U.S. View

- 24 million people have diabetes, 18 million are diagnosed, 6 million have it but have not yet been diagnosed.
- 90–95% of people have type 2 diabetes, 5–10% have type 1 diabetes.
- Women who have gestational diabetes (diabetes during pregnancy) have a 40–60% chance of developing type 2 in the next 5–10 years.
- Nearly 8% of the population has diabetes (all ages).
- 23% of people age 60 or older have diabetes.
- Diabetes affects nearly an equal number of men and women.
- 57 million people have pre-diabetes (many have not been diagnosed with this condition). Estimates suggest that up to 70% of these people (especially if they don't lose weight and control their blood glucose) will develop type 2 diabetes over time.

Source: National Diabetes Fact Sheet, 2007, Centers for Disease Control and Prevention (http://www.cdc.gov/diabetes/pubs/factsheet07.htm)

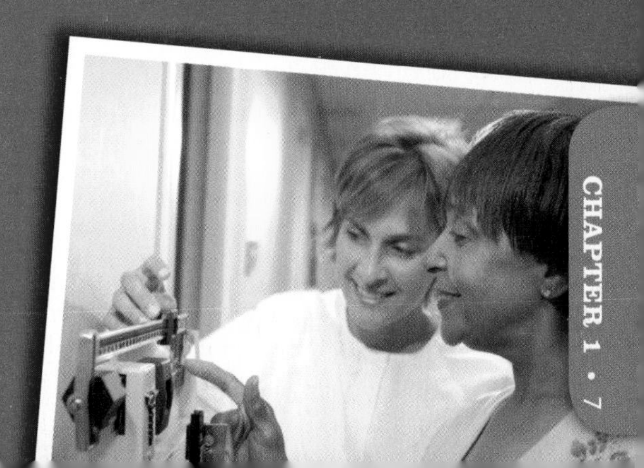

Wonder?

Does eating too much sugar and sweets cause diabetes?

Even after all these years, the causes of type 1 and type 2 diabetes are not fully understood; however, one thing is for sure: Eating too much sugar (from sugary foods and sweets) is not the sole cause of any type of diabetes. That being said, the negative health effects from eating a large amount of these foods over time cannot be ignored. Eating a lot of sugary foods and sweets, which contain calories from carbohydrate and fat, can lead to the consumption of too many calories and cause weight gain. Being overweight increases the likelihood of developing pre-diabetes and type 2 diabetes and related health problems if other risk factors (such as family history) are present.

Type 2 Diabetes

Type 2 diabetes is the most common form of diabetes. About 90 to 95% of people who have diabetes have type 2. People with type 2 diabetes, especially when they are first diagnosed, still produce at least some insulin in their pancreas. In fact, they may produce more insulin than a person who maintains a desirable body weight; however, due to insulin resistance, the large amount of insulin they make in their pancreas becomes a relatively insufficient amount to keep their blood glucose levels normal [also check out *Chapter 1: How Type 2 Diabetes Develops*, page 21].

Type 2 diabetes does not have a rapid onset. In fact, scientists report that people who are diagnosed with type 2 diabetes have often been developing it for more than a decade. This is why health experts now realize, and research has shown, that to prevent and/or delay the progression from pre-diabetes to type 2 diabetes, people need to prevent and control weight gain and promote weight loss. Slowly but surely, the beta cells in the pancreas that make insulin are no longer able to keep up with the demand for insulin, and blood glucose rises into the ranges that are used to diagnose diabetes [also check out *By the Numbers: Diagnosing and Managing Gestational Diabetes*, page 12]. Experts now estimate that up to 70% of people with pre-diabetes will develop type 2 diabetes over time, especially if they don't lose weight and control their blood glucose.

Type 2 diabetes and pre-diabetes are now considered progressive diseases, which means that over the years as blood glucose begins to rise (even before the diagnosis of type 2), there is a slow and steady loss of beta cells—the cells of the pancreas that make insulin. Research shows that by the time many people are diagnosed with type 2 diabetes (which may be 7 to 10 years after crossing the blood glucose level threshold from pre-diabetes to diabetes), they have already lost more than 80% of their beta cell function (insulin-making capacity).

If you are diagnosed with pre-diabetes, take action immediately to do what you can to delay the progression to type 2 diabetes. That means you must eat healthy, be active, and lose 5 to 7% of your body weight (about 10 to 20 pounds for many people) [also check out *Research Brief: Diabetes Prevention Program*, page 14]. At this point, the ADA guidelines do not recommend a blood glucose–lowering medication for pre-diabetes in addition to these action steps. This may change in the near future. Several large studies have shown the benefits of blood glucose–lowering medications called glitazones or TZDs in preventing and/or delaying the progression of pre-diabetes to type 2 [also check out *Chapter 8*, page 101].

Proper care and treatment can help slow the progression of pre-diabetes to type 2 diabetes. Don't be lulled into inaction thinking that type 2 diabetes is not as serious as type 1 diabetes...it is.

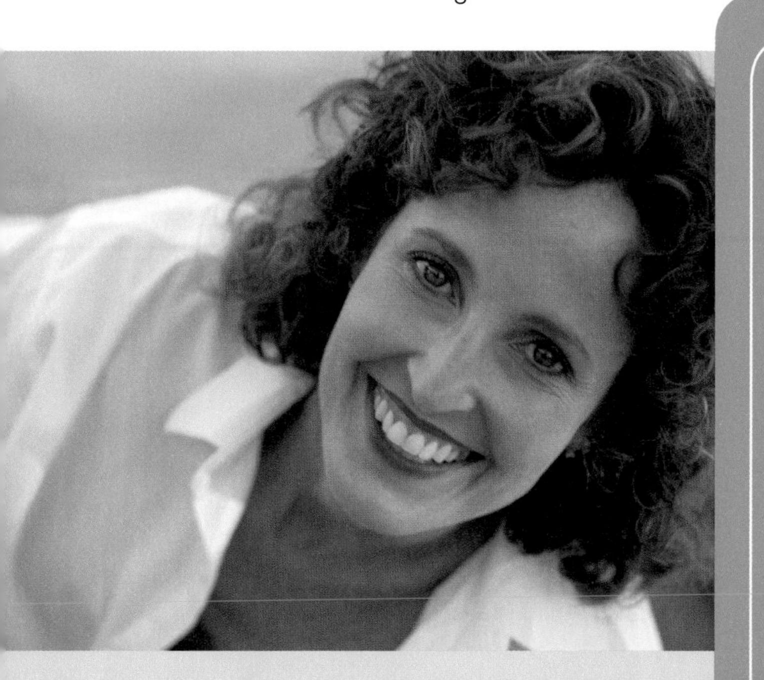

Common Symptoms of Diabetes

- Hunger
- Thirst
- Frequent urination
- Unusual weight loss or weight gain
- Irritability
- Fatigue
- Blurry vision
- Wounds that don't heal
- Numbness or tingling of your fingers and or feet
- Sexual problems: Men—difficulty achieving and maintaining an erection, Women—reoccurring yeast infections, vaginal dryness

It is not uncommon for people with type 2 diabetes to have no signs or symptoms of developing diabetes. This is why it is important to be aware of the risk factors for type 2 diabetes (refer to page 19 for this info) and follow the recommended guidelines for having your blood glucose checked.

DEFINITION:

beta cells: cells located in the islet cells of the pancreas that make two essential hormones in blood glucose control, insulin and amylin.

Wonder?

If you're an adult diagnosed with diabetes, how can you tell if it's type 1 or type 2?

If you and your health care provider are scratching your heads wondering whether you have type 1 or type 2 diabetes, your health care provider may order a blood test called C-peptide. The lab will also be asked to measure your blood glucose at the same time. This test will be done after an 8-hour fast. The C-peptide test can reveal how much insulin your pancreas is currently making.

Type 1 Diabetes

Type 1 diabetes occurs when the pancreas produces very little or no insulin. Type 1 used to be called juvenile onset diabetes, until it became known as insulin-dependent diabetes or type 1. It is diagnosed more often in children and teens but can be diagnosed well into adulthood. When diagnosed in adulthood, type 1 can have a slower onset and can sometimes be mistaken for type 2 diabetes. There are some telltale signs to determine if you have type 1. You are likely not overweight, and your signs and symptoms are similar to the onset of type 2 (refer to symptoms box on page 9). You probably are unable to control your blood glucose with oral blood glucose– lowering medication (though some health care providers may try these first). Your health care provider may want to measure your C-peptide level or your glutamic acid decarboxylase (GAD) antibodies (a marker of autoimmune beta cell destruction that is detected in the majority of type 1).

While the onset of type 1 diabetes appears to be rapid, scientists know that the development is actually a multi-year process. In fact, people who develop type 1 are born with a genetic predisposition to develop it. At some point, a currently unknown environmental injury occurs that causes an auto-immune response, which makes the body turn on itself and attack the beta cells of the pancreas. Possibilities for this environmental injury include Coxsackie virus, measles, and early introduction of cow's milk to an infant, among others

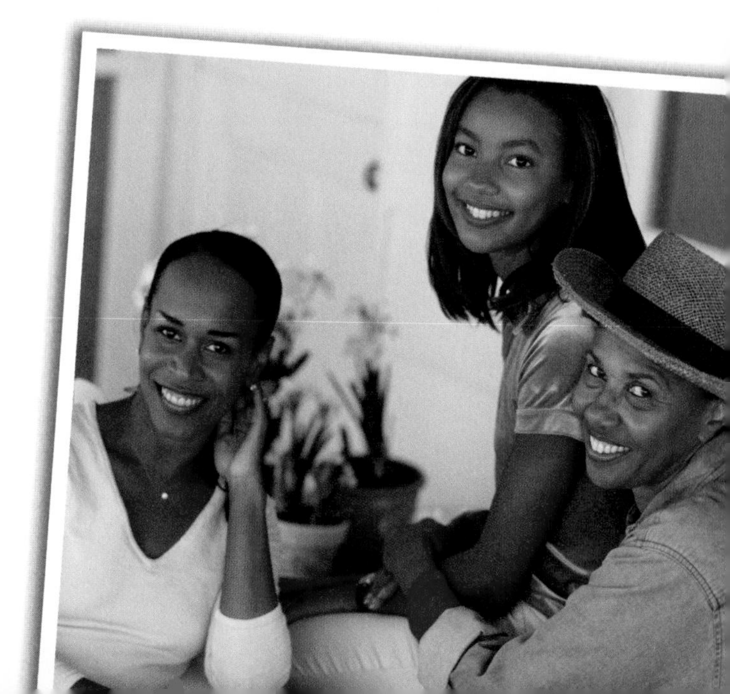

DEFINITION:

C-peptide: Abbreviation for "connecting peptide," a substance released by the beta cells into the bloodstream in amounts equal to that of insulin; testing levels of C-peptide reveals how much insulin is being made by the pancreatic beta cells.

that continue to be studied; however, no conclusive results have been reached yet.

After the environmental injury occurs, there is a phase where people's insulin-making capacity starts to dwindle slowly (but more quickly than in type 2 diabetes) and their blood glucose rises in response. Many studies are going on around the world to determine the causes of type 1 diabetes and also to determine how and when it may be possible and beneficial to intervene in the process to prevent or slow the progression of damage to the beta cells that result in type 1 diabetes.

People with type 1 diabetes need to take insulin the rest of their life to control their blood glucose levels. They need to balance their insulin doses with food intake and physical activity.

If a person is making nearly none of their own insulin, they will make very little or no C-peptide. Therefore, the level of C-peptide can be measured to give your health care provider a sense of whether you are or aren't making insulin in your pancreas.

A C-peptide test can be used to help clarify whether you have type 1 or type 2 diabetes; however, this test is not regularly done. Health care providers are more commonly beginning treatment based on your clinical situation and will change your treatment over time if they find that certain therapies, such as oral blood glucose–lowering medications, don't control your blood glucose sufficiently.

Wonder?

I was diagnosed with type 2, but now I take insulin. Do I now have type 1 diabetes?

No, you still have type 2 diabetes, but you now require insulin to keep your blood glucose levels under control. Just because you take insulin it doesn't mean you now have type 1. In addition to insulin, you may continue to need one or more medications that treat your insulin resistance. Insulin resistance, which is part of type 2 diabetes, continues over time. You may be surprised to learn that 30 to 40% of people with type 2 diabetes need to take insulin to manage their blood glucose levels.

Gestational Diabetes

Gestational diabetes occurs when the body is not able to make and use all the insulin it needs during the course of a pregnancy. Gestational diabetes is on the rise for two key reasons: more women are getting pregnant when they are older and women are more overweight when they get pregnant. About 1 in 15 women will develop gestational diabetes.

Gestational diabetes is more likely to develop during the second trimester of pregnancy, because the need for insulin rises as the pregnancy progresses. This is why most women who are pregnant should have an oral glucose tolerance test between 24 and 28 weeks of pregnancy (unless a higher-than-normal blood glucose level is detected earlier or if the woman has previously had gestational diabetes). If the results of this test are high, then they need to have an additional glucose tolerance test that lasts three hours.

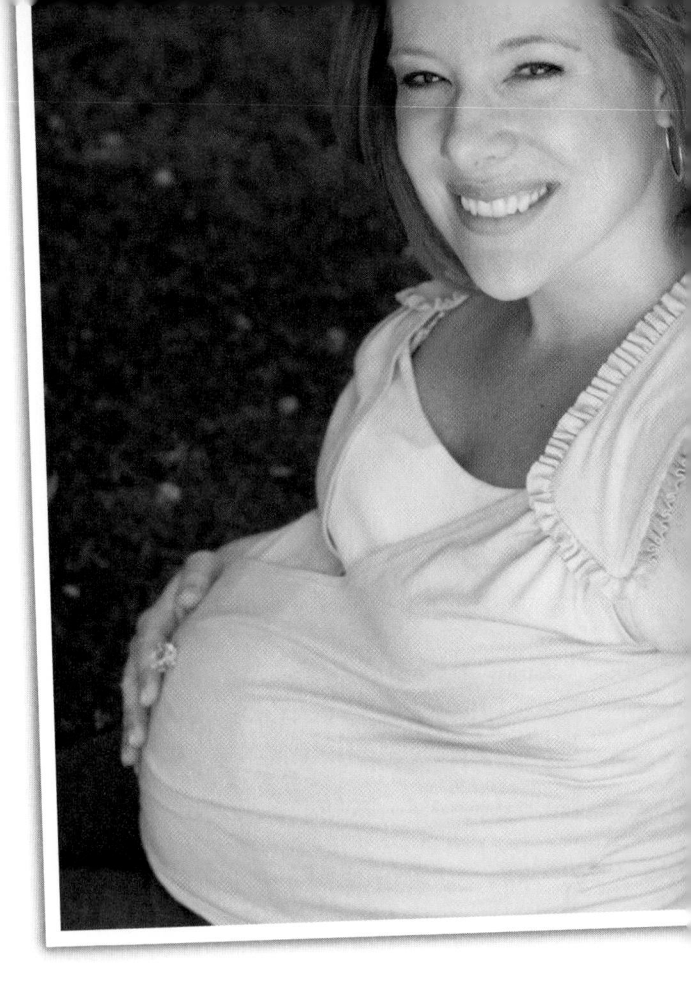

By the Numbers

Diagnosing and Managing Gestational Diabetes

Times of Tests	Diagnosis*	Management
Fasting	≥95 mg/dl	≤95 mg/dl
1 hour	≥180 mg/dl	≤140 mg/dl
2 hours	≥155 mg/dl	≤120 mg/dl
3 hours	≥140 mg/dl	

**Criteria for blood glucose levels after a 100 gram oral glucose tolerance test. Two or more of the glucose values must be met or exceeded for a positive diagnosis.*

Higher insulin needs during pregnancy are due to the hormones made by the pregnant woman. Several of these hormones are antagonistic to insulin. If a woman's body cannot keep up with the demand for insulin, then blood glucose levels can rise higher than desired to keep both mother and baby healthy. In fact, the blood glucose numbers used to diagnose gestational diabetes and manage it are lower than the diagnostic and target numbers for type 1 or type 2 diabetes [also check out *By the Numbers: Diagnosing and Managing Gestational Diabetes*, this page].

Blood glucose levels usually go back to normal after delivery; however, today more and more women are discovering that they had

DEFINITION:

impared glucose tolerance (IGT): a condition in which an oral glucose tolerance test shows one or more blood glucose levels that are higher than normal but not high enough for a diagnosis of diabetes. People with impaired glucose tolerance are at a higher risk for developing type 2 diabetes. IGT may be one indicator that a person has pre-diabetes.

type 2 diabetes prior to becoming pregnant, but it was just not diagnosed. Additionally, the ADA recommends that women with gestational diabetes should be screened for diabetes 6–12 weeks after delivery. If they continue to have higher-than-normal blood glucose levels, they should take steps to get their blood glucose under control. Once a woman has had gestational diabetes, she is at increased risk of it in future pregnancies, especially if she doesn't lose weight or gains more weight.

Developing gestational diabetes is a telltale sign that a woman has impaired glucose tolerance, which puts her at increased risk for developing type 2 diabetes later in life. Women who have developed gestational diabetes during a pregnancy have a 40–60% chance of developing pre-diabetes and type 2 in the next 5 to 10 years. Women who have or had gestational diabetes should follow the same recommendations as people with pre-diabetes—don't gain more weight, lose 10 to 20 pounds, and be physically active nearly every day.

Other Types of Diabetes

Other forms of diabetes can occur, though much less frequently than type 1 and type 2 diabetes. These types are typically brought on by another medical problem or disorder or from a treatment used for another condition. There are several categories: genetic disorders; disorders of the pancreas, such as pancreatitis; hormonal disorders, such as Cushing's syndrome; medical conditions, such as cystic fibrosis or Down syndrome; and the use of medications that raise blood glucose, such as steroids and protease inhibitors used to treat HIV and AIDS.

Pre-diabetes

Pre-diabetes is the term used to describe the common condition when blood glucose levels are higher than normal, but not high enough to be diagnosed as diabetes. About 70% of people diagnosed with pre-diabetes will develop type 2 over time; however, research has shown that with a small amount of weight loss (about 5–7% of body weight) and an increase in physical activity (about 150 minutes per week), the progression to type 2 can be delayed for several years or prevented altogether [also check out *Research Brief: Diabetes Prevention Program*, page 14].

Research Brief

CONFIDENTIAL

Diabetes Prevention Program

The Diabetes Prevention Program (DPP) was a large clinical trial conducted from 1998–2001 in the U.S. by the National Institutes of Health. The intent was to determine whether a combination of weight loss and physical activity (intensive lifestyle intervention) or the oral diabetes drug metformin could prevent or delay the onset of type 2 diabetes in more than 3,000 people with impaired glucose tolerance or pre-diabetes.

Participants in the intensive lifestyle intervention group (no medication) reduced their risk of developing type 2 diabetes by nearly 60%, nearly double the impact of using metformin without lifestyle intervention. This finding was true across all participating ethnic groups and for both men and women. The researchers concluded that weight loss improves the body's ability to use the insulin it makes and process glucose. People in the intensive lifestyle group also experienced a host of other health benefits: lowered blood pressure, improved blood lipids, and a reduction in medicines to control these conditions.

The DPP is being continued in a study called the DPP Outcome Study. The same researchers are continuing to offer intensive lifestyle intervention to all of the DPP participants—albeit not as frequently or intensively. They want to follow people over time to determine how many of them continue to be able to delay or prevent the diagnosis of type 2 diabetes. Stay tuned.

Source: *http://diabetes.niddk.nih.gov/dm/pubs/preventionprogram/*

How the body normally controls blood glucose

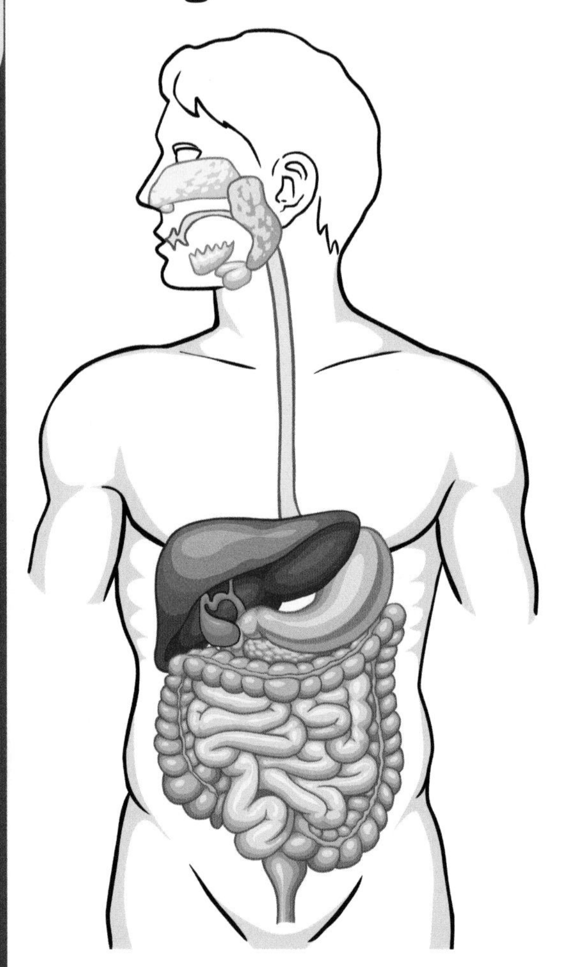

The purpose of eating is to build and nourish cells and provide the body with energy to keep it going and conduct daily activities. Foods are digested or broken down into small molecules that can be used by the body for energy (or glucose). Many organs, hormones, and enzymes are used in the process of turning what you eat and drink into useable energy.

Foods and beverages enter the body through

Diabetes Types: Know the Differences

	Type 2	Type 1
Usual onset	Slow. Can take many years (5–10) from the point that blood glucose first begins to rise to the point that it crosses the threshold for diagnosis. This is the road from pre-diabetes to diabetes.	Rapid. But the damage to beta cells and decline of insulin-making capacity is not overnight.
Usual age	Age 30 and above; however, due to current lifestyles, type 2 is being diagnosed starting in children and adolescents.	Age 30 and younger; however, people can develop type 1 at any age.
Causes	Combination of heredity, ethnic origin, excess weight, sedentary lifestyle, history of gestational diabetes and giving birth to a baby over 9 pounds. Insulin resistance develops over time, which leads to an inability to maintain normal blood glucose level.	Genetic set up to develop. Autoimmune reaction occurs that is caused by unknown environmental factors.
Diagnostic numbers	Same	Same
Symptoms	All, several, or none	All or several
Management	Healthy eating, physical activity, other healthy habits, and blood glucose–lowering medications (for many).	Insulin (exogenous), healthy eating, physical activity, other healthy habits.

the mouth. From the mouth, where you chew food into smaller particles, swallowed food proceeds into the esophagus. The esophagus connects the throat to the stomach. Once foods are mixed up in the stomach, they are moved through muscle action into the small intestine, which is 17 feet in length and has three sections—the duodenum, jejunum, and ileum. As the semi-digested food (chyme) enters the duodenum from the stomach, the duodenal lining releases intestinal hormones that stimulate the gallbladder and pancreas to release special digestive juices (bile and pancreatic juice), which help to further break down food molecules in the chyme.

It is in the small intestine that most nutrients are digested and absorbed, although different nutrients are absorbed at different speeds. Typically, carbohydrate are digested most rapidly, followed by proteins, and finally fats. The absorbed nutrients pass through the bloodstream to the liver where they are processed and either stored or distributed to other parts of the body.

In people without diabetes, blood glucose levels are controlled between about 70 mg/dl and 130 mg/dl, regardless of how little or how much one eats. For about four hours after eating, most of the glucose provided to, and used by, the cells is broken down from the last food intake. For the body's cells to use this glucose, insulin must be available.

Insulin levels always rise right after eating. Beyond four hours after eating, the amount of insulin secreted from the pancreas is minimal and the level of glucagon increases. Glucagon is a hormone, also secreted from the pancreas (the alpha cells), that breaks down glycogen (stored glucose) to provide the body with glucose (energy) when there is no new glucose coming from food.

Blood glucose control is an intricate balance of the production and secretion of nutrients, hormones, and enzymes, as well as myriad signals from the brain and other organs that maintain precise blood glucose control. It's no wonder why blood glucose is so hard to control when this intricate balance is disturbed by diabetes.

Normal Insulin Production and Secretion

Normal insulin production and secretion from the beta cells in the pancreas are critical features to keep blood glucose under

DEFINITIONS:

glucagon: a hormone produced by the alpha cells in the pancreas that raises blood glucose levels. An injectable form of glucagon, available by prescription, may be used to treat severe hypoglycemia. People with type 1 diabetes are encouraged to have injectable glucagon available for emergencies.

amylin: a hormone produced in, and secreted from, the beta cells in the pancreas; regulates the timing of glucose release in the bloodstream after eating by slowing the emptying of the stomach.

By the Numbers

Diagnosing Diabetes

	Normal Plasma Glucose Levels	Pre-diabetes^ Glucose Levels	Diabetes* Glucose Levels
Fasting	less than 100 mg/dl	≥100 and less than 126 mg/dl	≥126
2 hours after eating	less than 140 mg/dl	≥140 and less than 200 mg/dl	≥200 mg/dl
Any time of day			Symptoms of diabetes and casual plasma glucose ≥200 mg/dl

^It is more likely for a person with pre-diabetes and/or early-onset type 2 diabetes to have a normal fasting plasma [also check out Chapter 2, page 23] glucose level but a higher than normal two hour blood glucose level.

**A diagnosis of diabetes has to be confirmed with blood glucose measures taken on two different days with a measure of fasting plasma glucose, two hours after eating, or casual (any time of day) plasma glucose level.*

control. Insulin produced by the pancreas is called endogenous insulin. Endogenous insulin is put out into the bloodstream as needed based on blood glucose levels and other hormonal messaging.

Normally, insulin is secreted from the pancreas as needed in two bursts or phases. In the first phase, insulin is released in a quick burst, which lasts about 15 minutes. This insulin is ready and available in the beta cells. It control the rise of blood glucose from the first bite of food. In the second phase, insulin is released more slowly and for about 90 minutes. Additionally, insulin is secreted about one unit per hour around the clock to keep blood glucose normal through the day.

Another hormone, discovered in the 1980s, called amylin is co-released with insulin from the beta cells. It helps regulate blood glucose through the gut after eating.

People with either type 1 or 2 diabetes who take insulin by injection need it because their body no longer produces sufficient amounts of insulin to keep blood glucose under control. In the case of type 1 diabetes, people require insulin from the point at which they are diagnosed. In the case of type 2 diabetes, people may need to add insulin to other blood glucose–lowering medications they take when these medications are no longer able to control their blood glucose. (Learn more about all of the blood glucose–lowering medications in Chapter 8, page 101.) The injected insulin is called exogenous insulin. Considering the long history of diabetes, exogenous insulin has been available for human use for a relatively short time—since 1922.

Wonder?

Does diabetes skip generations?

No, this is a fallacy. Type 2 diabetes has a greater connection to hereditary than type 1 diabetes. Having a first-degree relative—a parent and/or sibling with type 2 diabetes—puts you at greater risk.

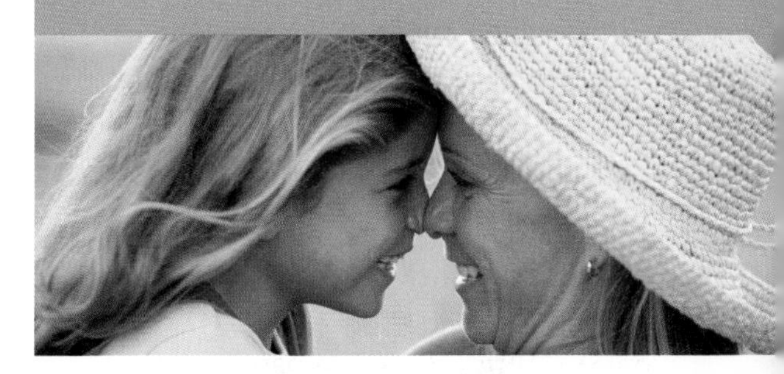

Today, the vast majority of exogenous insulin taken by injection is called human insulin. This doesn't mean it is extracted from humans as it was from cows and pigs years ago. Human insulin means it is manufactured through the use of recombinant DNA technology. It has almost the same structure as endogenous human insulin. Several types and brands of insulin are now available with more in development [also check out *Chapter 8*, page 101].

If you need insulin to keep your blood glucose levels in control, don't fight it. Taking insulin today is easier than ever before with new insulin, shorter and finer needles, and easy-to-use pens and insulin pumps.

Wonder?

Are the blood glucose numbers used to diagnose diabetes the same as the target goals to manage it?

No. The numbers you see for diagnosing diabetes are not the same as the target goals for management; however, the numbers are not very different. The diagnostic numbers are based on research that considers the levels of blood glucose at which people begin to develop diabetes complications, such as eye or heart disease. The management numbers are based on what blood glucose levels research shows help people who have diabetes prevent and/or delay diabetes complications. Additionally, the management numbers consider whether the numbers are realistic to achieve, while still minimizing low blood glucose or hypoglycemia. These numbers will undergo changes as new research is published and recommendations are changed. The most recent numbers can be found in the ADA Standards of Care at *www.diabetes.org/for-health-professionals-and-scientists/cpr*.

Risk Factors for Type 2 Diabetes and Pre-Diabetes

Research reveals that a number of risk factors put you at risk of developing pre-diabetes and/or type 2 diabetes. Several of these risk factors are related to your genes, while others are related to your age, ethnic group, and current health status. Read the two sets of risk factors in the tables on the next page. In the first table, think about whether your answer is yes or no. The second table provides risk factors about your health status and the healthy target for that risk factor. Review the risk factor and determine whether you are in a healthy target range or not. If you have pre-diabetes or type 2 diabetes, you will quickly see why you are at risk.

Psst...

Know Someone at Risk?

Do you have family members you believe are at risk of pre-diabetes and type 2 diabetes? If so, have them scan through the risk factors on the next page. If they have a significant number of risk factors, encourage them to ask their health care provider to check their blood glucose level. Also encourage them to take action now by making healthy changes to their lifestyle.

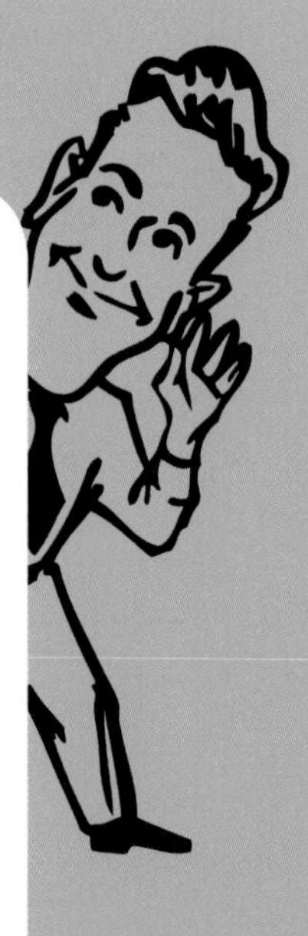

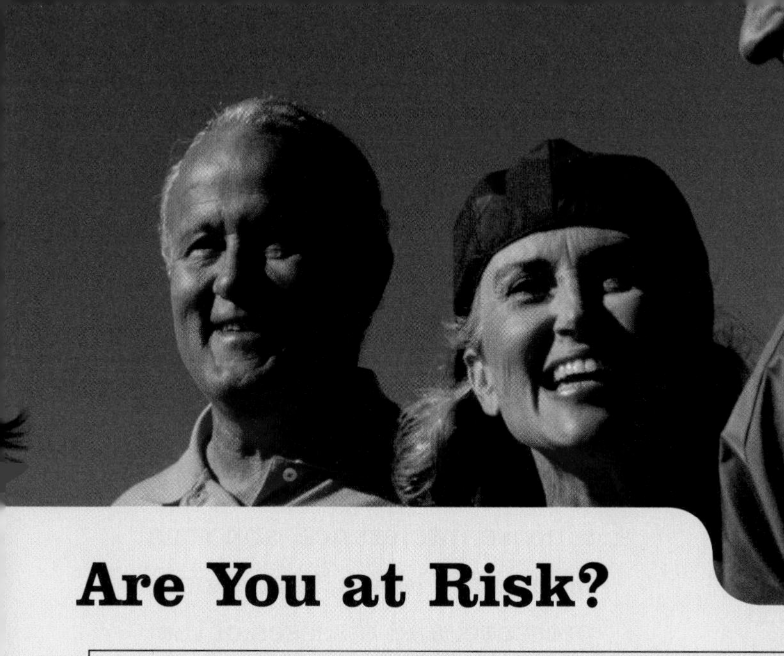

Are You at Risk?

Risk Factor	Answer
WOMEN AND MEN	
Parent or sibling who has or has had diabetes	Yes
You are over 45 years old	Yes
Member of an ethnic group that, likely due to genetic makeup mixed with current lifestyle habits, has a greater-than-average incidence of diabetes: African American, American Indian, Asian American, and Pacific Islander	Yes
WOMEN ONLY	
Have had gestational diabetes	Yes
Have delivered a baby weighing more than 9 pounds at delivery	Yes

Risk Factor	Healthy Target or Range
Overweight or obesity	Body Mass Index between 19 and 25
Waist circumference	Less than 35 inches for women, 40 inches for men
High LDL (bad) cholesterol	Less than 100 mg/dl
Low HDL (good) cholesterol	Greater than 60 mg/dl
High total cholesterol	Less than 200 mg/dl
High triglycerides	Less than 150 mg/dl
High blood pressure	Less than 120/80 mmHg
High blood glucose (goes up last)	Less than 100 mg/dl
Smoking cigarettes	No safe level
Physical inactivity	At least 30 minutes of moderate activity most days

Source: *www.diabetes.org/diabetes-prevention/checkup-america/unhealthy-cholesterol.jsp*

How the Shape of Your Body Can Determine Your Health

Are you an apple or a pear shape, and why should you care? Having an apple shape, or carrying your excess weight in your gut, puts you at greater risk of insulin resistance and type 2 diabetes than if you are shaped like a pear and carry your excess weight in your hips and butt [also check out *Apple vs. Pear Shape*, below]. Research shows that people with an apple shape have more visceral fat—more fat around their abdominal organs. This fat contains more capillaries and blood flow, which makes the fat more metabolically active than fat around the hips and thighs. Research shows that certain populations of people, such as Asians, American Indians, and Hispanics have a propensity to put on weight in their abdomen, which is a reason for their increased presence of type 2 diabetes.

Experts talk about measuring your waist-to-hip ratio. Simply measuring your waist circumference, the number of inches around at your umbilicus (navel) and determining whether you are at or below these numbers, will help you determine whether your waist-to-hip ratio means you have excess visceral fat. A measurement of less than 35 inches for women and less than 40 inches for men is recommended.

DEFINITION:

visceral fat: also known as fat around your vital organs, visceral fat is located inside the peritoneal abdominal cavity, packed in between internal organs. Visceral fat accumulation is associated with insulin resistance, glucose intolerance, abnormal blood lipid levels, high blood pressure, and diseases of the heart and blood vessels.

Apple vs. Pear Shape

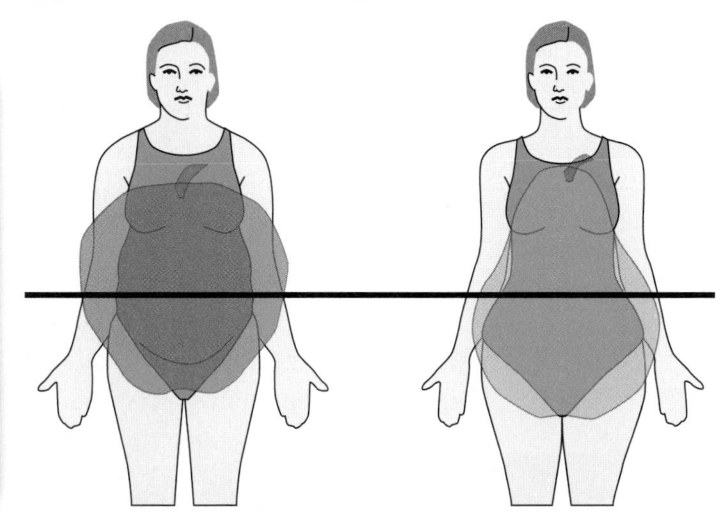

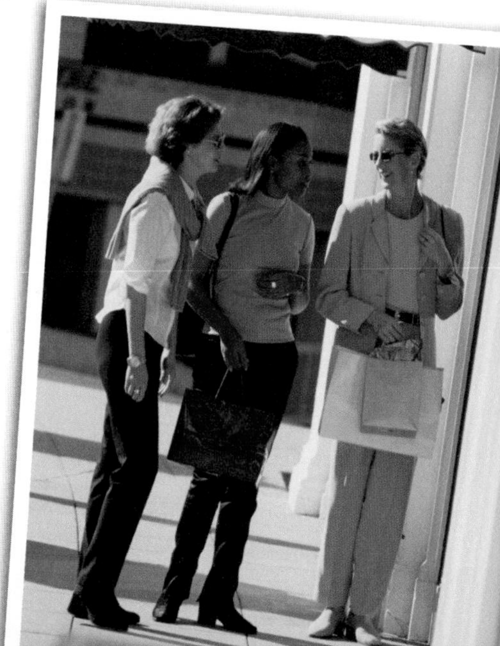

How Type 2 Diabetes Develops

Type 2 diabetes doesn't just happen in an instant. For many people, it takes 5 to 10 years to go from normal blood glucose levels to levels high enough for the diagnosis of diabetes. If symptoms don't present themselves right away, it can be another few years before diabetes is even diagnosed.

Follow the cascade of events that insulin resistance and chronic inflammation trigger due to excess weight.

- Excess weight and inactivity stoke the flame. Excess weight leads to extra fatty tissue, which releases cytokines (inflammatory markers) into the blood stream, causing inflammation.
- Inflammation causes insulin resistance to escalate. Inflammation inhibits the action of insulin made in the pancreas, which leads to the ineffective use of your body's insulin and increases the demand for insulin. These changes happen unnoticed, yet damage is occurring to the body's tissues.
- With ongoing inflammation and insulin resistance, your body powers up your pancreas' beta cells to crank out more insulin. Larger amounts of insulin are delivered to the blood stream to keep blood glucose normal; however, your lipid levels begin to go askew. Triglycerides rise, and good cholesterol (HDL) decreases. Blood pressure often rises, too.
- First-phase insulin production dwindles. Blood glucose levels rise after meals, but fasting and before-meal blood glucose numbers remain normal.
- Blood glucose climbs. The pancreatic beta cells can't make enough insulin to keep blood glucose at normal levels. Blood glucose rises to pre-diabetes levels [also check out *By the Numbers: Diagnosis Diabetes*, page 16].
- When your pancreas is no longer able to keep up with the demand for insulin, blood glucose rises to levels that are high enough to diagnose diabetes. When most people are diagnosed with type 2 diabetes, they've already lost about 80% of their insulin-making capacity.
- Insulin-making capacity continues to dwindle, causing you to need a blood glucose–lowering medication. You'll also need to continue to treat your insulin resistance with medication.

Body Mass Index

Body Mass Index (BMI) measures weight in relation to height and relates to a measure of body fatness. Use this formula to calculate your BMI, or go to *www.diabetes.org/bmi* for a quick calculation. BMI = weight (pounds) × 703 divided by height squared (inches^2).

BMI Categories

BMI Categories
Underweight = <18.5
Normal weight = 18.5–24.9
Overweight = 25–29.9
Obesity = BMI of 30 or greater
Extreme obesity = BMI of 40 or greater

Note: Research shows that people of Asian decent have a risk of type 2 diabetes and heart disease at a BMI above 23.

Progression From Normal Blood Glucose to Pre-Diabetes and Type 2

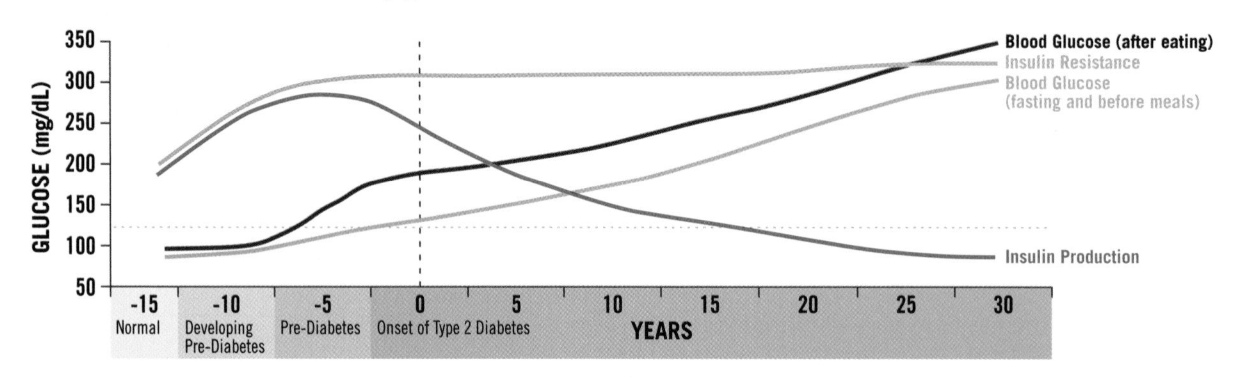

- Over time, insulin production dwindles further, so many people who have type 2 diabetes eventually need to take insulin by injection or through a pump to have enough insulin to control their blood glucose.

Managing Diabetes Today and in the Future

At this point in time, neither type 1 nor type 2 diabetes can be cured; however, a person diagnosed with diabetes can, with effort, stay healthy for many years to come. Through research on many different fronts, much is being done to learn how to prevent both type 1 and type 2 diabetes. Cures and management solutions are being sought. It is more probable that there will be a cure for type 1 sooner than for type 2.

Research into the prevention of type 1 diabetes is focusing on identifying the environmental injury and identifying people at risk (usually family members of people diagnosed with type 1 diabetes) to offer treatments to prevent or delay the disease onset. In the case of type 2 diabetes, one significant way to minimize the incidence is to get to, and stay at, a healthy weight, eat healthy, and be physically active. These actions can prevent insulin resistance and the ensuing medical problems.

Managing diabetes today is a balancing act between doing what needs to be done to care for your diabetes to stay healthy and accomplishing your life goals day to day. There will be days when managing diabetes will be more center stage and others where the commitments you have as an employer, employee, father, mother, wife, husband, student, grandparent, grandchild, and many other life roles, will not allow you to be as on-track with your healthy eating or physical activity plan. As the saying goes, such is life!

In the pages ahead, you will gain knowledge about diabetes and how to manage it ideally. You will also gather plenty of tips, tricks, and tools to make managing your diabetes realistic and practical as you strive to live well as manage your diabetes.

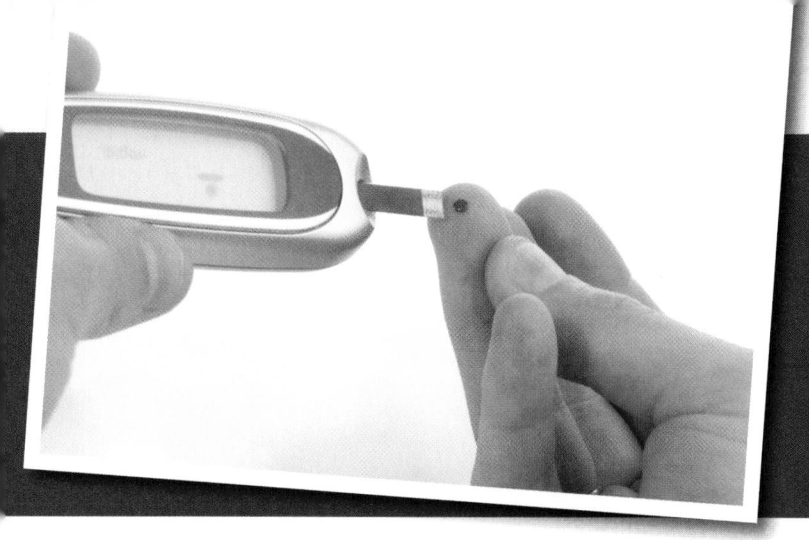

CHAPTER 2

Know and Control Your ABCs

Diabetes can have devastating effects on your overall health, so it's important to take the disease seriously starting now. Research shows that damage to the heart, kidneys, and other organs can be prevented and/or delayed by knowing and managing some key numbers that make up the ABCs of diabetes control. You learned in Chapter 1 that type 2 diabetes is not only about high blood glucose levels, but is also about insulin resistance and inflammation that usually leads to high blood pressure and abnormal lipids before you even see an elevated blood glucose level. This is the diabetes-heart connection, also called cardiometabolic syndrome [also check out *Chapter 1*, page 5].

What You'll Learn:

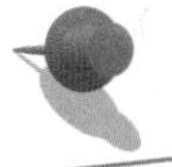

- The ABCs of diabetes control
- What lab tests you need to manage your diabetes
- How to compare your A1C test to your average blood glucose
- The importance of recording your numbers

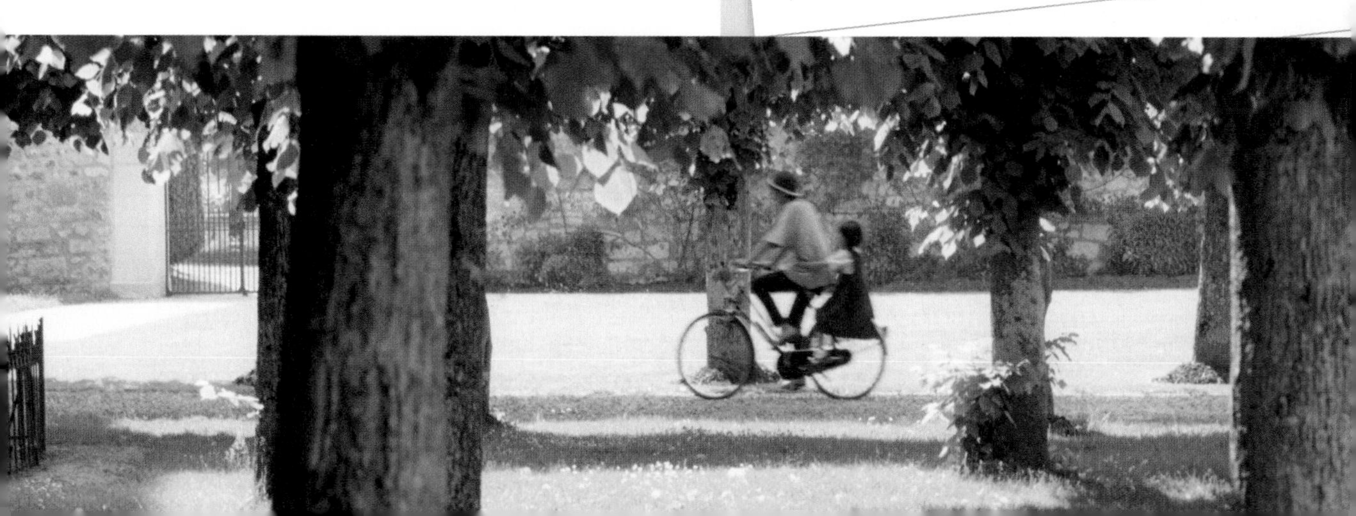

The ABCs of Diabetes

Because managing diabetes is more than just about controlling blood glucose levels and is so closely related to heart disease, the ADA and the American College of Cardiology (ACC) encourage people with diabetes to know and manage their ABCs. The ABCs of diabetes include management goals to help you live healthy and prevent the complications of diabetes.

Understanding Your Blood Glucose Numbers

As you learned in Chapter 1, your blood glucose level is not the same at all times and is affected by many things. It's important to keep track of your blood glucose throughout the day to see how food, exercise, medications, sleep, stress, and other factors in your daily life effect your levels [also check out *Chapter 1*, page 5, and *Chapter 13*, page 163].

Your health care professionals look at your blood glucose numbers in relation to when

Goals for Control: The ABCs of Diabetes

A is for...
A1C or average blood glucose

- A1C: < 7%*
- Fasting and before-meal blood glucose: 70–130mg/dl
- 1–2 hours after the start of a meal: < 180mg/dl
- ADA specifies different goals for children:
  - < 6 years old: 7.5–8.5%
  - 6–12 years old: < 8%
  - Adolescents: 7.5%

B is for...
Blood pressure

- < 130/80mmHg

C is for...
Cholesterol or lipid profile

- Triglycerides: < 150mg/dl
- LDL Cholesterol: < 100mg/dl
  If heart disease: < 70mg/dl
- HDL Cholesterol
  - Men: > 40mg/dl
  - Women: > 50mg/dl

**This result is based on the normal range of 4–6% based on the DCCT Assay method*

DEFINITIONS:

A1C test: A test that shows a person's average blood glucose level over the last 2–3 months, shown as a percentage.

cholesterol: A type of fat produced by the liver and found in the blood; it is also found in foods that are from animal origins; used by the body to make hormones and build cell walls.

you eat, so it's important to write down the times you eat to help evaluate your blood glucose numbers [also check out *Chapter 13, page 163*]. In the United States, blood glucose is measured in milligrams of glucose per deciliter of blood, or mg/dl. If your doctor wants to check your blood glucose, they will often recommend a plasma glucose test.

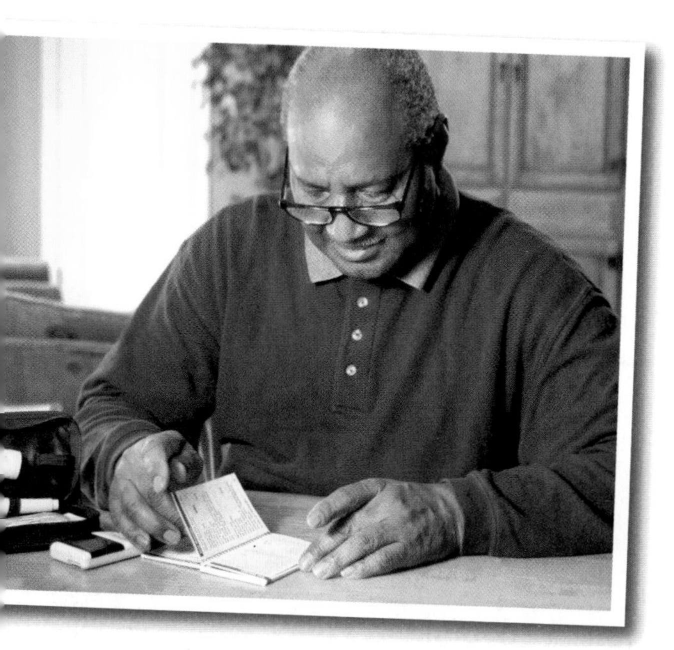

Wonder?

What is the difference between blood sugar and blood glucose?

There is no difference. You will see the words blood sugar and blood glucose used interchangeably. Don't be confused. They mean the same thing; however, we will use blood glucose in this book.

Your Target Glucose Numbers

Although this book uses the general recommendations of the ADA, these recommendations also take into consideration the fact that you will have your own unique goals and requirements. For example, although the general recommendation for the A1C test is $< 7\%$, your provider might suggest an even lower goal if it can be achieved without significant hypoglycemia or other adverse effects of treatment.

Work with your health care provider to determine your personal targets. Once you know what your targets are, you can work together to reach your target numbers. It may take adding more physical activity, eating less, sleeping better, taking a yoga class for stress management, or taking more medication, but whatever it takes, you can do it. Until you have your personal blood glucose targets, the goals provided in this book are reasonable targets.

TIPS + TACTICS

If you are instructed to be fasting for a medical test, ask your health care provider how long you need to fast, if you can drink water, and if you should take your medications prior to your test or procedure.

ADA's Recommendations for Blood Glucose Monitoring

- If you take more than one insulin injection a day or use an insulin pump, check your blood glucose three or more times a day.
- If you take one insulin injection per day or other medications to lower your blood glucose, or manage your diabetes with medical nutrition therapy (MNT) alone, blood glucose monitoring may be useful in achieving glycemic goals.
- To reach your after-eating (postprandial) glucose targets, check your blood glucose one to two hours after your start eating.
- Continuous glucose monitoring (using a monitoring device that measures your glucose levels every one to five minutes, 24 hours a day) may be a supplemental tool to blood glucose monitoring for some people, especially those with hypoglycemia unawareness [also check out *Chapter 13*, page 163 and *Chapter 15*, page 195].

DEFINITION:

blood glucose monitoring: the process by which a person with diabetes checks, records, and evaluates his or her own blood glucose levels.

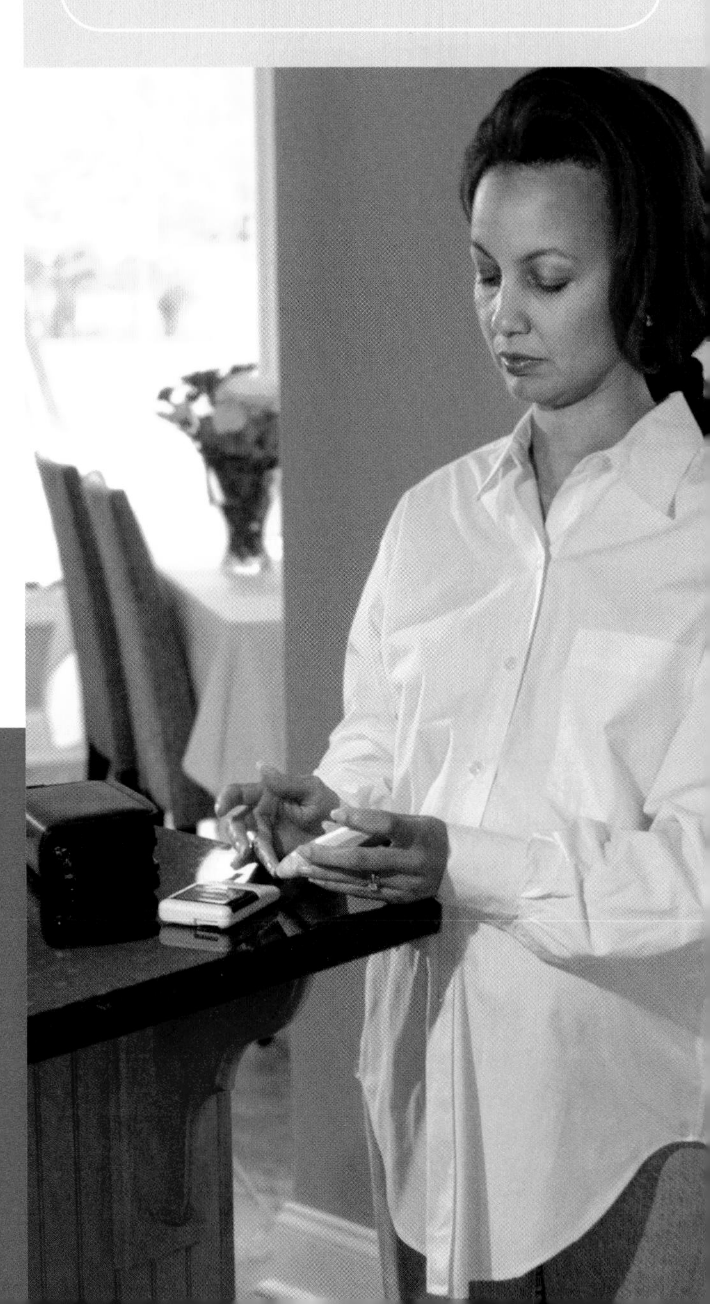

By the Numbers

ADA Recommendations for Blood Glucose Levels to Manage Diabetes

Fasting and Before Meals	70–130 mg/dl
1–2 Hours After Eating	<180 mg/dl

Research Brief

ACCORD, ADVANCE, and VADT

In 2008, there was breaking news about three major clinical studies concerning the relationship between blood glucose levels and heart disease in people who have type 2 diabetes. Since people with diabetes are at increased risk for heart disease, each study examined whether intensive glucose lowering to near-normal levels would prevent cardiovascular (heart) disease.

ACCORD studied the effects of intensive blood glucose, blood pressure, and cholesterol management, as compared to standard management in people who had heart disease or were at risk for getting it. The ADVANCE study compared the cardiovascular effects of lowering blood glucose and blood pressure in people 55 years old and older who had a history of either heart disease or microvascular (small blood vessel) disease, or at least one risk factor for vascular disease. The VADT sought to determine the effect of intensive glucose control on cardiovascular risk in people with type 2 diabetes.

The results:

ACCORD: The intensive blood glucose management part of the study was stopped due to a small increase in death rates. Experts don't agree on the reason for this, but it could have been due to the side effects of medications, weight gain, hypoglycemia, or other factors.

ADVANCE: No difference was noted in the two arms for the risk of heart disease, but the study did identify a 14% reduction in microvascular complications with intensive therapy. The blood pressure component of the study ended in 2007. It found a significant benefit in getting people's blood pressure to even lower levels than currently recommended.

VADT: Cardiovascular events were slightly lower in the intensive glucose arm, but the results were not conclusive.

You may wonder what this means for you. It means you should strive to meet the recommended targets in this book and work with your health care provider to determine whether you should have more personalized targets.

CONFIDENTIAL

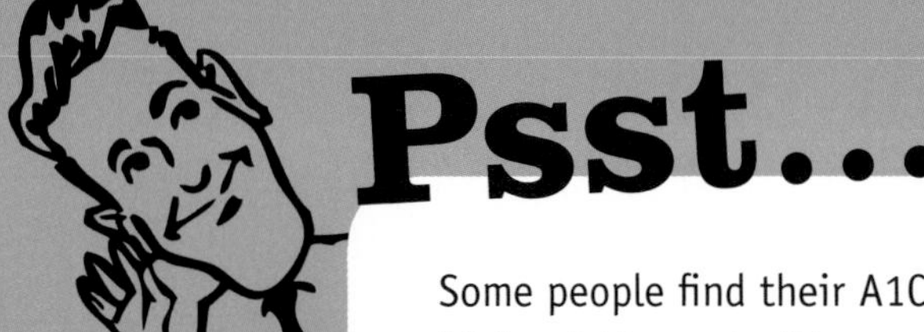

Some people find their A1Cs vary with the seasons. With colder weather comes higher A1Cs, and with warmer weather comes lower A1Cs. Although some might think the swing to higher A1Cs in colder weather is related to the long holiday, this has not been proven. Maybe the warmer weather alone causes better insulin sensitivity, or maybe you're more physically active. Check your A1C results to see whether the weather seems to affect your test. If so, try to figure out why that is. And stay tuned. The verdict is not in yet.

The A1C Test

The A1C is a blood test that shows your average blood glucose level over the past 2–3 months and is shown as a percentage. The A1C test measures the amount of glycosylated hemoglobin in your blood. Other terms used for the A1C test are hemoglobin A1C, glycated hemoglobin, or HbA1c.

The A1C blood test is usually taken from blood drawn and read in the lab. Some health care offices and clinics have a machine that can read it from a blood sample taken from your finger. There are also kits you can buy over the counter. You do not need to fast for this test.

A1C testing methods are currently not all standardized, as different labs use different methods of testing. A1C testing methods should be standardized to ensure that a 7% reading on one method is a 7% on another. At this time, there is a collaborative effort of the International Federation of Clinical Chemistry and Laboratory Medicine (IFCC)—with support from the ADA, the European Association for the Study of Diabetes, and the International Diabetes Federation, to adopt worldwide standardization of A1C measurement. This means that an A1C in one lab will mean the same thing in another lab. Ask which method is being used in your lab, and how your A1C compares to your average blood glucose.

Estimated Average Glucose

To make the comparison of your blood glucose levels and your A1C a bit easier, health care providers may begin to give you another number along with your A1C. This number is called the estimated average glucose (eAG). The readings will be reported in mg/dl just like a blood glucose result is reported.

For example, if your A1C is 7%, you'll also receive the eAG that tells you what your average glucose level is.

DEFINITIONS:

glycosylated hemoglobin: a form of hemoglobin to which glucose has joined; in people with diabetes, the amount of glycosylated hemoglobin may be increased and can be measured to determine average blood glucose levels over the last two to three months.

estimated average glucose: The eAG is an estimate of your average blood glucose derived from your A1C test.

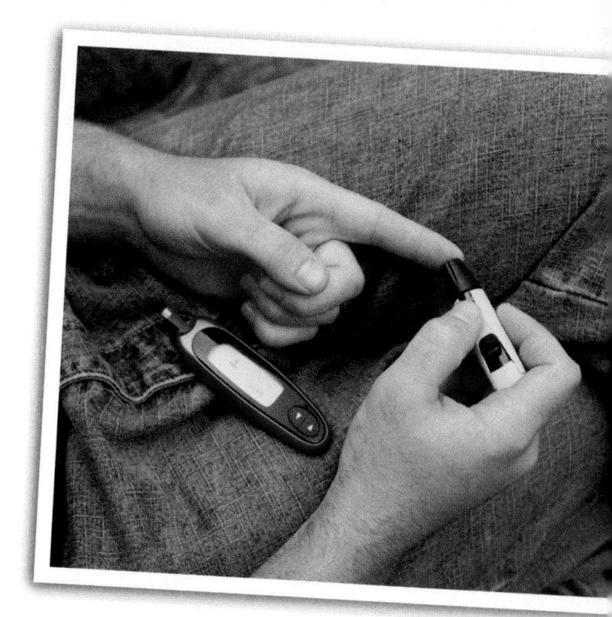

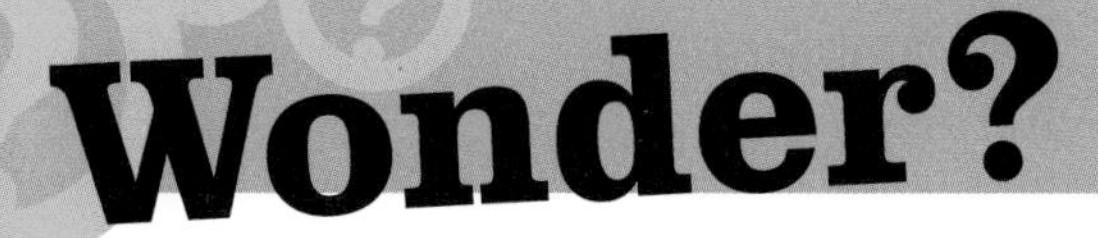

How often should my A1C be checked?

- At least two times per year (every six months) if you are meeting your targets and your blood glucose is stable.
- Quarterly (every 3 months) if you are not meeting your treatment goals.
- Use point-of-care testing for A1C. This allows for timely decisions for therapy changes when needed. Point-of-care testing means you have your A1C taken at your health care provider's office the same time as your visit, so it can be interpreted during your visit.

Calculating Your eAG

If your A1C is (%)	Then your eAG is (mg/dl)
5	97
5.5	111
6	126
6.5	140
7	154
7.5	169
8	183
8.5	197
9	212
9.5	226
10	240
10.5	255
11	269
11.5	283
12	298

Wonder?

Why doesn't my A1C seem to reflect the readings on my blood glucose meter?

Some people check their blood glucose at the same time every day. When they get their A1C result, there doesn't seem to be a correlation. This is because the A1C is an average of all the ups, downs, and in-betweens from the whole day, every day, for 2–3 months. To get a better picture with your meter, check your blood glucose more often per day, including 1–2 hours after meals. Some people find that their blood glucose can fluctuate between 60 mg/dl and 400 mg/dl, but their A1C could be 6.5%. Once again, the A1C test shows an average blood glucose level over a period of time. If you know you are having wide blood glucose swings, but your A1C seems to be within target range, talk with your health care team to come up with a plan to stabilize your blood glucose.

Research Brief

CONFIDENTIAL

Diabetes Control and Complications Trial (DCCT), Epidemiology of Diabetes Interventions and Complications (EDIC) Study, and the United Kingdom Prospective Diabetes Study (UKPDS)

The DCCT was a nine-year study completed in 1993. It showed that for people with type 1 diabetes, keeping blood glucose levels as near normal as possible slows the onset and progression of eye, kidney, and nerve diseases caused by diabetes.

The EDIC followed the DCCT study population to investigate whether the short-term blood glucose control during the DCCT affected the long-term incidence of complications. The conclusion was that even short-term intensive therapy reduces the risk of complications in people who have type 1 diabetes.

The UKPDS was a 20-year study that studied people with type 2 diabetes. It proved that, by using more intensive glycemic management, complications of type 2 diabetes could be reduced.

Impact of Glycemic Control from DCCT and UKPDS: Reducing Diabetes Complications

	DCCT	UKPDS
A1C	9–7%	8–7%
Retinopathy (Eye Disease)	63%	17–21%
Neuropathy (Nerve Disease)	54%	24–33%
Nephropathy (Kidney Disease)	60%	–
Macrovascular (Large Vessel Disease)	41%*	16*

*Not statistically significant

Source: National Diabetes Education Program *www.ndep.nih.gov/diabetes/WTMD/impact.htm*

Managing Blood Pressure

Research has proved that if you manage your blood pressure—which you can—you greatly reduce the complications associated with hypertension, also known as high blood pressure. Many people are diagnosed with high blood pressure long before they are diagnosed with diabetes [also check out *Chapter 1*, page 5].

To decrease your risk of complications from diabetes, it is important that you also know and manage your blood pressure [also check out *Chapter 13*, page 163]. The ADA recommends you have your blood pressure measured at every medical visit. If your top number (systolic blood pressure) is › 130mmHg or your bottom number (diastolic blood pressure) is › 80mmHg, you should have your blood pressure checked on a different day. If your blood pressure reaches those numbers again, you will be diagnosed with high blood pressure.

Because there is such a high correlation between diabetes and high blood pressure, many things you learn to do in this book to manage your blood glucose will also help you manage your blood pressure [also check out *Chapter 4*, page 49; *Chapter 5*, page 59; *Chapter 7*, page 89; *Chapter 9*, page 121; *Chapter 11*, page 141; and *Chapter 14*, page 181].

Cholesterol and Blood Fats (Lipids)

Although most people are familiar with the word cholesterol, a better term to use is lipid profile (lipids), which measures one of your risks of developing cardiovascular disease. The lipid profile is a blood test that measures the various types of lipids (total cholesterol, triglycerides, LDL cholesterol, and HDL cholesterol) in your blood.

In order to understand your lipid profile, it's helpful to first understand the types of lipids that make up the profile. These include total cholesterol, triglycerides, LDL (or bad) cholesterol, and HDL (or good) cholesterol. Total cholesterol is a rough measure of all the cholesterol and triglycerides in your body. Triglycerides are the storage form of fat in the body. Sometimes, high triglyceride levels may occur when diabetes is out of control. Low Density Lipoprotein (LDL) is a fat found in the blood that moves cholesterol around the body to where it is needed for cell repair and also deposits it on the inside of artery walls. High Density Lipoprotein (HDL) is a fat found in the blood that removes extra cholesterol from the blood via the liver.

Psst...

Knowing Good Cholesterol From Bad

An easy way to remember the difference between LDL and HDL cholesterol is:

L is for "lowsy" cholesterol; you want it low.

H is for "healthy" cholesterol; you want it high.

Abnormal lipid values are related to cardiovascular disease and cardiovascular disease is closely related to diabetes. As you learn more about managing your diabetes, you will learn more about how to manage your lipids as well. The good news is you can change your lipid profile and decrease your chances of getting cardiovascular disease [also check out *Chapter 21*, page 257].

By the Numbers

ADA Recommendations for Lipid Profile

Triglycerides	< 150 mg/dl
HDL Cholesterol	Men > 40 mg/dl Women > 50 mg/dl
LDL Cholesterol	< 100 mg/dl < 70 mg/dl if you have overt cardiovascular disease

Wonder?

How often should I have my lipid profile tested?

The ADA recommends most adults with diabetes have their fasting lipid profile tested at least annually. In adults with low-risk lipid values (LDL cholesterol <100mg/dl, HDL cholesterol > 50mg/dl, and triglycerides < 150mg/dl), lipid profiles may be repeated every two years. Although you hear a lot about the dangers of a high LDL, it is important to know that many people with type 2 diabetes have a normal LDL, but have elevated triglycerides and a lower-than-recommended HDL. This dangerous duo can change the type of LDL you have to a dense LDL that can cause more damage to your arteries [also check out *Chapter 1*, page 5, and *Chapter 21*, page 257].

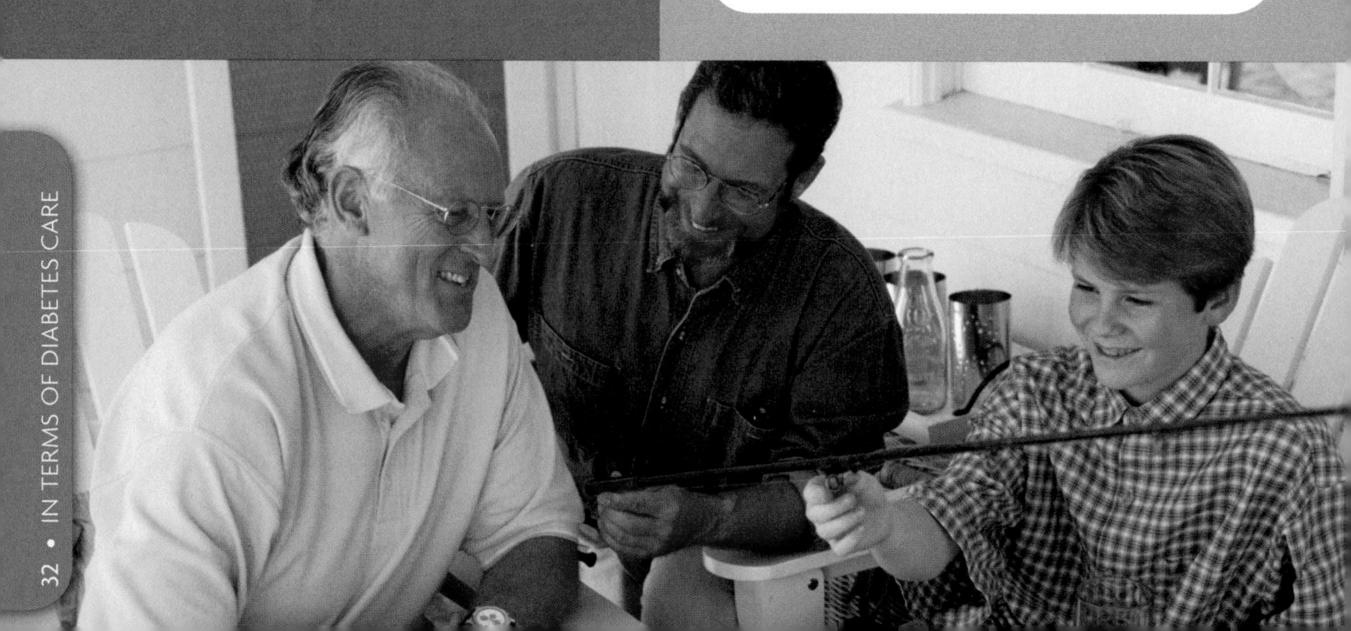

TIPS + TACTICS

When it comes to your laboratory test results, as well as other tests and treatments, always ask for a copy. Keep these forms in a folder so you can take them to all your health care exams. This is a great way to communicate with your health care provider, and also a great way for you to track your progress.

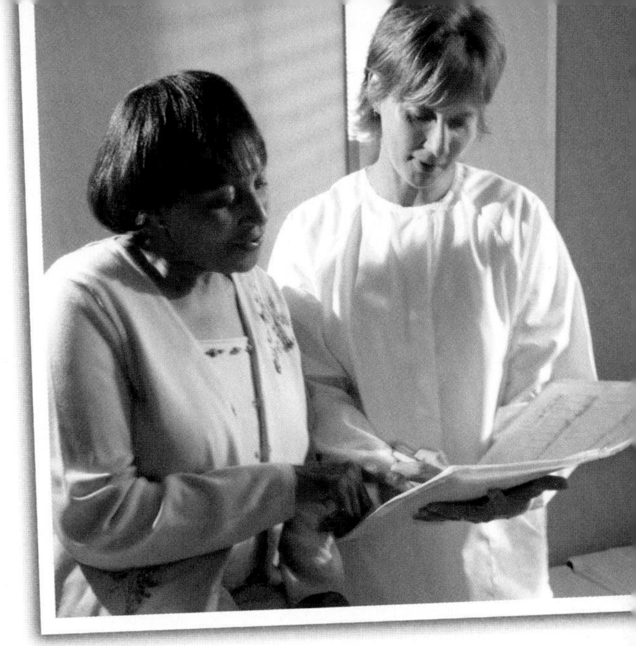

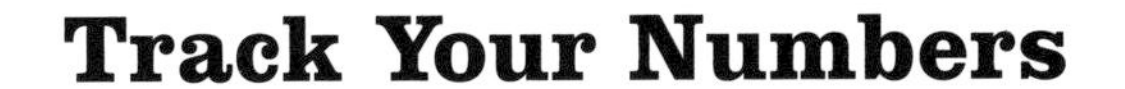

Track Your Numbers

There is a saying, "If you didn't write it down, it's as though you didn't do it." You'll find that true with your diabetes numbers. You may think you'll remember what your fasting blood glucose was this morning; however, if you don't have some sort of record of it, you won't remember it three months from now when you evaluate your overall care with your health care provider.

At the very least, record the time of day and your test results. Don't forget to note when you ate last. From here, you can add your weight, your physical activity, your stress level, your food log, and when you take medications. The more information you include, the easier it is to evaluate how to best manage your diabetes [also check out *Chapter 13*, page 163].

Evaluating Your Records

It's one thing to record, and another thing to learn to evaluate this information. As you read and learn more, you will learn that diabetes management is really a balancing act. The best way for you to manage this delicate balance in your life is to learn as much as you can about diabetes, look at your information, evaluate it, then make decisions and changes if needed [also check out *Chapter 3*, page 35].

Don't make decisions on one number at one time of the day. Instead, look at your patterns. This is called pattern management. What you do is check out the big picture over a period of 3–5 days, which should give you enough information to see what your numbers are at certain times of the day in relation to your food, physical activity, medications, stress, sleep, and any other information you think might be affecting your diabetes management. If you don't see a pattern emerge in 3–5 days, you may need to look at a longer period of time. Continue to evaluate your information every few days. Armed with this information, you and your health care team can make the necessary adjustments to fine-tune your diabetes management. It's very motivating to see how what you do (or don't do) affects your numbers [also check out *Chapter 13*, page 163].

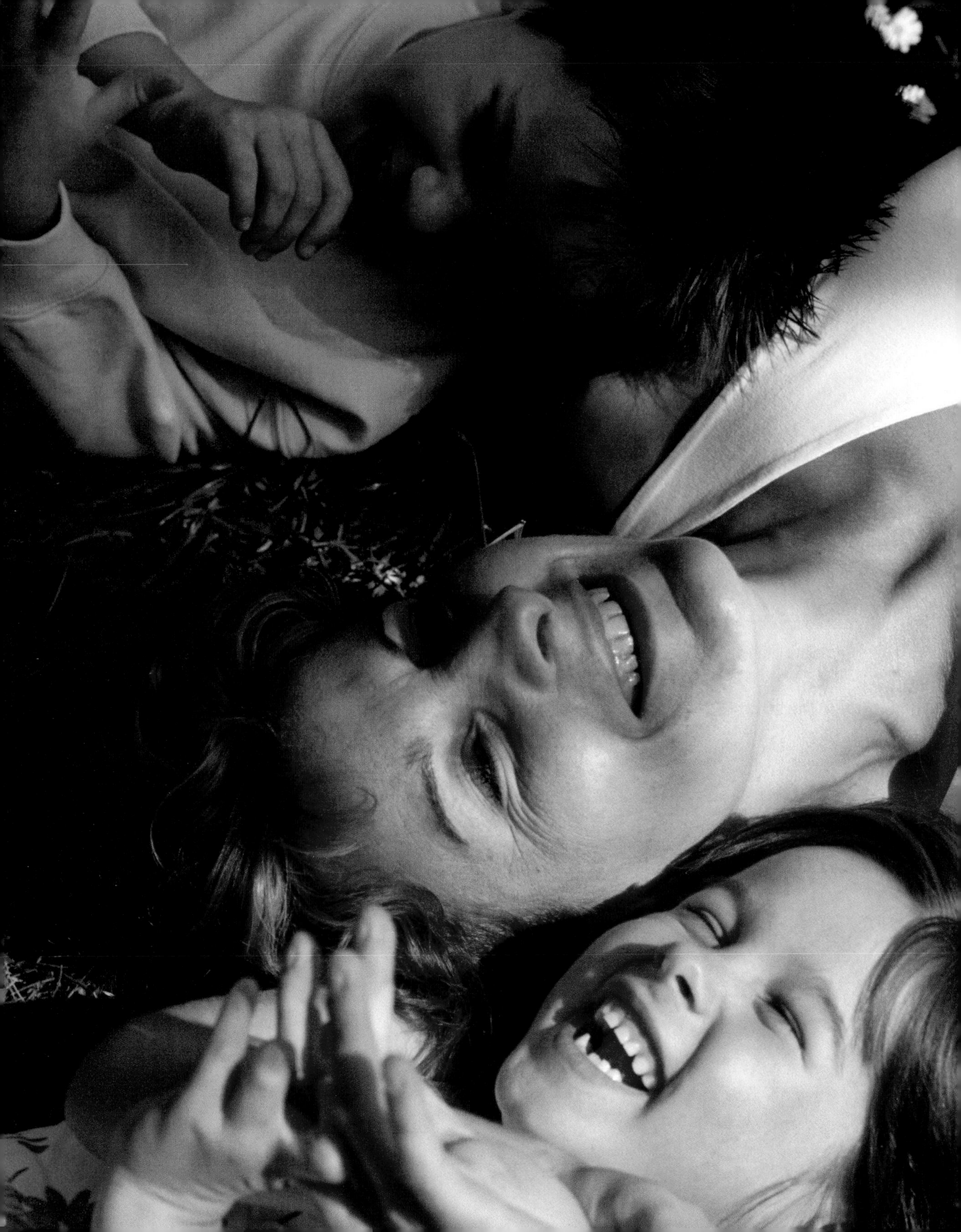

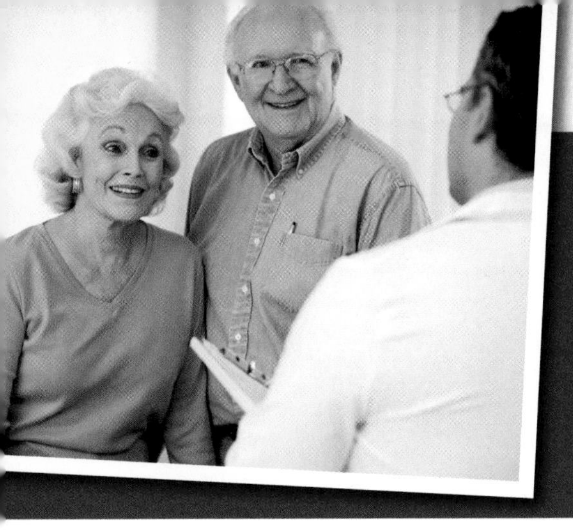

CHAPTER 3

Seek and Find Care and Support

Diabetes is a disease that puts you in the driver's seat—steering your daily activities in the direction of health and well-being. You'll spend time figuring out how to manage your diabetes within the framework of your pre-existing lifestyle and schedule. You'll want to seek out and work with health care providers with whom you can be open and honest and form a positive and supportive partnership. You'll also want to seek social support when you are ready, from loved ones, a school or work friend with diabetes, a local support group, or an online global diabetes community. Step by step, you'll begin to figure out the best way for you to manage your diabetes.

What You'll Learn:

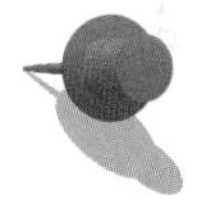

- To take care of yourself and your diabetes your way
- The diabetes health care providers you may need to help you care for your diabetes
- How to find and develop a true partnership with your providers
- How to find and nurture support from family, friends, and other social and community networks
- How healthy coping and ongoing support can help you manage successfully
- Access routes to diabetes support from local to global

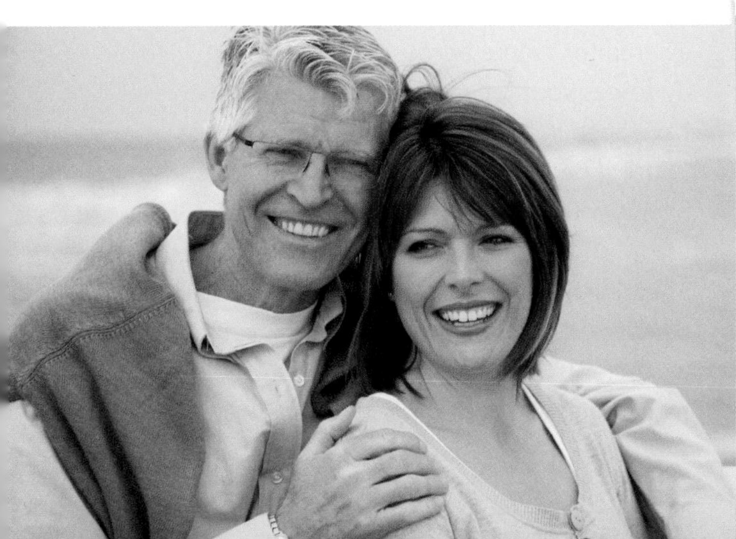

Fit Diabetes Care into Your Life, Your Way

YOU are at the center of managing your diabetes. Think about and work toward developing your support networks within each of these three categories: health care providers; loved ones, social, spiritual, and community networks; and local and global diabetes community. Developing your supports in one category might come more easily than another, and initially you may need to put your emphasis on your health care providers. Over time, developing and nurturing all three of these networks will serve you well.

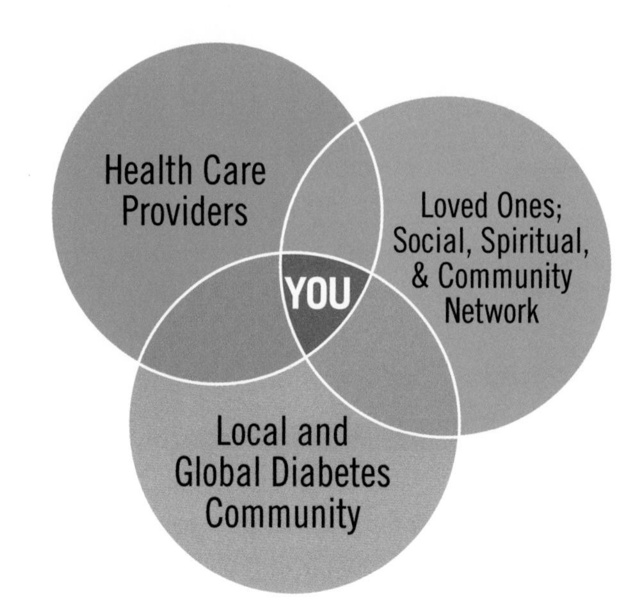

If I Only Knew . . .

When my husband and I were first dating (in our 40's), he asked me how I felt about having diabetes. We were in the car driving home after a hike on which I experienced a low blood glucose reaction. After an hour of heart to heart, I turned the tables and asked him, "What do you think about me having diabetes?" He told me that my diabetes was just part of my total package. Wow! I had felt so broken and alone until that moment, having never expressed my inner feelings about having diabetes. I didn't want to worry anyone or let them think I couldn't manage my diabetes on my own. Now I had someone in my corner—someone I could trust to listen to me and support me through the highs and lows of living with diabetes.

As you build your knowledge and determine the elements involved in your care, you'll begin to figure out how to fit diabetes care into your life. You need to fit your diabetes care into your pre-existing life and not the reverse. Don't let health care providers push you into turning your life upside down in order to manage your diabetes. This is a setup for failure because it unnecessarily forces you to change a lifestyle you may have been in for years. Research shows that you will be more successful over the long haul if you slowly, but surely, set and accomplish incremental lifestyle changes, such as eating fewer sweets and more fruit each day or walking during your lunch time. Plus, it's easier than ever before to find a diabetes care plan that works for you.

Wonder?

Diabetes team—reality or illusion?

You may hear the phrase "your diabetes team" as you read countless articles about managing diabetes. A diabetes team is a group of health care providers consistently consulting about your situation and working with you as a team to manage your diabetes. For some people, this was more of a reality years ago, but it is even less so today due to the health care system that doesn't usually cover this level of service. You are likely to find a team of diabetes experts only at the diabetes centers of university medical centers.

Your Diabetes Care Health Care Partners

To help you take good care of your diabetes through the years, seek the expertise of health care providers. You'll see your primary care provider or endocrinologist on a regular basis. This health care provider should help you get the tests and checks that you need to prevent and/or delay the complications of diabetes [also check out *Chapter 21*, page 257].

There are other health care providers who may play an intricate role in your diabetes management. Certified diabetes educators, pharmacists, eye doctors, and psychologists are just a few examples of these specialists. Get to know the ones you need. Let them help you in your quest for better diabetes control and long-term health.

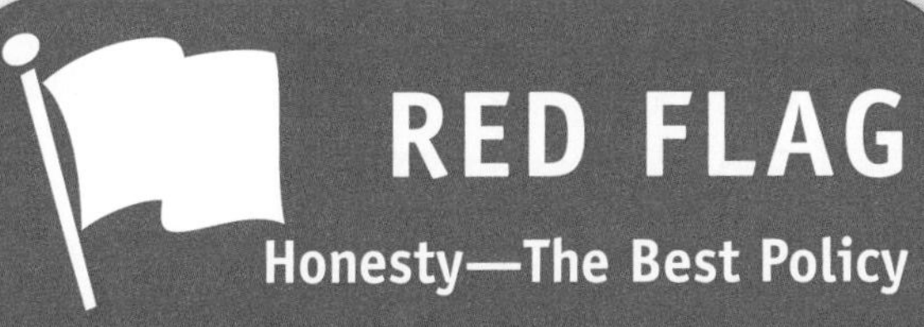

RED FLAG

Honesty—The Best Policy

Set a policy of honesty with your health care providers and your supporters. Be honest and clear about what you are willing and able to do to manage your diabetes. If you feel they are loading your days with too many tasks, making your care plan too complex, or asking you to complete tasks at times you can't, speak up. Let them know your schedule and lifestyle and that their plan for you isn't something you can do. Let them know what will work for you *[also check out* Research Briefs: Diabetes Attitudes, Wishes, and Needs (DAWN), *page 40]*.

DEFINITIONS:

endocrinologist: a doctor who treats people who have endocrine gland problems, such as diabetes.

certified diabetes educators: a health care professional who has expertise in diabetes education and has met eligibility requirements and completed a certification exam.

Endocrinolgists and primary care physicians

Endocrinologists are physicians who specialize in working with people who have diseases of the endocrine system, such as diabetes, or thyroid, adrenal, or parathyroid gland problems. Some endocrinologists call themselves diabetologists, meaning as an endocrinologist they specialize solely in treating diabetes. It is more common for a person with type 1 diabetes to see an endocrinologist, even a pediatric endocrinologist in the younger years, because managing type 1 is thought to be more challenging; however, the management of type 2 is becoming more complex as more treatment options are approved and data about the importance of intensive blood glucose, blood pressure, and blood lipid control are published.

Your primary care provider could be a physician, physician's assistant, nurse practitioner, or clinical nurse specialist. Your primary provider should be up to date in diabetes management and should be willing to form a healthy and honest working partnership with you.

If you believe it is in your best interest, to consult with an endocrinologist, talk to your primary care provider about getting a referral. You may or may not need a referral depending on the rules and regulations of your health plan.

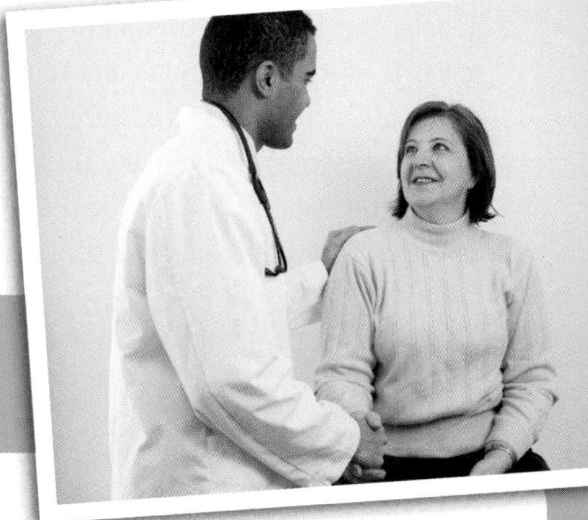

Psst...

Routes to Diabetes Specialists

Several directories of primary care providers and endocrinologist exist. The ADA and the National Committee for Quality Assurance (NCQA) in Washington, D.C., joined forces to develop and offer the Diabetes Physicians Recognition Program (DPRP). This is a voluntary program designed to recognize physicians who use evidence-based measures and provide excellent diabetes care. Call toll-free to 888-275-7585, or search on *www.recognition.ncqa.org* for a physician or group of physicians who have obtained this provider recognition in diabetes. Many endocrinologists in the U.S. belong to the American Association of Clinical Endocrinologists (AACE). You can search the AACE website (*www.aace.com/resources/memsearch.php*) to locate an endocrinologist in your area.

DIABETES NCQA ADA RECOGNIZED PHYSICIAN

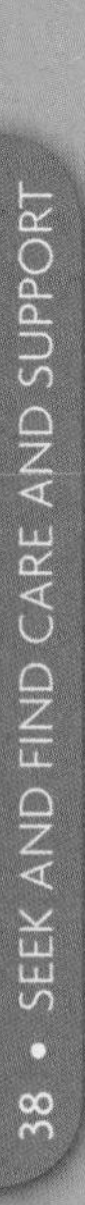

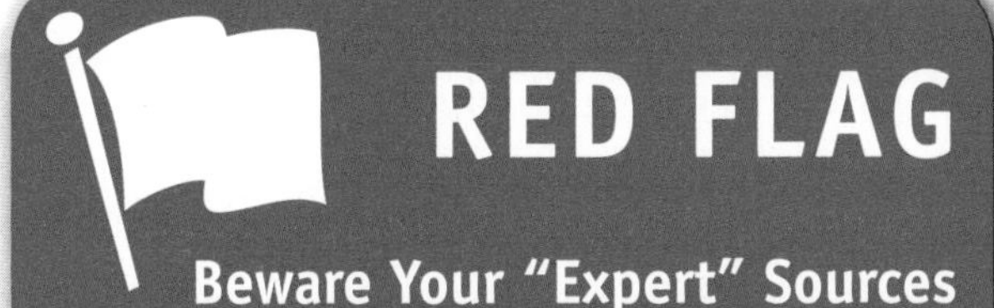

RED FLAG

Beware Your "Expert" Sources

Diabetes is a disease that runs in families; so many people have it or know someone who does. Keep in mind that diabetes is a disease for which the treatments and management have changed dramatically in just a few decades. You'll be offered a lot of advice from friends, family, co-workers, and others who know you have diabetes. A word of advice: listen, consider the advice, and then consult with medical experts and trusted resources before you initiate or make a change in your diabetes care plan.

Specialists

Along with your primary care physician or endocrinologist, there are a slew of specialists who may become a regular player in helping you care for your diabetes. Pick the specialists who will help you manage your diabetes in the way you want it to be managed.

DIABETES EDUCATORS are most often nurses, dietitians, and pharmacists who have specialized training and expertise in diabetes. These health care providers may have achieved and maintained the credential CDE (certified diabetes educator). Individually, or within a group setting, diabetes educators provide knowledge, skills, support, and counsel as you work to manage your diabetes. If you haven't been referred to a diabetes educator or a diabetes self-management education program, ask your primary care provider or endocrinologist for a referral.

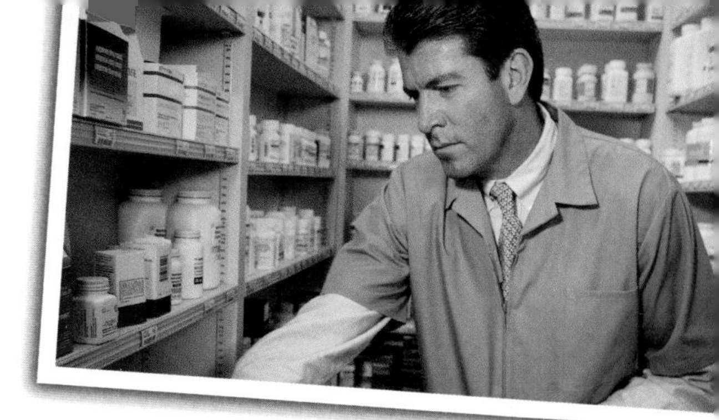

PHARMACISTS are trained to know how drugs, both prescription and over-the-counter products, affect the body. A word to the wise: develop a trusting relationship with a knowledgeable pharmacist who is current on diabetes care. This can serve you well.

EXERCISE PHYSIOLOGISTS, PHYSICAL THERAPISTS, and **PERSONAL TRAINERS** can help you design a safe and effective activity plan that will help you manage your diabetes more effectively. Very few people have the benefit of working directly with one of these health care providers within the context of basic diabetes care or their health care plan. In all likelihood, your other health care providers will most likely be your advisors when it comes to physical activity.

DEFINITION:

diabetes self-management education program:
a program that aims to teach and support people with diabetes how to address and care for the daily demands of a chronic disease like diabetes.

A **COUNSELOR, SOCIAL WORKER,** or **PSYCHOLOGIST** can help ease the distress of dealing with the diagnosis and ongoing effort of managing diabetes. Some people find that working with a counselor who has skills to help you manage your feelings or assist you in making behavior changes can be beneficial. Check with your health plan to determine coverage for these services.

An **EYE DOCTOR** should be among your health care providers from early on, and your visits should be annual. Ophthalmologists are medical doctors who detect and treat eye diseases. Optometrists are not medical doctor, but are trained to examine eyes for vision problems and write prescriptions for glasses and contact lenses. People with diabetes should have an annual dilated retinal eye exam [also check out *Chapter 21*, page 257] done by an optometrist or ophthalmologist.

PODIATRISTS or **FOOT DOCTORS**, may be needed on occasion due to temporary foot problems. Some people need to see a podiatrist regularly because of ongoing foot care needs or the inability to adequately take care of their feet themselves.

DENTISTS and **DENTAL HYGIENISTS** should check your teeth for problems and do X-rays to check for bone loss or gum disease [also check out *Chapter 21*, page 257]. Let your dental care experts know you have diabetes. With diabetes, it becomes even more important that you have your teeth cleaned and checked at least every 6 months.

CONFIDENTIAL

Research Brief

Diabetes Attitudes, Wishes, and Needs (DAWN)

The Diabetes Attitudes, Wishes, and Needs study (DAWN) is an initiative that was started in 2001 by the International Diabetes Federation (IDF) and Novo Nordisk Pharmaceuticals. The goal of DAWN is to help improve the outcomes of diabetes care by gaining insights into the psychosocial and behavioral barriers to effective diabetes management from people with diabetes and health care providers. Overall, the DAWN survey observed that not enough attention is paid by health care providers to the psychosocial impact of diabetes on a person's life.

The DAWN project is encouraging these five actions by health care providers who care for people with diabetes around the world. As you work with your health care providers, consider these actions and reflect on whether your providers are taking these actions.

1. Involve the person with diabetes in decisions about their care and encourage them to take responsibility for their actions.
2. Promote communication and collaboration with other health care providers involved in the person's diabetes care.
3. Promote active self-management by the person with diabetes by developing an individualized treatment plan based on their abilities, wishes, needs, and psychosocial barriers.
4. Reduce barriers to effective therapy by helping the person with diabetes understand the consequences of inadequate diabetes care by providing sufficient information to make informed decisions about treatment options.
5. Provide better psychological care by informing people that positive feelings and emotions are important elements of active self-management. Consider referring people for psychological support when it is warranted.

Source: *www.dawnstudy.com*

If I Only Knew . . .

My voice was important, too . . .

Just after I was diagnosed with diabetes, it was easier to let my health care provider take the lead. "Don't worry," was my doctor's mantra at each appointment, and that's what I did. In my gut, however, I had doubts every time I left my doctor's office. For example, my personal schedule was always changing, yet his guidance was to keep my daily schedule for meal times and amounts of foods to eat static. I eventually did some research and changed providers. My new provider encouraged me to ask lots of questions. She encouraged me to do more blood glucose checks beyond just before meals. We reviewed and interpreted the results together and made adjustments to better fit my schedule. She even encouraged me to learn more about my diabetes — to feel more in control.

How to Find a Diabetes Educator or Diabetes Education Program

Diabetes education programs are usually staffed by diabetes educators who are most commonly nurses and dietitians. Some programs also have exercise physiologists, pharmacists, or behavioral counselors on staff. To promote quality diabetes education, the ADA endorses the National Standards for Diabetes Self-Management Education (*http://care.diabetesjournals.org/cgi/content/extract/31/Supplement_1/S97*). The ADA uses these standards to recognize diabetes education programs for quality. This is called the ADA Education Recognition Program (ERP). ERPs are among the few programs covered by Medicare; however, some rural health centers, where access to diabetes education is challenging, receive coverage for this service. Locate diabetes education programs near you by calling toll free 800-DIABETES (800-342-2383) or go to *www.diabetes.org/education/edu.asp*.

Wonder?

Will my health plan cover diabetes education and/or medical nutrition therapy?

Like many questions about health care coverage, there's no simple or single answer to this question. The answer depends on your health coverage and the state or federal regulations that apply to this plan. Today, many people who have a health care plan can get coverage for diabetes self-management education [also check out *Chapter 19*, page 237].

Locate a diabetes educator through the American Association of Diabetes Educators (AADE). Call 800-TEAMUP4 (832-6874) or go to *www.diabeteseducator.org* to find a diabetes educator.

In addition, you may want to seek the services of a dietitian who has expertise in diabetes, referred to as medical nutrition therapy (MNT). You will find dietitians who offer this service at the above-mentioned ADA diabetes education programs as well as other places dietitians practice.

By the Numbers

ADA Recognized Diabetes Education Programs

Don't expect to find a diabetes education program in every health care setting across the country. Today, there are only about 3,000 ADA Education Recognition Programs (ERPs) nationwide, which are concentrated in urban and suburban areas.

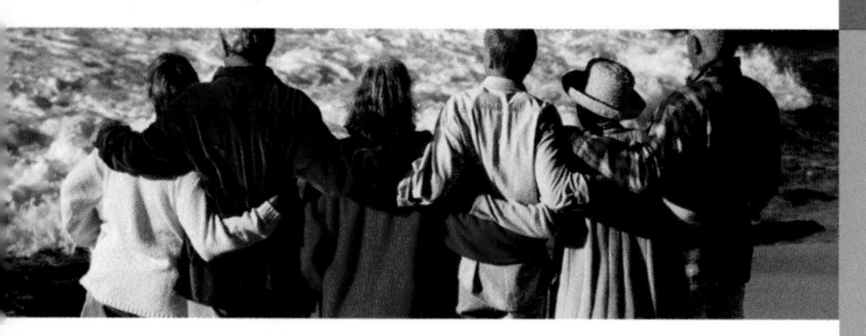

The Five Stages of Grief

In the late 1960s, Dr. Elizabeth Kubler-Ross introduced the five stage of grief—denial, anger, bargaining, depression, and acceptance. These stages, though initially intended to apply to death and dying, define the process people typically go through when they face the diagnosis of a chronic disease like diabetes. All of these stages are the normal process of moving to acceptance of your condition. And because you will have diabetes for the rest of your life, you will probably revisit one or more of these stages from time to time. Be kind to yourself. Allow yourself to feel your feelings and, if need be, seek counsel from a loved one, spiritual leader, or a mental health professional to work through these stages.

Stage of Grief	Definition
DENIAL	The conscious or unconscious refusal to accept facts, information, or reality about the current situation, such as the diagnosis of diabetes.
ANGER	People can be inwardly angry, taking the anger about the diagnosis out on themselves, or they can direct the anger outward, at family members or others even more external to their lives.
BARGAINING	This is the stage in which there is a negotiation about the diagnosis. In the case of diabetes, a common area for bargaining is blood glucose-lowering medication. For example, a person with type 2 diabetes may bargain with their health care provider to more closely adhere to their healthy eating plan to delay starting insulin therapy.
DEPRESSION	In this stage, a person begins to move toward acceptance; however, there are sadness, anxiety, hopelessness, fear and other feelings of uncertainty [also check out *Chapter 12*, page 149].
ACCEPTANCE	This is the final stage and indicates that the person has gained a level of acceptance and willingness to become involved in their management plan.

Myth

Once you learn what you need to do, managing diabetes is a snap.

Fact

Don't let anyone try to convince you that managing diabetes is easy. It's simply not! This doesn't mean you throw up your hands, cast caution to the wind, and give up trying. It means that you take a step-by-step approach and make small changes, tackling what you feel you can handle first. There will be days when you handle your diabetes more successfully and others when you don't. Don't beat yourself up for what you didn't get done. Learn from all of your experiences. Managing diabetes isn't easy, but with effort and perseverance you can do it!

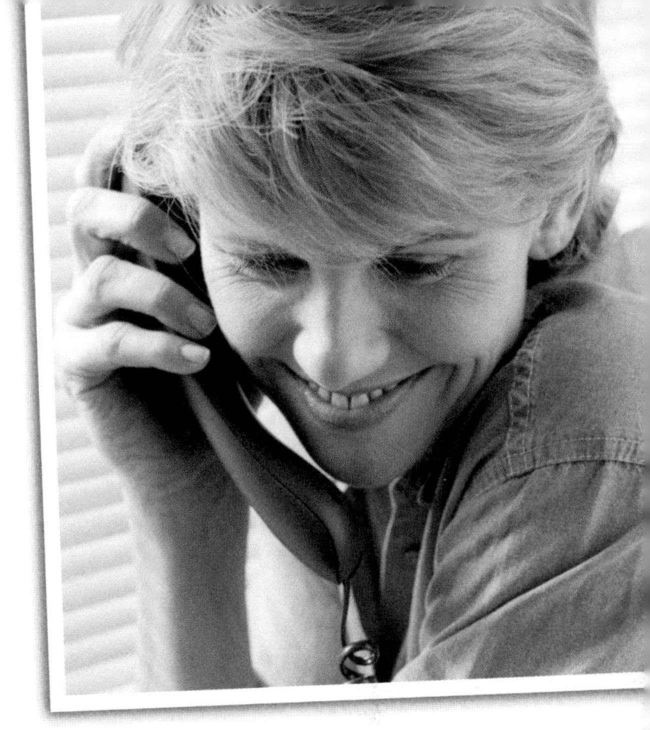

Get the Support You Need—Near and Far

Don't feel you need to go it alone! You'll want and need people to support you with the challenges of managing diabetes. Beyond support from friends and loved ones, you'll find both local support groups and support networks via the Internet. The Internet is filled with plenty to read; however, make sure the information is reliable. Because so many people have diabetes, be open to finding support in surprising places [also check out *If I Only Knew: Support takes time and comes from surprising places*, page 45].

With all this support and information at hand, your job is to figure out what resources and support you need, how and from whom you want to receive it, and when. Scroll through this list and consider who has helped you get through stressful times in your past. Also, think about new avenues for support and information that fit your current time availability and lifestyle.

- Your spouse
- Your siblings, parents, or other family
- A religious or spiritual leader
- Close friends
- Co-workers or classmates
- A counselor
- Support from people with your type of diabetes
- An online support network
- A pet

Find Support Groups On and Offline

Today, diabetes support groups are available both locally and globally via the Internet. Local support groups are usually available through a diabetes education program [also check out *How to Find a Diabetes Educator or Diabetes Education Program*, page 41]. Support groups may also be available through your local ADA office or other local diabetes organizations. Typically, support groups are free or only charge a small fee.

The availability of the Internet has opened up communication among people globally. You'll find diabetes blogs, social networking opportunities, chatrooms, message boards, and more. You'll also have opportunities to stay up to date with e-newsletters and more. For starters, connect through the ADA at *www.diabetes.org*. If you like what you see, you may want to consider becoming a member. ADA membership includes 12 monthly issues of ADA's magazine for people with and affected by diabetes, *Diabetes Forecast*; a discount on all ADA books and cookbooks; and a network of diabetes support and information that will help you stay up to date on new diabetes research and get you connected to other people with diabetes.

TIPS + TACTICS

Find Your Healthy Ways to Cope

People cope with the stress and strains of life in varied ways. Research shows that the more you put healthy coping skills into practice, the better you'll care for your diabetes.

The activities you can engage in to cope healthfully are endless. If you are on a search, give some of the options below a try.

- *Chatting with a friend or close relative*
- *Seeing a silly movie*
- *An early morning, lunch time, or late evening walk*
- *Reading a pleasure book*
- *Going to a gym*
- *Scheduling a massage*
- *Joining a book club*
- *Learning and playing a musical instrument*
- *Attending a religious service or event*
- *Volunteering in schools, a homeless shelter, or for others in need*
- *Cooking a gourmet meal*
- *Traveling*
- *Visiting a museum or exhibit*

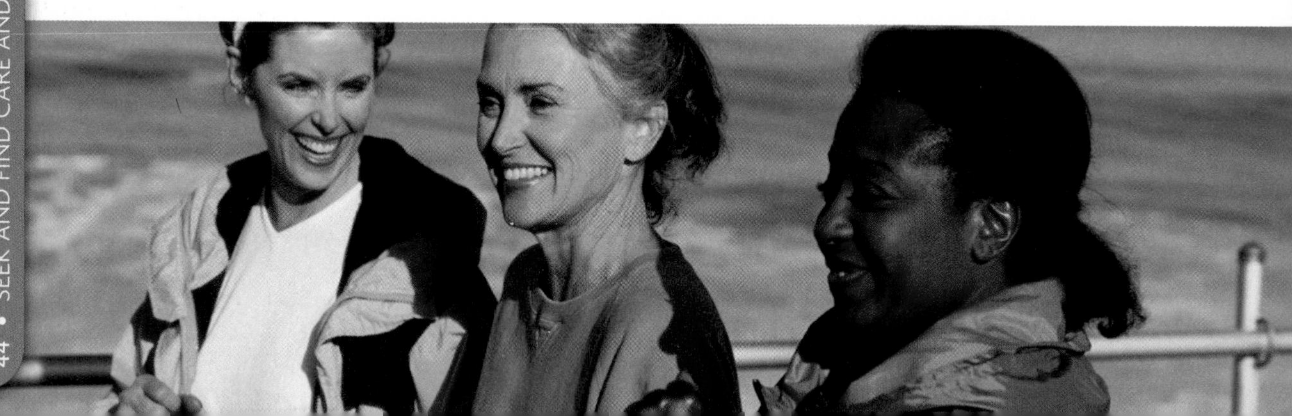

Myth

Once you learn what you need to do, managing diabetes is a snap.

Fact

Don't let anyone try to convince you that managing diabetes is easy. It's simply not! This doesn't mean you throw up your hands, cast caution to the wind, and give up trying. It means that you take a step-by-step approach and make small changes, tackling what you feel you can handle first. There will be days when you handle your diabetes more successfully and others when you don't. Don't beat yourself up for what you didn't get done. Learn from all of your experiences. Managing diabetes isn't easy, but with effort and perseverance you can do it!

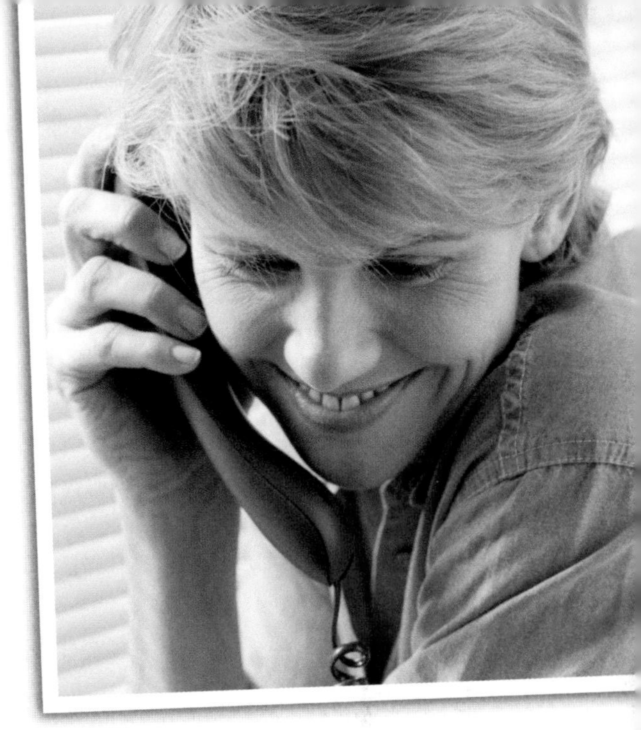

Get the Support You Need—Near and Far

Don't feel you need to go it alone! You'll want and need people to support you with the challenges of managing diabetes. Beyond support from friends and loved ones, you'll find both local support groups and support networks via the Internet. The Internet is filled with plenty to read; however, make sure the information is reliable. Because so many people have diabetes, be open to finding support in surprising places [also check out *If I Only Knew: Support takes time and comes from surprising places*, page 45].

With all this support and information at hand, your job is to figure out what resources and support you need, how and from whom you want to receive it, and when. Scroll through this list and consider who has helped you get through stressful times in your past. Also, think about new avenues for support and information that fit your current time availability and lifestyle.

- Your spouse
- Your siblings, parents, or other family
- A religious or spiritual leader
- Close friends
- Co-workers or classmates
- A counselor
- Support from people with your type of diabetes
- An online support network
- A pet

Find Support Groups On and Offline

Today, diabetes support groups are available both locally and globally via the Internet. Local support groups are usually available through a diabetes education program [also check out *How to Find a Diabetes Educator or Diabetes Education Program*, page 41]. Support groups may also be available through your local ADA office or other local diabetes organizations. Typically, support groups are free or only charge a small fee.

The availability of the Internet has opened up communication among people globally. You'll find diabetes blogs, social networking opportunities, chatrooms, message boards, and more. You'll also have opportunities to stay up to date with e-newsletters and more. For starters, connect through the ADA at *www.diabetes.org*. If you like what you see, you may want to consider becoming a member. ADA membership includes 12 monthly issues of ADA's magazine for people with and affected by diabetes, *Diabetes Forecast*; a discount on all ADA books and cookbooks; and a network of diabetes support and information that will help you stay up to date on new diabetes research and get you connected to other people with diabetes.

TIPS + TACTICS

Find Your Healthy Ways to Cope

People cope with the stress and strains of life in varied ways. Research shows that the more you put healthy coping skills into practice, the better you'll care for your diabetes.

The activities you can engage in to cope healthfully are endless. If you are on a search, give some of the options below a try.

- *Chatting with a friend or close relative*
- *Seeing a silly movie*
- *An early morning, lunch time, or late evening walk*
- *Reading a pleasure book*
- *Going to a gym*
- *Scheduling a massage*
- *Joining a book club*
- *Learning and playing a musical instrument*
- *Attending a religious service or event*
- *Volunteering in schools, a homeless shelter, or for others in need*
- *Cooking a gourmet meal*
- *Traveling*
- *Visiting a museum or exhibit*

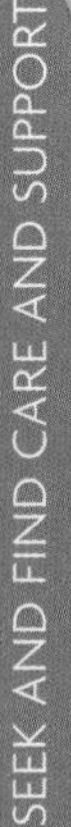

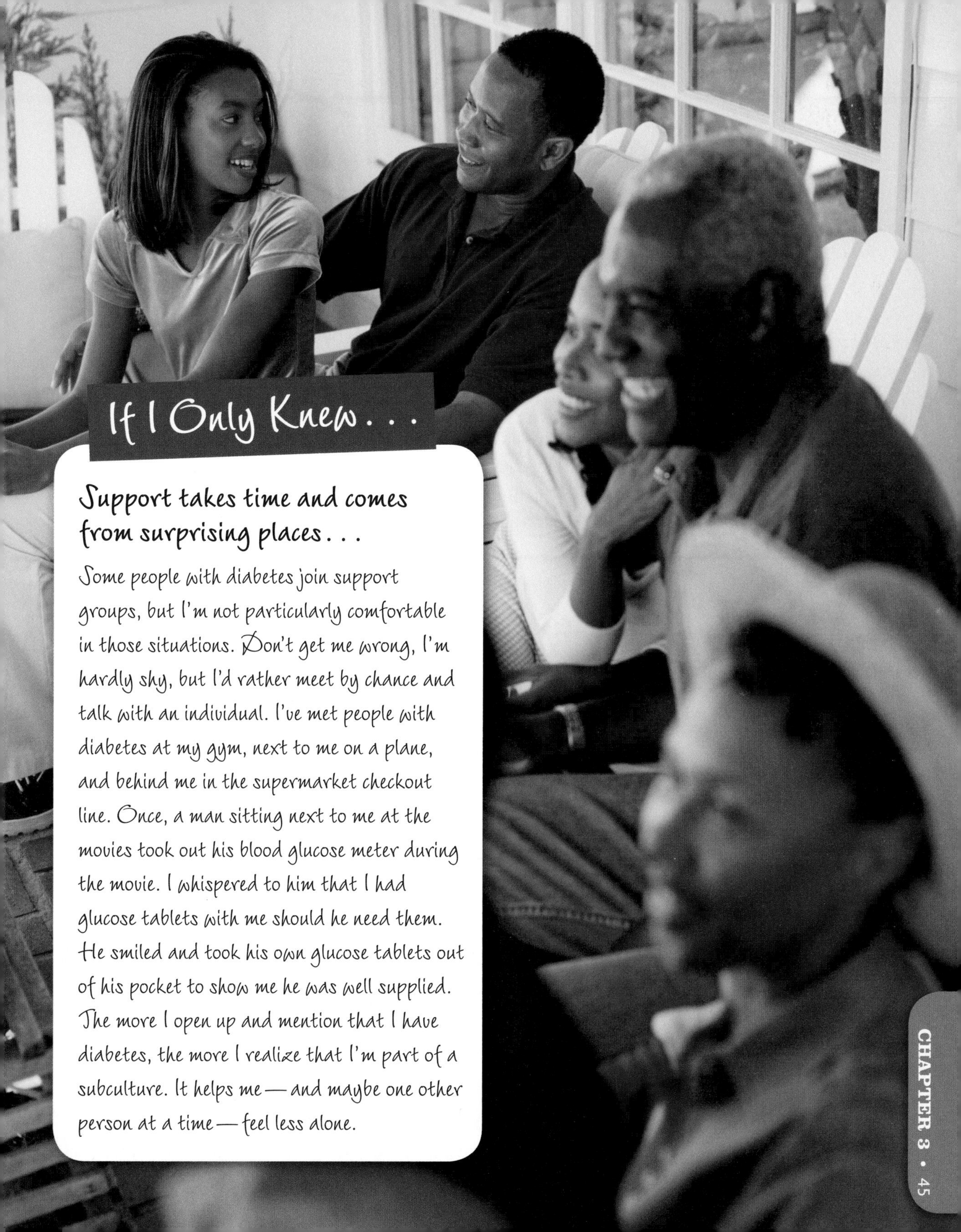

If I Only Knew . . .

Support takes time and comes from surprising places . . .

Some people with diabetes join support groups, but I'm not particularly comfortable in those situations. Don't get me wrong, I'm hardly shy, but I'd rather meet by chance and talk with an individual. I've met people with diabetes at my gym, next to me on a plane, and behind me in the supermarket checkout line. Once, a man sitting next to me at the movies took out his blood glucose meter during the movie. I whispered to him that I had glucose tablets with me should he need them. He smiled and took his own glucose tablets out of his pocket to show me he was well supplied. The more I open up and mention that I have diabetes, the more I realize that I'm part of a subculture. It helps me — and maybe one other person at a time — feel less alone.

Section 2

Create Your Real-Life Diabetes Plan

Section 2 focuses on the meat of the matter—the key elements of daily diabetes self-care. From choosing healthy foods to being physically active, taking blood glucose–lowering medication and other medications to controlling blood pressure and preserving your heart's health, you'll learn all you need to know about the key diabetes self-care plan elements and figure out how to put this plan into action in your real life.

A real-life plan doesn't call for perfection but aims to help you balance the demands of real life with those of diabetes care. It accepts that you can't change everything at once and encourages you to work on making the behavioral changes necessary to live a healthier lifestyle.

Your priorities will depend on your current habits along with how you and your providers choose to manage your diabetes and progress your management over time. The good news is that even a few small behavioral changes can produce BIG positive health impacts. Try a few and you'll see.

Chapter 4

Realistic Behavioral Changes for Success: Consider this chapter a primer on how to slowly change your behaviors to successfully live a healthier lifestyle and implement your diabetes self-care plan. You'll learn that no matter what behaviors you choose to change, the same goal-setting and evaluation processes apply.

Chapter 5

Eat Healthy—The Basics: You'll learn the key concepts for eating with diabetes and that these principles echo the healthy eating guidelines for everyone. You'll gather plenty of tips and tactics to help you make realistic behavioral changes to eat healthier one step at a time.

Chapter 6

Eat Healthy—Real-Life Challenges and Solutions: Learn how to deal with daily food dilemmas, such as shopping, meal planning, and portion control. You'll learn the meaning of nutrition claims, read about sugar substitutes, and get tips to eat restaurant foods with success.

Chapter 7

Get Up, Get Active: Learn both the general and diabetes-specific benefits to being physically active. Get ready...the list is long. You'll learn the specific exercise recommendations for people with diabetes and gather tips on new ways to fit physical activity into your already busy life.

Chapter 8

Medications That Lower Blood Glucose: Today, there are more categories of blood glucose–lowering medications than ever before. Though lowering blood glucose is their goal, the categories of medications work differently. Learn their actions and common combinations and how your health care provider may start and progress these medications over time.

Chapter 9

Other Medications to Manage Diabetes: Managing diabetes today often entails preventing or managing high blood pressure and abnormal blood lipids. Learn about the categories of blood pressure and lipid-management medications and check out whether you

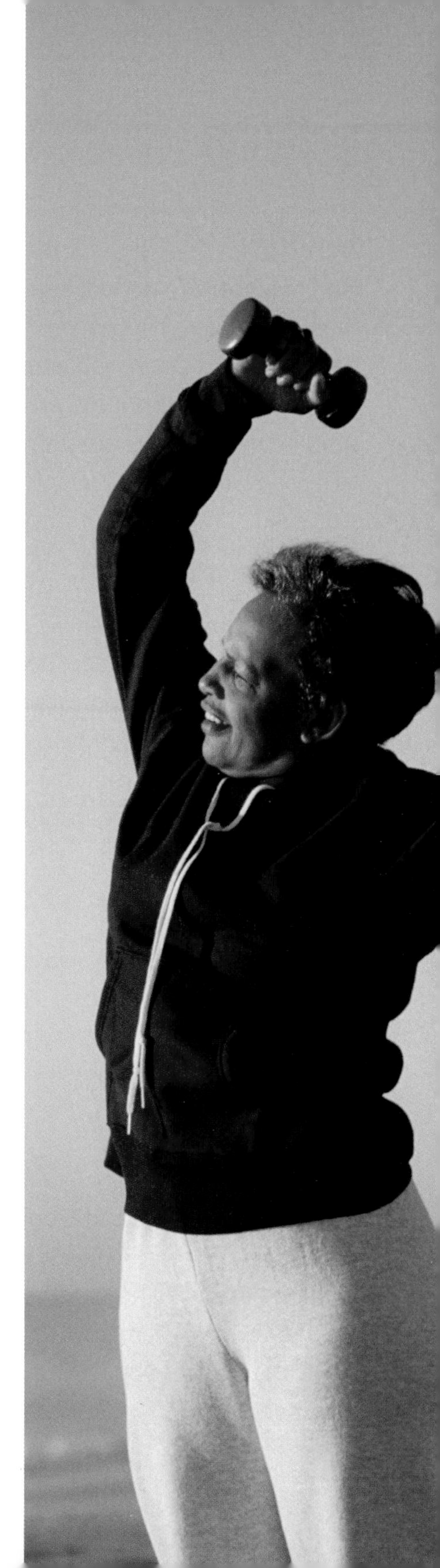

should be on one or more of them. Plus, check out whether you should pop an aspirin every day.

Chapter 10

No Prescription Needed: Beyond prescription medication, you may wonder about whether you need certain dietary supplements or other alternative therapies. Learn about the pros and cons of dietary supplements and the questions to ask before you begin to use any alternative therapies.

Chapter 11

The Importance of Catching Your Z's: The correlations between insufficient sleep, being overweight, and developing type 2 diabetes (and its related diseases) are growing stronger. Make the connection, learn how much sleep you need, and determine whether you should be checked out for a sleep disorder.

Chapter 12

Stress, Depression, and Diabetes: Learn how stress can impact your blood glucose, strategies to use to manage your stresses and strains, and about the available treatments—from counseling to medications.

Chapter 13

Monitoring Glucose and Blood Pressure Matters: Checking your glucose levels and blood pressure are key ways to determine how well your real-life diabetes care plan is working. Learn about the monitoring tools you need, the choices you have, and what technologies fit your needs.

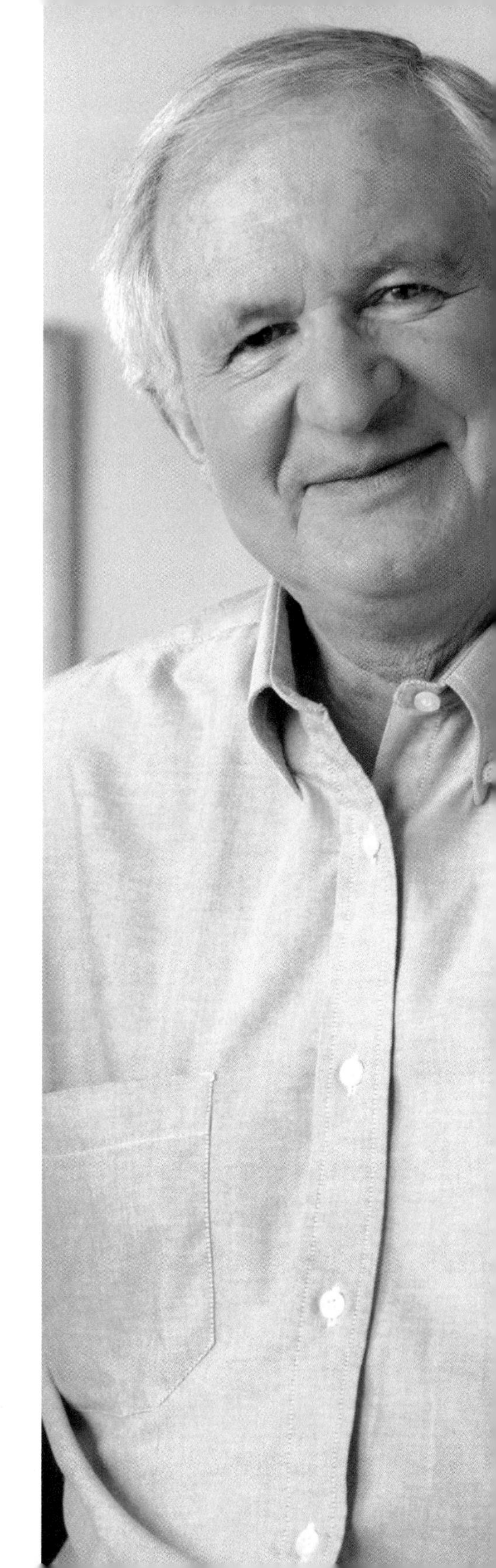

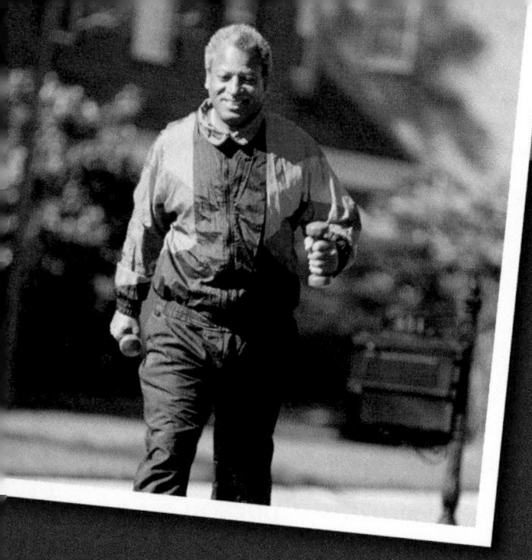

CHAPTER 4

Realistic Behavioral Changes for Success

There are loads of to-dos on the list of daily diabetes self-care tasks your health care providers want you to complete. You may feel particularly overwhelmed if you've attempted to make changes in the past and weren't successful. Take a deep breath! In this chapter, you'll learn that making permanent behavioral changes is a slow and steady process—truly a lifetime of effort. The good news, however, is that even small changes produce BIG results. Give yourself a pat on the back for any successes. Don't expect perfection. And don't let other people in your support networks expect too much of you either. Strive to do the best you can each day.

What You'll Learn:

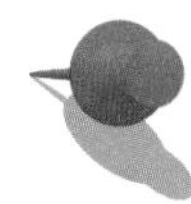

- Diabetes self-care has evolved over the decades from a health care provider-centered to person-centered approach
- How to identify your unhealthy lifestyle behaviors
- How to make behavioral changes step by step
- Two behavioral change theories that can help you realistically and practically change your behaviors
- Changing behavior for good is a slow and steady process that requires time, energy, and commitment
- The SMART format for setting realistic behavioral changes

Get to Know YOU

Before you start making behavioral changes, take a closer look at your current habits. Get to know yourself and your current lifestyle habits. For example: to change your eating habits, you need to have a clear picture of what you currently (and honestly) eat and drink. The same is true for physical activity and other key diabetes self-care behaviors. Recording these details pushes you to be honest with yourself and your providers. A simple chart for tracking what you eat and drink works well (see the one below for an example). If paper and pen aren't right for you, consider the use of an online food log from a diabetes- or weight-control website. Getting in the habit of recording the details of your life will be good practice. You'll discover that keeping records is a key skill for behavioral change and diabetes self-care [also check out *Record Keeping Matters*, page 58].

Myth

Your health care provider directs your diabetes care, not you.

Fact

Years ago (and still too often today) health care providers dictated how a person was to take care of their diabetes. A shift has occurred over the last several decades to a person-centered approach. Knowing how to implement your plan, change behaviors, obtain support from providers, and keep a positive attitude are also important factors. Are you receiving person-centered care, or is your health care provider dictating what you must do and how you must manage your diabetes? Your provider should be asking you what behavior changes you are willing to make and how you want to manage your diabetes. You should have a partnership with your provider in which you can be open and honest.

Sample food tracking form

Time	Food or Drink	Amount*	How Prepared	Calories	Carbohydrates (g)	Fat (g)

** Weighing or measuring foods and beverages raises your awareness of the quantities you consume. This new-found awareness helps you set realistic goals for controlling portions of foods and beverages.*

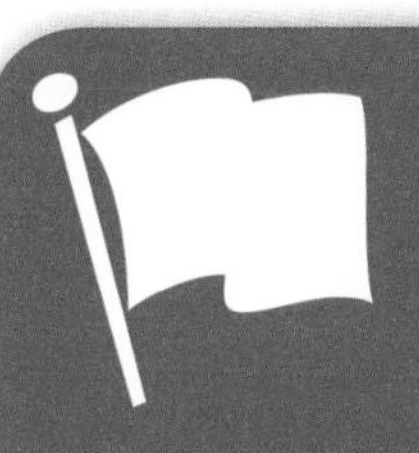

RED FLAG

Stop Chasing those Magic Potions and Pills

Whether it's the new diet that promises to help you magically shed pounds, an exercise gizmo that will melt away your spare tire, or an herb from an African plant that will make your blood glucose plummet, don't buy it! Quick fixes are everywhere you turn and almost never work. The reality is that making and maintaining the behavior changes essential for long-term health and diabetes control are hard work and take time.

Multiple Approaches to Behavioral Change

The art and science of achieving behavioral change are based on a variety of researched approaches, or theories, that continue to evolve. As your health care providers work with these approaches to help people with diabetes successfully change their behaviors, they may emphasize the use of one approach or integrate the strengths of several to create a customized approach just for you.

Two behavioral-change theories used in diabetes self-management education today are the Empowerment Model and the Transtheoretical

The Empowerment Model: 5 Steps for Making Behavior Changes

Step	Associated questions to consider *(with examples)*
STEP 1: DEFINE THE PROBLEM	What is it about your diabetes self-care that makes it a challenge for you to manage? • *Checking my blood glucose levels several times a day.*
STEP 2: IDENTIFY THE FEELINGS	What are your thoughts or feelings about the problem? • *It is painful and time consuming.* • *Results that are too high make me feel bad.*
STEP 3: IDENTIFY LONG-TERM GOALS	What are your options? What barriers will you face? • *Vary times I check my blood glucose and check less often.* • *Think of results as information for learning rather than value judgment.*
STEP 4: IDENTIFY SHORT-TERM BEHAVIORAL CHANGE PLAN	What are steps you can take to problem solve? What are you going to do and when? • *Research other finger-pricking devices that hurt less.* • *Make sure I'm using the quickest meter.*
STEP 5: IMPLEMENT AND EVALUATE PLAN	What did you learn? What would you do differently next time? • *I wasn't using the most up-to-date equipment so the checks were taking longer and hurting more. This has taught me to stay abreast of new blood glucose–monitoring products.* • *Ask more questions of my pharmacist about the quickest and easiest devices to monitor.* • *I can vary the times of day I check from day to day.* • *I can check less often and learn more.*

Model (more simply known as the Readiness to Change Model). The Empowerment Model and Readiness to Change Model are designed for you to use with your health care providers or on your own to set behavioral change goals and evaluate your progress. Think about using one of these models to work through your concerns and issues. Set goals to change your behaviors. Try it out!

The Empowerment Model

The Empowerment Model of behavior change was introduced into the diabetes lexicon in the early 1990s by diabetes experts at the Michigan Diabetes Research and Training Center, including Robert Anderson, PhD, and Martha Funnell, MS, RN, CDE. This model helps people discover and develop their inherent ability to take responsibility for their lives and their diabetes self-care. As the developers of the model explain, the Empowerment Model is based on the key characteristics of diabetes as a chronic illness vs. an acute illness and state the following:

- Your self-care choices have the greatest impact on your health outcomes vs. the treatment choices of the health care provider.
- You are in control of your self-care vs. the health care provider being in control.
- You have the right and responsibility to be the primary decision maker, because the consequences (both positive and negative) of self-care decisions happen to you (not the health care provider).

DEFINITIONS:

chronic: a medical problem that is long lasting (diabetes is a chronic disease).

acute: something that happens suddenly and for only a short time.

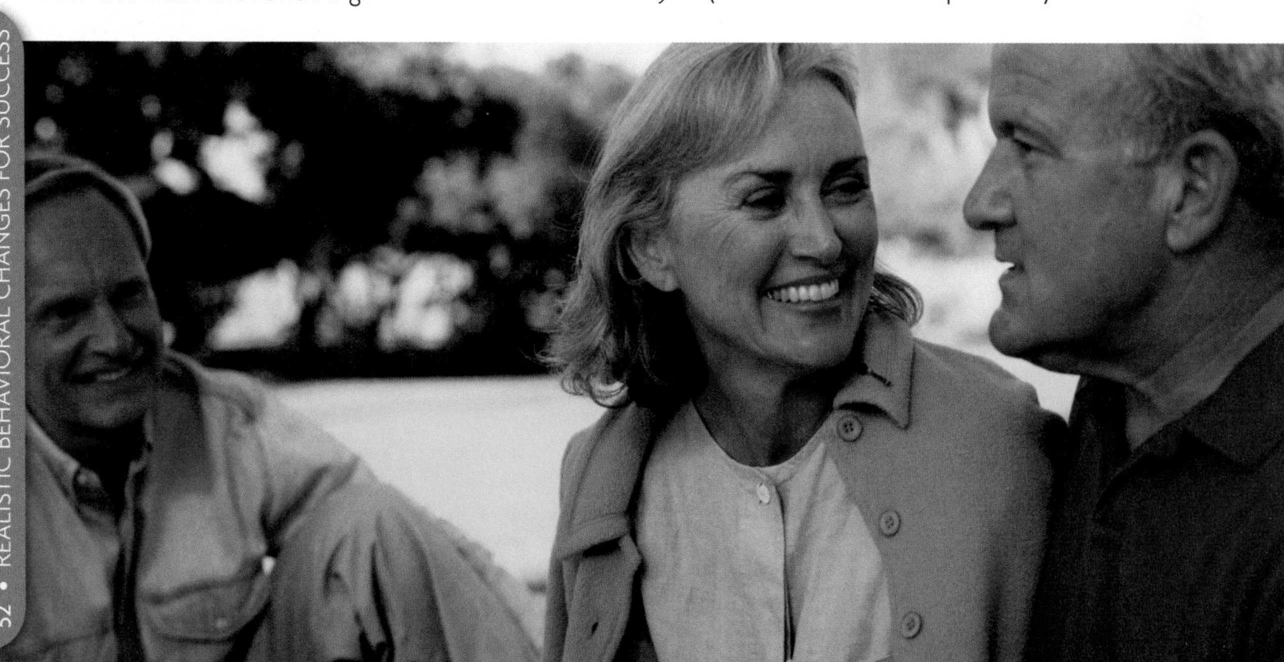

The Readiness to Change Model

The Transtheoretical Model, or more commonly known as the Readiness to Change Model, was originally developed by behavioral researchers for the purpose of helping people quit smoking. Over the years, it's been successfully used to help people change many other health behaviors, including the ones central to diabetes self-care.

The Readiness to Change Model is a good fit with diabetes care. It helps you focus first on the behaviors that will be easiest for you to change. This model uses six so-called "stages of change" to help people identify where they are along this continuum of change for behaviors. For example, you may be in the "action stage" to become more physically active, but in the "pre-contemplation stage" to quit smoking. The model factors in forward

The Readiness to Change Model: 6 Stages of Behavioral Change

Stage	Definition of stage *(with examples)*
STAGE 1: PRE-CONTEMPLATION	The person is not aware that the behavior in question is a problem. They have no intention of changing this behavior. • *My doctor has never told me that smoking cigarettes is hazardous to my health or to my diabetes care.*
STAGE 2: CONTEMPLATION	The person is aware that the behavior in question is a problem, but they are in a state of ambivalence—between recognizing the benefits of changing this behavior vs. awareness of the downsides. • *I realize that smoking is hazardous to my health and that it's even more harmful to my circulation and other organs, now that I have diabetes. I know I should quit, but I've tried quitting before, and I'm not pleasant for anyone to be around.*
STAGE 3: PREPARATION	The person begins to put a plan in place to change this behavior in the near future (several months). • *After I get through the stress of my wife's impending surgery in two months, I will sign up for the smoking-cessation program at our local hospital.*
STAGE 4: ACTION	The person puts the plan they assembled during the preparation stage into action. • *I just signed up for the smoking-cessation program at our local hospital.*
STAGE 5: MAINTENANCE	The person's plan is working and they are able to maintain the behavioral change over time. • *I have been tobacco-free for six months and am still attending my monthly smoking-cessation group. This is the longest I have ever gone without smoking. I'm not coughing and can walk a mile without feeling winded.*
STAGE 6: EVALUATION	The last (and repeating) lap in this cycle is to measure your success. Once the time period you set with your goals is over, reflect on how you have done. Ask yourself these questions: *Did I meet my goals? If not, why not? Were they unrealistic? Was the time frame too long?* Once the time period you set with your goals is over, reflect on how you have done. If you have succeeded, that's great! If not, make your goals easier or choose a new goal.

and backward motion in making changes. It also acknowledges that behavioral change is a time- and energy-consuming proposition.

What's your next step? You guessed it! Start the behavioral-change cycle again. If you were successful, choose a couple of new goals to work on. Keep in mind that practicing a new behavior for two weeks or a month does not mean that this new behavior has become a lifelong habit. Experts believe it takes about six months of practice to cement new behaviors. It's very human to slip back to old behaviors, particularly in times of stress or a crisis in life. If you use the behavioral-change process provided here, it won't be long before you find yourself a few pounds lighter on the scale, and your blood glucose, blood lipids, and blood pressure numbers moving in the right directions.

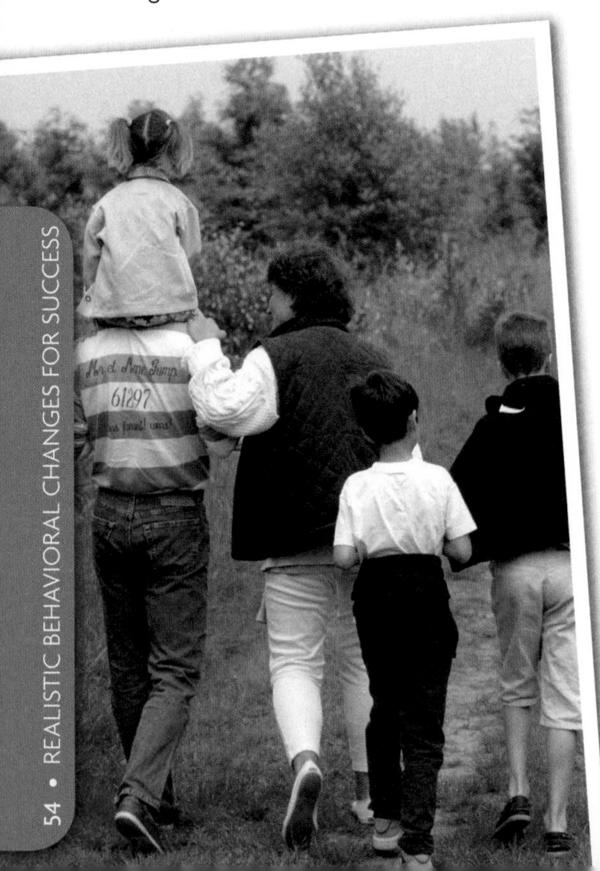

RED FLAG

Change One Step at a Time

A word to the wise: don't try to tackle too many behavior changes at one time because you won't be successful and will get frustrated fast. Focus on setting two to three realistic goals [also check out Set SMART Goals, *page 56] that you are confident you can accomplish. Start with behaviors for which your importance and confidence ratings are 7 or above. The good news is that making just a few behavioral changes to eat healthier and be more physically active can have a huge effect on your weight and your diabetes numbers. Changing your behaviors will get easier over time. You'll have the best shot at keeping your diabetes under control once your new healthy behaviors become lifelong behaviors.*

Success Breeds Success

The success-breeds-success notion is easy to get: start with small realistic goals—behaviors that are important to you to change and that you have confidence that you can change—and make these changes successfully. Step by step, you'll create your history of successful behavioral changes. With success, you'll build confidence in yourself and your ability to make changes toward living a healthier lifestyle and managing your diabetes.

Positive behavioral change doesn't just happen, it takes time, energy, and effort. Try these suggestions for success:

- **Think positive thoughts out loud.** "I think I can, I think I can." Research shows that if you hear yourself state your goals out loud either to yourself, a loved one, or a friend, you are more likely to follow through.
- **Write down your goals.** Keep them handy, and place them where you will see them often—on the refrigerator, on your bathroom or bedroom mirror, in your purse, or on your dashboard.
- **Think about how you need to change your environment to promote success.** Does your desk at work have a candy bowl? Is the vending machine on your current route to the restroom? Are there places for you to work out conveniently, or should you buy a piece of equipment? Set your environment up for success!
- **Be a pre-planner.** Take a few minutes to think through your day. What do you need to have in place to put your behavioral change into practice? Do you need to pack a lunch to eat healthier? Do you need to resupply your blood glucose–monitoring case to have sufficient supplies? When will you fit in a few minutes of being active?

Wonder?

Are you ready, willing, and able to change?

According to behavioral-change experts, in order to make changes to your lifestyle, you must believe that it is **important** for you to make and maintain these changes and have **confidence** that you can do it. If making the behavioral change is important to you, and you have confidence that you can do it, then you are more likely to succeed. Behavioral experts and diabetes educators use a scale from 0 to 10, like the ones below, to help you flesh out your internal dialogue.

What numbers on the importance and confidence scales predict success?

On this scale of 0 to 10 (0 being not important and 10 being highly important), how important is it for you at this point to make (fill in the blank with a certain behavior change)?

0 1 2 3 4 5 6 7 8 9 10

On this scale of 0 to 10 (0 being not confident and 10 being very confident), how confident are you now that you can make (fill in the blank with a certain behavior change)?

0 1 2 3 4 5 6 7 8 9 10

Good question! Here's what the experts say:

- 7 or greater predicts that you will successfully be able to change a certain behavior.
- 4–6 suggest that you are probably in a contemplation mode about making the change.
- 3 and below suggests that this is not a behavioral change to focus your efforts on at this point because you are unlikely to be successful.

Set SMART Goals

When you set behavioral-change goals, it's important to make them realistic. If your goals are too general or overly ambitious, you won't achieve them. Consider setting your goals using the SMART format. SMART stands for **s**pecific, **m**easurable, **a**ttainable, **r**ealistic, and **t**ime-frame specific.

As you read about the importance of becoming more physically active, eating healthier, taking your medications, checking your blood glucose, and quitting smoking (if need be), begin to set your behavioral goals to change for good. Put the SMART format for goal-setting into action.

S • Specific
Narrowly define your goal.

M • Measurable
Choose a frequency for the goal. How many times a day or week will you do this?

A • Attainable
Make the goal challenging, but something that you can accomplish.

R • Realistic
Make the goal something you can do within the confines of your current life.

T • Time-frame Specific
Limited in time frame—set short-term goals that help you achieve them.

If I Only Knew . . .

Small steps eventually build big results and rewards . . .

I was determined to be the perfect patient when I was diagnosed with diabetes. Regarding food, I eliminated many favorite foods and all desserts and wine. It didn't take long for me to feel deprived and resentful. My response was to stop recording my blood glucose numbers, and I began to "cheat," particularly at my favorite breakfasts on Sunday mornings. It was time to take small steps to make this a healthier brunch. I started by ordering an egg white omelet with little or no cheese. Next, I ordered the toast unbuttered and spread on a smidge of strawberry jam. Now, I order a salad instead of potatoes. It took a long time to take that final step. These incremental changes have resulted in much better glucose results afterward. If I only knew, I would have started making small changes earlier—and been healthier and happier sooner.

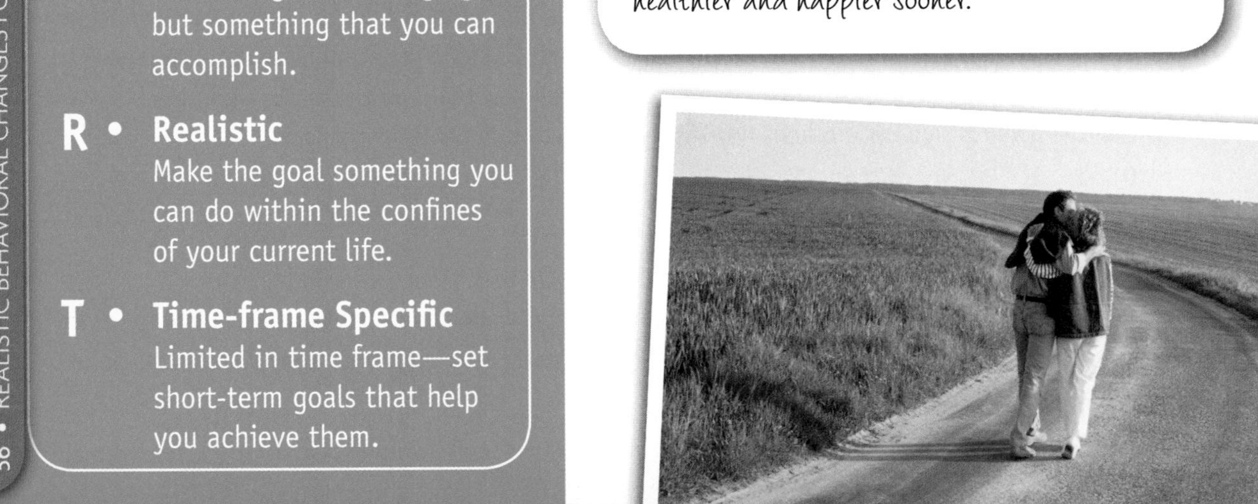

Sample Behavior Changes Using SMART

Find a few examples of behavioral-change goals set using the SMART format in the table below. Letters in parenthesis represent the five aspects of SMART: specific, measureable, attainable, realistic, and time-frame specific.

Behavioral Change Category	Current Behavior	Behavioral Change Goal Using SMART
Healthy Eating	You eat breakfast on the run from a fast-food spot, or the cafeteria at work Monday through Friday. Your usual choices are a sausage biscuit, a bagel with a thick layer of regular cream cheese, or a mega muffin and a banana.	For the next two months (T), three days each week (M) I will choose one of these healthier breakfasts: an English muffin with jelly and a small banana, or a bagel with light or fat-free cream cheese with an orange or half grapefruit (S,R,A).
Taking Medications	You manage to take your blood glucose–lowering medication most mornings but often forget to take your bedtime dose.	For the next two weeks (T), I will remember to take my bedtime blood glucose–lowering medication four days each week (M) by laying out the dose by my toothbrush in the morning when I take my morning dose (S,R,A).
Being Active	You currently get no physical activity outside of your daily life activities.	For the next three weeks (T), three days each week (M) I will get off the bus I take to work one stop before my current stop and walk the rest of the way (S,R,A).
Coping Healthfully	You feel angry about your diagnosis of diabetes and are yelling at your spouse more than usual.	During the next week (T), I will make three phone calls (M): to my doctor's office, the diabetes education program, and the local ADA (S) to determine where I can attend a local diabetes support group each month (R,A).

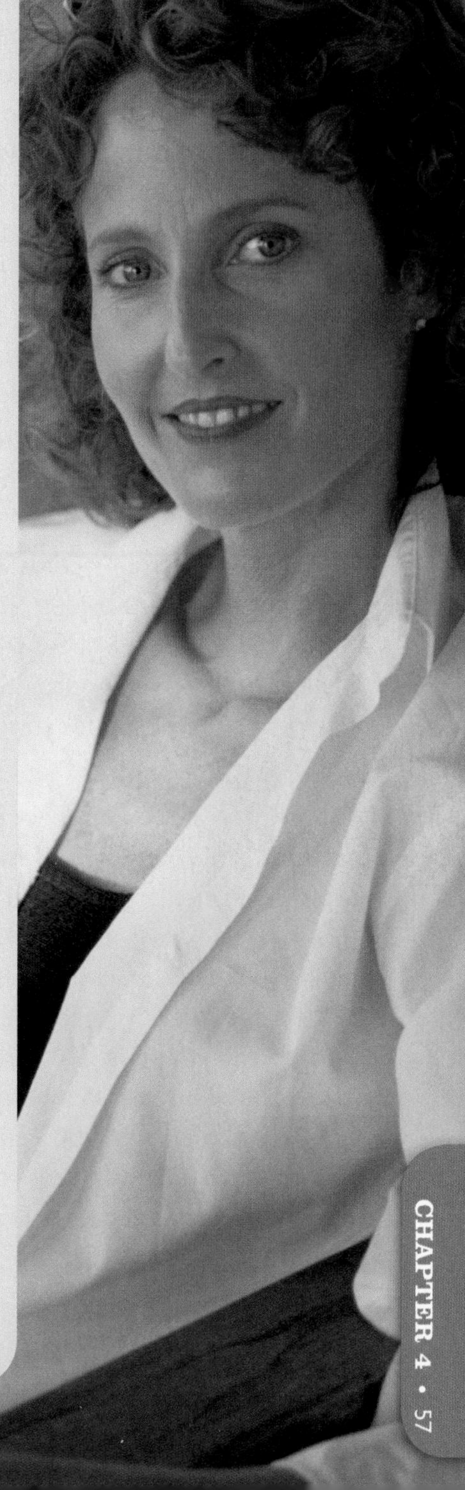

Record Keeping Matters

Studies show that regular record keeping helps people make and maintain their behavioral changes by getting and keeping them aware of their progress. It's valuable to keep records of your glucose checks, the foods and amounts you eat, the physical activity you do, and whatever else you and your providers feel will help you achieve your health and diabetes care goals. Use records to see whether you are successfully making the behavioral changes you set or whether you need to revise your goals. Use the records to understand your stumbling blocks, actions that you find helpful, and the effects of tweaks in your diabetes-care plan.

Take two copies of your records when you visit your health care providers, so you each have one to look at. Talk about any patterns you see in your records, and get a few suggestions from your health care provider to help accomplish your goals.

If you want and are able to check and record other aspects of your self-care, ask your health care provider whether you should be recording anything else. For instance, if you are only checking your blood glucose levels before meals, and they are always between 80 and 160, you might be surprised to find that your A1C is 8.4%. This number shows that your average blood glucose is near 200. Perhaps you should check your blood glucose two hours after meals to see what the results are then.

Record keeping is an ongoing process. Think about what you want to learn and what changes you want to make.

Wonder?

How long will it take me to make all of the necessary behavioral changes to stay healthy and manage my diabetes?

Living a healthy lifestyle and managing diabetes is a life-long proposition; however, to be successful, set short-term SMART goals. Research shows that there's no need for you to be perfect all the time to stay healthy and manage diabetes. It's the actions you take the majority of the time that will count the most. Small changes make BIG impacts. Don't beat yourself up for not doing things right every day. Give yourself positive strokes for all the positive actions you do take. Try to maintain a perspective of balance...and enjoy your real life.

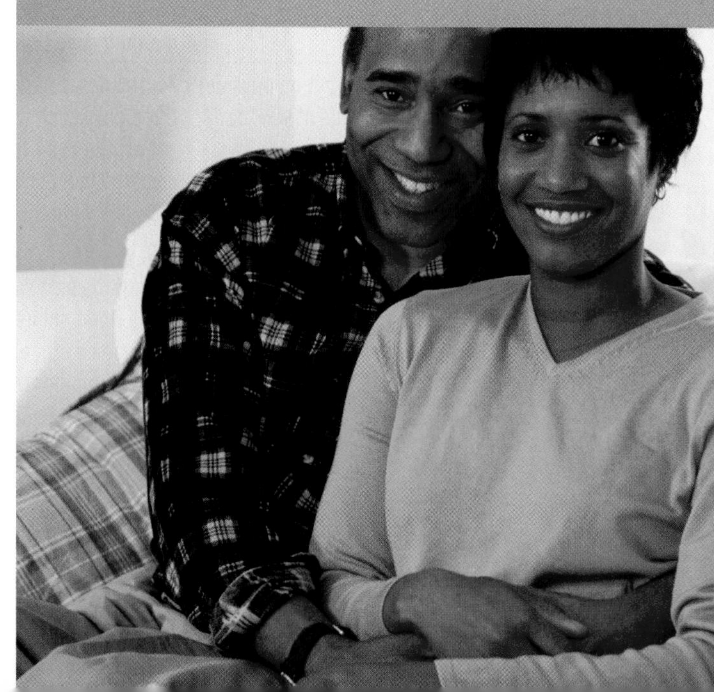

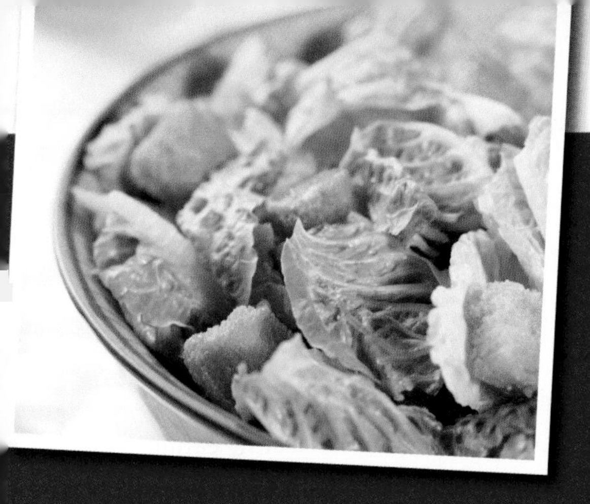

CHAPTER 5

Healthy Eating— The Basics

Hands down, healthy eating is often the most challenging part of managing diabetes. Research continues to show that eating healthy is an essential component of diabetes care—whether you take blood glucose–lowering medications or not. Times have changed when it comes to diabetes nutrition recommendations. The notion of a "diabetic diet" no longer exists. No special foods, meals, or menus are called for, and sugary foods and sweets are no longer forbidden. While this all makes life easier, eating healthy is by no means a simple task. This is especially true in today's fast-paced fast-food world. The best way to become a healthier eater is to make small, steady behavioral changes toward your healthy eating goals. Observe your current eating habits, and start to change them one by one. Over time, new habits will become second nature.

What You'll Learn:

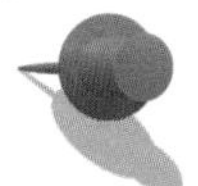

- Healthy eating goals to manage diabetes
- Recommendations for how much carbohydrate, protein, and fat to eat
- The truth about sugary foods and sweets
- The role of sodium and potassium in blood pressure control
- The number of meals and snacks to eat each day and why
- Common methods of diabetes meal planning

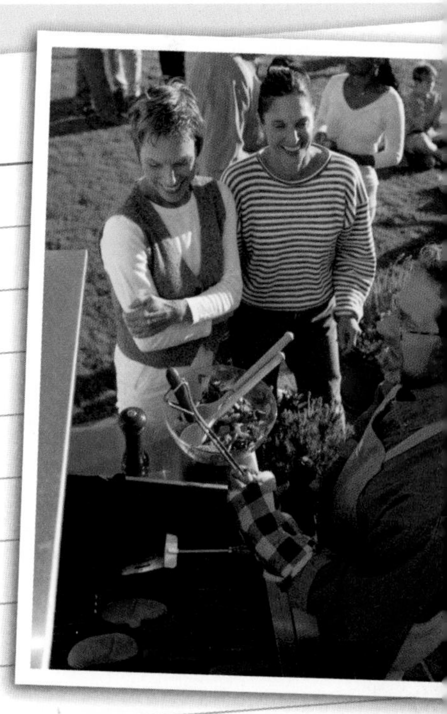

Wonder?

I already have to manage my high blood pressure and high cholesterol. Does the nutrition advice for diabetes conflict with that advice?

Good news! Today's nutrition recommendations for diabetes focus on disease prevention and management—that includes high blood pressure and abnormal blood lipids (fats), which are very common in people with pre-diabetes and type 2 diabetes. As you'll learn, the healthy eating guidelines for diabetes advise you to limit saturated and trans fats and eat minimal salt and sodium. These echo the recommendations to prevent and manage heart disease and high blood pressure.

DEFINITION:

sodium: a mineral and nutrient in foods that helps maintain the balance of water in the cells and keeps nerves functioning.

Today's Healthy Eating Goals

Whether you have pre-diabetes or diabetes, or just want to prevent developing type 2 diabetes, today's healthy eating goals are in sync with the healthy eating guidelines from worldwide health organizations, including the ADA's nutrition recommendations, the American Heart Association's recommendations, and the federal government's Dietary Guidelines for Americans.

The nutrition recommendations from the ADA suggest that you follow the same healthy eating guidelines as the general public in the Dietary Guidelines for Americans. These guidelines promote six key healthy eating goals.

TIPS + TACTICS

Tips to Eat More Vegetables

- *Take advantage of all the ready-to-eat or easy-to-fix vegetables in the supermarket.*
- *Keep some frozen and low-sodium canned vegetables on hand so that you always have vegetables ready to eat.*
- *Make a big salad to last a few days; store it in a plastic container.*
- *Don't buy frozen or canned vegetables in butter or flavor sauces.*
- *Make double and triple portions at one time, and spread them out over a few meals.*

Six Key Healthy Eating Goals

Goal	Which means...
Eat a variety of foods within and among the basic food groups while you stay within your calorie needs.	Make your calories count. Choose foods packed with vitamins and minerals. Don't use your calories up on foods that are high in added fats and sugars.
Control the amount of calories you eat to get to or stay at a healthy body weight.	Get to or stay at a healthy body weight. To achieve and maintain a healthy body weight, eat only the calories you burn each day. If your weight is creeping up, shave off calories by choosing healthier foods, and burn more calories with physical activity.
Increase the amount of fruits, vegetables, whole grains, and fat-free or low-fat milk and milk products you eat each day.	These foods provide essential vitamins and minerals to keep your body functioning properly. Choose more of these healthy low-fat foods to get the vitamins and minerals you need.
Choose fats wisely for good health.	Keep the amount of saturated fat and trans fats you eat low. Choose healthier fats and oils—those with mainly polyunsaturated and monounsaturated fats.
Choose carbohydrate wisely for good health.	Get about half the calories you eat each day from healthy carbohydrate—whole grains, legumes, dried beans, fruits, vegetables, and low-fat dairy foods. Eat fewer processed foods and foods with added sugars and fat.
Choose and prepare foods with little salt.	Limit your sodium intake to no more than 2,300 milligrams a day by eating fewer processed and prepared foods and not shaking the salt on when you prepare foods and eat them.

Wonder?

Do I need to prepare my food separately from my family?

No. The foods that are healthy choices for you will also be healthy choices for your family members who don't have diabetes. The easier you make it for everyone to eat healthy together, the more likely it is that you'll be able to continue practicing these important lifestyle changes over the years. Plus, it's more likely you'll raise your children and grandchildren with healthy eating habits. Keep in mind that if you have diabetes, your family members—children and grandchildren—are at risk, too.

Nutrition Nuts and Bolts—Calories

Food supplies energy in the form of calories to help the body function and move. Your body's need for calories never stops, even when you sleep. Calories in food come from one of three nutrients: carbohydrate, protein, and fat. The number of calories you need each day depends on many factors, including whether you are male or female, short or tall, younger or older, active or sedentary, have lost and gained weight many times, and others.

Here's a quick way to get a ballpark figure on how many calories you should consume daily.

Step 1: Calculate your basic energy needs.

These are the calories you need if you are doing nothing but lying in bed all day—just the calories to keep your organs functioning.

Women: Multiply your current or desired weight in pounds by 10 (pounds x 10).

Men: Multiply your current, or desired, weight in pounds by 11 (pounds x 11).

Step 2: Add the calories you need for activity.

Multiply basic calorie needs (from step 1) by the following, based on your level of physical activity. Add the two numbers together.

Sedentary (don't do much): x .2 (or 20%)

Moderately active: x .3 (or 30%)

Active: x .4 (or 40%)

Very active (your job involves physical work): x 0.5 (or 50%)

DEFINITION:

calories: a unit of measurement for the energy provided by food and alcohol; carbohydrate, protein, fat, and alcohol provide calories.

The number you get is your recommended daily calorie allowance. It's important to recognize that you won't eat the same precise number of calories each day. Instead, aim for a calorie range. For example, if the calculation above tells you that you should be consuming 1,800 calories, shoot for a daily range of 1,600–1,900 calories. The number of calories you eat each day depends greatly on the fat content of the foods you select.

Another BIG factor that plays into your calorie count is how precise you are about measuring your portions. Research shows that people can be off in their calorie counts by 500 calories at the end of a day simply by guessing at portions rather than weighing and measuring them precisely.

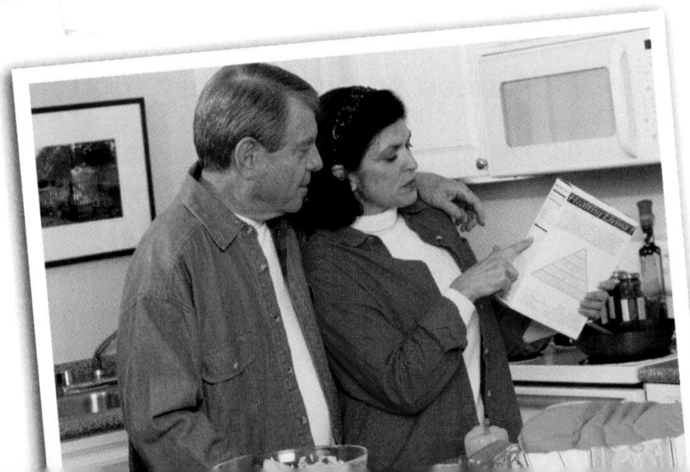

Wonder?

How many calories do I need to lose weight?

To figure out how many calories you need to lose weight, first figure out your total daily calories you should have using the formula on the previous page. To lose about one pound per week (which is a realistic goal for long-term weight loss), subtract 500 calories from the figure you obtained in the calculation. So, if you should be eating 2,000 calories a day, reducing your intake to 1,500 calories a day should allow you to lose up to a pound per week.

Foods That Contain Carbohydrate

The carbohydrate found in foods fall into three general categories: sugars, starches, and fibers:

- STARCHES: breads, cereals, pasta, and starchy vegetables (corn, potatoes)
- SUGARS: regular soda, gum drops, and syrup
- SWEETS: dessert, ice cream, and candy
- VEGETABLES (non-starchy): lettuce, broccoli, and carrots
- FRUITS: apples, oranges, fruit juice, and raisins
- DAIRY: milk and yogurt (cheese contains just a small amount of carbohydrate)

Carbohydrate

Carbohydrate are the main source of calories that provide your body with energy. They are your body's preferred source of energy because they provide that energy in a form that's easy for your body to break down and use. After you eat, your body breaks down carbohydrate into glucose that travels to your bloodstream. To help the cells use this glucose, the body normally releases insulin from the pancreas. This is where people with diabetes, depending on the type, level of control, and other factors, have varied responses to carbohydrate.

TIPS + TACTICS

Tips to Eat More Fruit

- *Take advantage of the precut, ready-to-eat fruit available in today's supermarkets to always have fruit at the ready.*
- *Keep a plastic container full of cut-up fruit, so you can have it any time.*
- *Take one or two pieces of fruit from home each day to eat with lunch, as an afternoon snack, or on your way home to take the edge off your hunger.*
- *Stock canned or jarred fruit with no sugar added in the pantry—applesauce, peaches, pears, and pineapple for starters.*
- *Serve fruit with the main course at dinner.*

Remember to eat fruit in moderation because too much fruit can increase your blood glucose.

TIPS + TACTICS

Tips to Choose Whole-Grain, High-Fiber Starches

- *BREADS: Choose breads that list whole-wheat flour, rather than enriched white flour, as one of the first ingredients.*
- *CRACKERS: Choose low-fat or fat-free crackers made from whole grains instead of butter crackers made from enriched flour.*
- *CEREALS: Pick whole-grain dry cereals made from bran that contain at least 3 to 5 grams of fiber per serving.*
- *RICE AND PASTA: Choose brown rice. Buy a whole-wheat or whole-grain pasta.*

Wonder?

How many grams of carbohydrate do people with diabetes need?

The Dietary Guidelines for Americans recommend that people get 45 to 65% of their calories from carbohydrate. As a frame of reference, Americans eat about 50% of their calories as carbohydrate—a moderate amount of carbohydrate. For example, a sedentary woman who wants to lose weight should limit her calories to 1,400 to 1,600 a day, so she should consume 700 to 800 calories from carbs daily. At 4 calories per gram of carbohydrate, this translates to 175 to 200 grams of carbohydrate per day.

Carbohydrate are the main nutrient that raises blood glucose levels after eating. Both the amount and the type of carbohydrate you eat affect your blood glucose, but the amount of carbohydrate seems to have a greater effect than the type. It's important to eat similar amounts of carbohydrate at your meals and snacks to keep your blood glucose under control.

If you are not able to keep your blood glucose levels on target by eating a healthy and balanced amount of carbohydrate throughout the day, you may need a blood glucose–lowering medication. Decreasing the amount of carbohydrate you eat to an unhealthy level (meaning you will not eat enough of the wide array of vitamins and nutrients you need) will probably not bring your blood glucose back to normal. If you are not hitting your blood glucose goals, and you aren't taking a blood glucose–lowering medication, talk with your health care provider about starting on one or more medications to get your blood glucose under control.

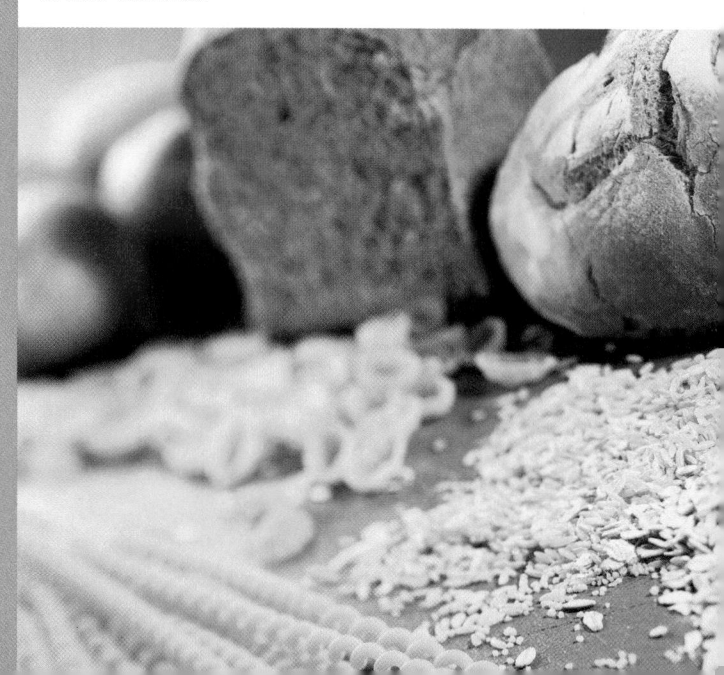

DIETARY FIBER

The fiber in foods, called dietary fiber, is a source of carbohydrate. The main sources of fiber are foods that contain most of their calories from carbohydrate—whole grains, breads, cereals, beans and peas, and fruits and vegetables. Fiber can affect how quickly your food is digested and can have an effect on your blood glucose level as well. Some research shows that very high-fiber diets (excess of 50 grams per day) can also improve total and LDL cholesterol. The reality is that most Americans eat an average of 10–13 grams a day, which is nowhere near the amount of fiber you need, let alone the amount you would need to improve blood glucose and lipids. The U.S. Government nutrition recommendations suggest you eat 20 to 35 grams of dietary fiber per day—just about double what you might be currently consuming [also check out *Chapter 6*, page 75]. There are two main types of dietary fiber—insoluble and soluble.

DEFINITION:

dietary fiber: fiber contained in the diet, consisting of both soluble and insoluble fiber. General recommendations are for 20–35 grams of fiber per day.

TIPS + TACTICS

Tips to Eat More Low-fat and Fat-free Milk and Yogurt

- *Gradually switch to fat-free milk to lower your saturated and trans fats and calories. Start with reduced-fat (2%), then low-fat (1%), and finally fat-free.*
- *Choose fat-free milk when you order a fancy coffee or tea drink.*
- *Don't limit cereal and milk to breakfast; it can be a quick and easy lunch, dinner, or snack.*
- *Use plain yogurt as a substitute for sour cream on potatoes.*
- *Keep containers of light yogurt to use as a quick snack or part of a meal.*

INSOLUBLE FIBERS. Insoluble fiber grabs onto liquid as it travels down the gastrointestinal tract, pushing food through the gastrointestinal tract more quickly. If you eat a good supply of insoluble fiber to promote a bulkier and softer bowel movement, you also reap other health benefits—preventing hemorrhoids, diverticulosis, and colon and rectal cancer. Foods that contain insoluble fiber include whole-grain cereals and breads.

SOLUBLE FIBER. Soluble fiber dissolves during digestion but remains gummy and thick. It is thought that eating a lot of soluble fiber can, by binding onto cholesterol during digestion, lower blood cholesterol a small amount. It is also thought that eating a lot of soluble fiber can slightly lower the rise of blood glucose by slowing down the absorption of glucose. Food sources of soluble fiber include beans, peas, and some grains, such as oats and barley.

Wonder?

What are resistant starches?

Resistant starches are a third type of dietary fiber. There are several types of resistant starch—some are naturally found in carbohydrate-containing foods like legumes, cooked and cooled potatoes, pasta, and rice. Resistant starches are digested in the large intestine, not, as most carbohydrates are, in the small intestine. When resistant starches are digested, they produce a type of fat (fatty acid) that has been shown to have health benefits, such as lowering blood glucose after eating and increasing insulin sensitivity.

DEFINITION:

resistant starches: starches that escape digestion in the small intestines but are digested in the large intestine, which provides some health benefits; they are considered a third type of fiber.

If I Only Knew . . .

How easy it is to fit in more vegetables . . .

Yes, I know, I should eat more vegetables, but do I have time and do I want to prepare them? No way! So, I've invented all sorts of one-dish wonders using as many shortcuts—with as many varied vegetables—as possible. I find salads are the easiest and most versatile. I buy lettuce in a bag (pre-washed), sliced mushrooms, and grape tomatoes that I can just toss on top. I buy artichoke hearts in a can, red peppers in a jar, and grated Parmesan cheese to sprinkle on top for flavor and texture. Canned tuna or salmon, garbonzo and kidney beans, or a handful of chopped walnuts or almonds provide a bit of protein. I also make a mean stir-fry with pre-cut vegetables—peppers, mushrooms, and broccoli. And if I'm out and a sub sandwich or pizza is the healthiest I can manage, I get either loaded with sliced tomatoes, mushrooms, onions, and green peppers. "Pack on the veggies" I tell them.

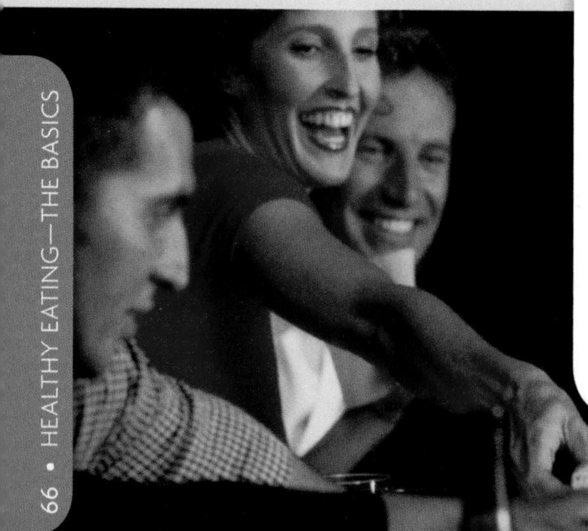

GLYCEMIC INDEX/GLYCEMIC LOAD

The glycemic index (GI) measures the increase in blood glucose levels during the two hours after you eat a particular kind of carbohydrate-containing food. Research has shown that some foods that contain carbohydrate create a quick and more dramatic rise in blood glucose, while others cause a slower rise. Glucose itself is the standard for the GI, and it is assigned an arbitrary number of 100. Other foods are assigned GI numbers—relative to the glucose standard of 100—either higher or lower. The GI doesn't consider typical food portions. Glycemic load (GL) takes the GI of a food and factors in a common serving size to give a more practical indicator of the glycemic impact or effect of that food on blood glucose.

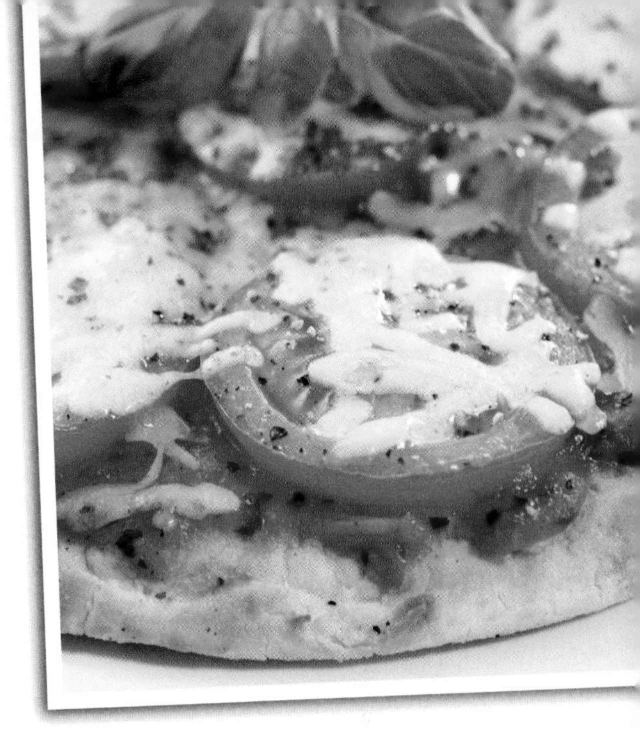

Keep in mind that GI numbers are available only for a small number of commonly eaten foods and non-mixed dishes (such as lasagna or enchiladas). In other words, carrots, watermelon, and potatoes have GI numbers, but casseroles and soups do not. It's also important to note that the type of carbohydrate (e.g., starch or sugar) does not consistently predict the GI. For example, some fruits have a lower GI, and others have a higher GI.

The use of the GI and GL in diabetes meal planning has been an area of debate for several decades. The ADA now suggests that GI and GL may be valuable concepts for people with diabetes if these measures are used in addition to careful monitoring of your total carbohydrate intake at meals and snacks. For example, you might decide to eat beans or barley instead of white rice because beans and barley have a lower GI. Think of GI and GL as two more factors to consider when you choose which foods to eat.

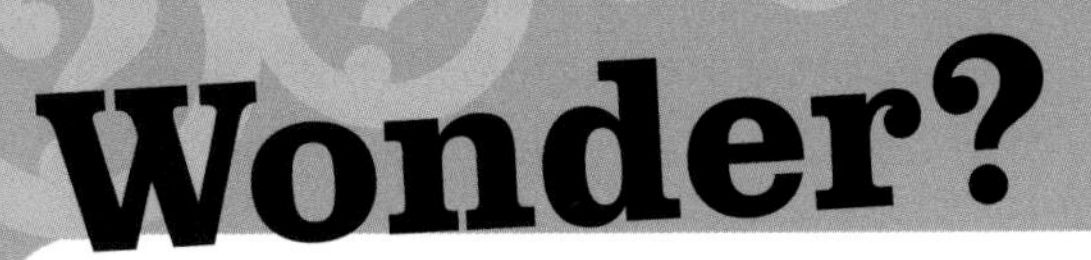

Wonder?

What's the difference between whole grains and dietary fiber?

Whole grains and grain products contain the entire grain seed of a plant, while dietary fiber is found in more foods than just those that supply whole grains. Fiber is also found in fruits; starchy vegetables, such as corn and peas; legumes, such as beans, peas, and lentils; and nonstarchy vegetables, such as broccoli, green beans, and carrots. They are rich in fiber, vitamins, minerals, and more.

Wonder?

How much protein do people with diabetes need?

Both the Dietary Guidelines for Americans and the ADA recommend that you eat 15–25% of your calories from protein. For a frame of reference, 20% protein for a woman who needs 1,400 calories a day would be 70 grams. Most Americans eat more protein than they need. Plus, Americans in general also eat more sources of protein that are high in total and saturated fat—meats and cheeses. To lighten up on protein and total and saturated fat, choose lean cuts of meat, prepare foods in healthy ways, and eat smaller amounts of these foods. Choose more low-fat and non-meat sources of protein, such as beans and peas, whole grains, low-fat dairy foods, and fruits and vegetables.

Also, keep in mind that myriad factors can affect how slowly or quickly foods raise your blood glucose levels, such as:

- your blood glucose at the time you eat
- how much blood glucose–lowering medicine you take, when you take it, and when you eat
- the amount of fiber and whole grains in a meal (these can slow the rise of blood glucose)
- how ripe a fruit or vegetable is when you eat it (the riper the food, the more quickly it can raise blood glucose)
- the variety of the food (for example, long-grain or short-grain rice, Idaho vs. Yukon Gold potatoes)
- the other foods you eat along with the carbohydrate (a meal that is mainly carbohydrate with a small amount of fat will raise your blood glucose more quickly than a meal with more fat)

Protein

Protein is a source of calories from foods that provides energy, but unlike carbohydrate, protein isn't your body's preferred source of energy. Once you eat protein, the body breaks it down into amino acids, which are used to build, repair, and maintain the body's tissues. Like carbohydrate, protein contains 4 calories of energy per gram. Protein eaten in reasonable amounts does not generally cause a rise in glucose levels.

These foods provide most of their calories from protein:

- Red meats (beef, lamb, pork, and veal)
- Seafood, fish, and shellfish
- Poultry
- Cheese
- Eggs

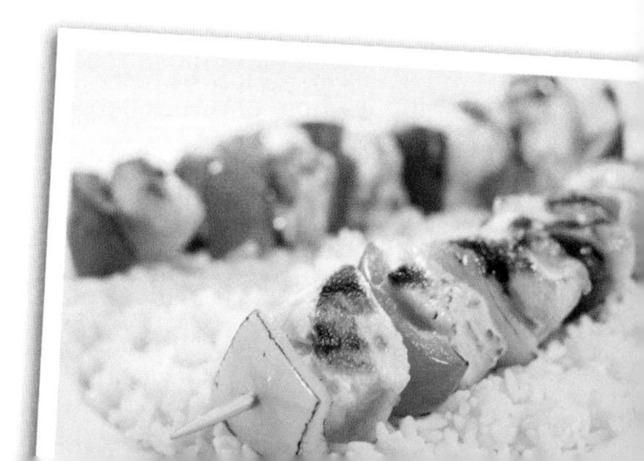

TIPS + TACTICS

Tips to Eat Less Protein

- *Buy and prepare smaller quantities (just what you need for the recipe) so that you eat less.*
- *Cook dishes that stretch the meat portion—Chinese stir-fry, pasta with meat sauce, beef and bean burritos.*
- *Split a meat or meat-substitute entrée in restaurants. If you need more food, fill the meal out with an extra salad or cooked vegetables.*
- *In fast-food restaurants, order single, regular, or junior-size sandwiches, and stay away from the doubles and triples.*

Tips to Eat Less Total Fat

- *Use less of these, and take advantage of reduced-fat versions (as long as you enjoy the taste!): butter, margarine, oil, salad dressing, mayonnaise, cheese, cream cheese, and sour cream.*
- *Prepare foods using low-fat preparation methods, including broiling, baking, braising, barbecuing, grilling, poaching, and steaming.*
- *Eat fried foods only once in a while.*

Wonder?

What should my main focus be when it comes to fats and my health?

Today, nutrition experts agree that your main focus should be on choosing and eating healthy fats. Your secondary focus should be on eating less total fat, especially if you believe you eat more than the American average of 35% of your calories as fat. Keep in mind that all fat—whether from a healthy or unhealthy source—still rings in at about 50 calories per teaspoon. If you want to eat fewer calories to lose weight, research shows that you will be most successful keeping your percentage of calories from fat between 25 to 30% of calories. For someone who needs about 1,500 calories a day, that's about 42 to 50 grams of fat a day.

Fat

Calories from fat are used for energy if the body doesn't have enough calories from carbohydrate. Insulin plays a role in helping your body store fat in your cells. Fat does not tend to cause a rise in glucose levels. In fact, higher-fat meals can delay the rise of glucose from carbohydrate in the meal.

Fat provides a concentrated source of calories at 9 per gram, regardless of whether it's healthier or less healthy fat [also check out *Types of Fats: The Healthy and the Not So Healthy*, page 70]. That's more than double the calories per gram for carbohydrate and protein. Some of the fat you eat is in the food itself, like the fat in meat, chicken, and cheese. Some fat is added to foods, such as margarine on a potato, cream cheese on a bagel, dressing on a salad, or the fat used in frying.

These foods provide many or nearly all of their calories from fat:

- oils
- margarine, butter, and cream cheese
- salad dressings, mayonnaise, and sour cream
- nuts and seeds
- sausage and bacon (regular)
- cheese (reduced-fat and part-skim cheese contains less fat)

TYPES OF FATS: THE HEALTHY AND THE NOT-SO-HEALTHY

If you have diabetes, you are at risk for, or may already have, abnormal blood lipids [also check out *Chapter 2*, page 23, and *Chapter 9*, page 121], so it's important to lighten up on the unhealthy fats you eat. The chart to the right defines the four types of fat and provides tips to eat more or less.

One other component in this heart-healthy mix is dietary cholesterol—which is not fat, but a wax-like substance that is part of some foods from an animal origin. The recommendation for people with diabetes is to keep your intake of cholesterol to no more than 200 milligrams each day.

TIPS + TACTICS

Tips for Limiting Cholesterol Intake

- *Eat small portions (no more than 3 ounces cooked) of red meat, poultry, and seafood.*
- *Choose reduced-fat or part-skim cheeses.*
- *Select fat-free milk or yogurt.*
- *Limit foods that are high in cholesterol—organ meats and some shellfish (calamari, shrimp).*

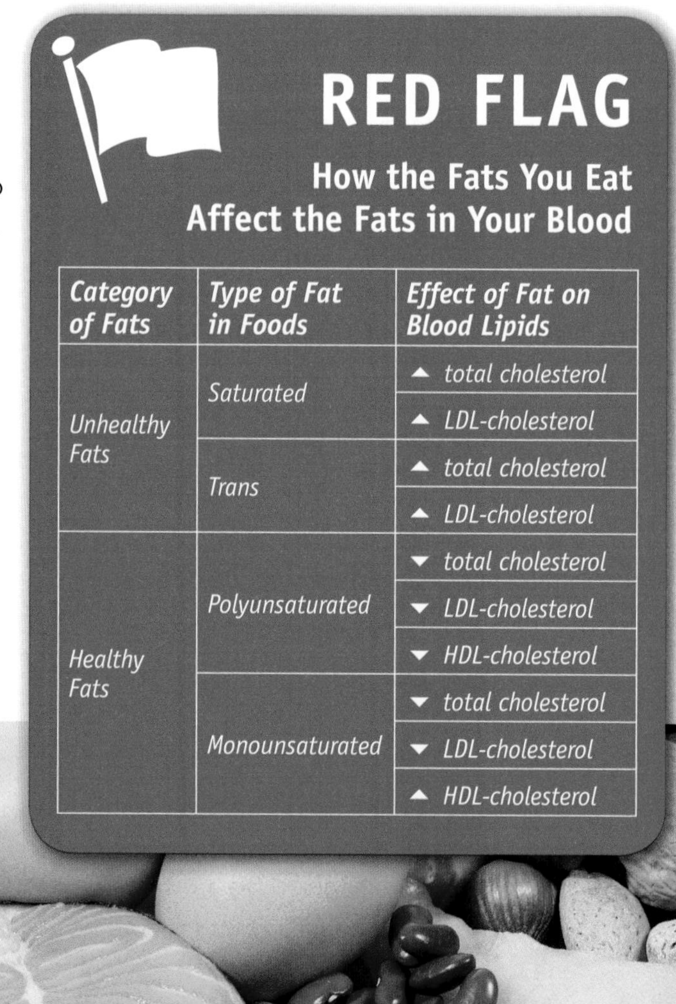

RED FLAG

How the Fats You Eat Affect the Fats in Your Blood

Category of Fats	*Type of Fat in Foods*	*Effect of Fat on Blood Lipids*
Unhealthy Fats	*Saturated*	▲ *total cholesterol*
		▲ *LDL-cholesterol*
	Trans	▲ *total cholesterol*
		▲ *LDL-cholesterol*
Healthy Fats	*Polyunsaturated*	▼ *total cholesterol*
		▼ *LDL-cholesterol*
		▼ *HDL-cholesterol*
	Monounsaturated	▼ *total cholesterol*
		▼ *LDL-cholesterol*
		▲ *HDL-cholesterol*

Salt, Sodium, High Blood Pressure, and Diabetes

Research suggests that an increased intake of salt causes the body to hold on to more fluid. More fluid retained in the blood vessels can contribute to high blood pressure. Some people—especially those who are over age 50, who are African American, or who have high blood pressure or diabetes—are known to be "salt sensitive." In other words, they are especially sensitive to the blood pressure–raising effects of sodium and salt. The good news is that salt-sensitive people have a better response to eating less sodium and salt than people who aren't salt-sensitive. The only way to tell whether you are salt sensitive is to see whether your blood pressure responds to a lower-sodium eating plan.

Unfortunately, high blood pressure and diabetes go hand in hand. Nearly three quarters of people with diabetes have high blood pressure greater than or equal to the ADA's goal of 130/80 mmHg [also check out *Chapter 2*, page 23, and *Chapter 9*, page 121]. High blood pressure plays a role in heart and blood vessel diseases. Many people with diabetes take one or more blood pressure medications to lower blood pressure. Cutting down on salt and sodium may help you reduce and control your blood pressure. Other changes in your eating plan that are in line with healthy eating can also help you control your blood pressure.

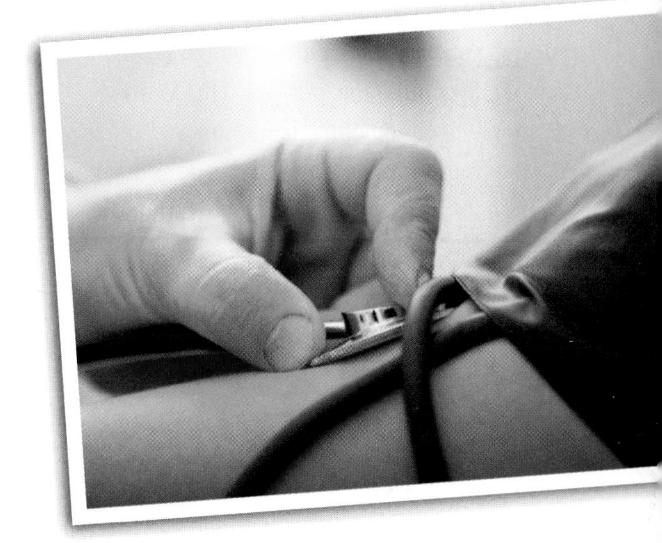

TIPS + TACTICS

Tips for Lowering Blood Pressure: Beyond Salt and Sodium

- *Eat more potassium. Potassium plays a role in the proper functioning of the heart. Research shows you can counterbalance the effects of too much salt and sodium by eating enough potassium.*
- *Consume more dairy foods for calcium. Several studies, including the well-known Dietary Approaches to Stop Hypertension (DASH), have shown that getting enough dairy foods can help lower blood pressure.*
- *Keep alcohol intake to moderate amounts. Excess consumption of alcohol—more than three drinks a day for both men and women—has been shown to raise blood pressure.*
- *Trim a few pounds. Research shows that losing even 10 pounds can lower blood pressure.*

Wonder?

Should I limit sodium?

Most Americans eat too much sodium—between 4,000 and 6,000 mg a day. That's nearly double, sometimes triple, the amount of 2,300 milligrams per day that the ADA and the healthy eating guidelines suggest. This is the amount recommended for people who don't have high blood pressure. If you have high blood pressure, it is suggested that you get your sodium count down to no more than 1,500 milligrams per day. This is an extremely small amount of sodium and quite challenging unless you use all fresh and unprocessed foods and say no to restaurant meals, especially fast food.

Psst...

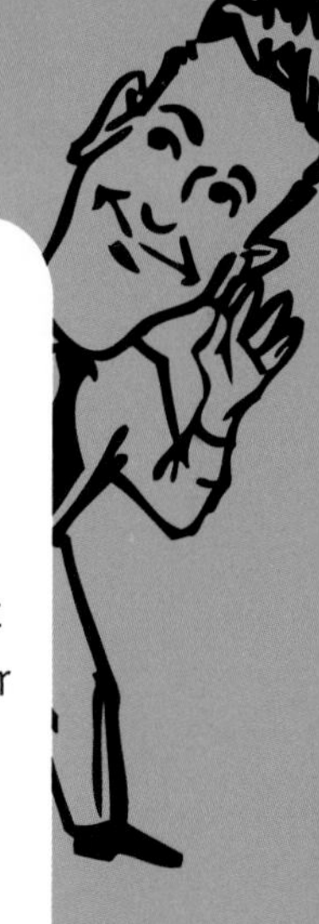

Biggest Sodium Culprits

Salt is the most common condiment added to foods in preparation and used at the table. That's why it's easy to understand why you may think that salt puts a lot of people's sodium count over the top; however, this isn't true. The largest sodium culprit is convenience, processed, and restaurant foods, which add up to nearly 75% of the sodium in the American diet. Sodium finds its way into foods because it both flavors and preserves. Manufacturers are being encouraged to reduce the amount of sodium in foods and are doing so slowly.

Meal Planning Methods for Diabetes

Over the years, various meal-planning methods have been used by health care providers to teach people with diabetes about how to eat healthier with diabetes. Today, there are a variety of approaches used. Keep in mind that no single meal-planning approach works for everyone with diabetes. Today, more health care providers are using a mix of meal-planning approaches.

Exchange Lists for Meal Planning

The Exchange System came into being back in 1950, when the ADA, The American Dietetic Association, and the United States Public Health Service joined forces to develop it. The goals? To make meal planning easier for people with diabetes and to develop a consistent approach so health professionals could have a common language. Foods are divided into six groups based on their macronutrient profile—the amount of carbohydrate, protein, and fat in them. A meal plan is created around eating a set number of food servings from the six different food groups. Since 1950, the Exchange Lists for Meal Planning have been revised numerous times. The latest resource is *Choose Your Foods: Exchange Lists for Diabetes* (ADA, 2007).

Carbohydrate Counting

For years, carbohydrate counting was the method of choice in the United Kingdom.

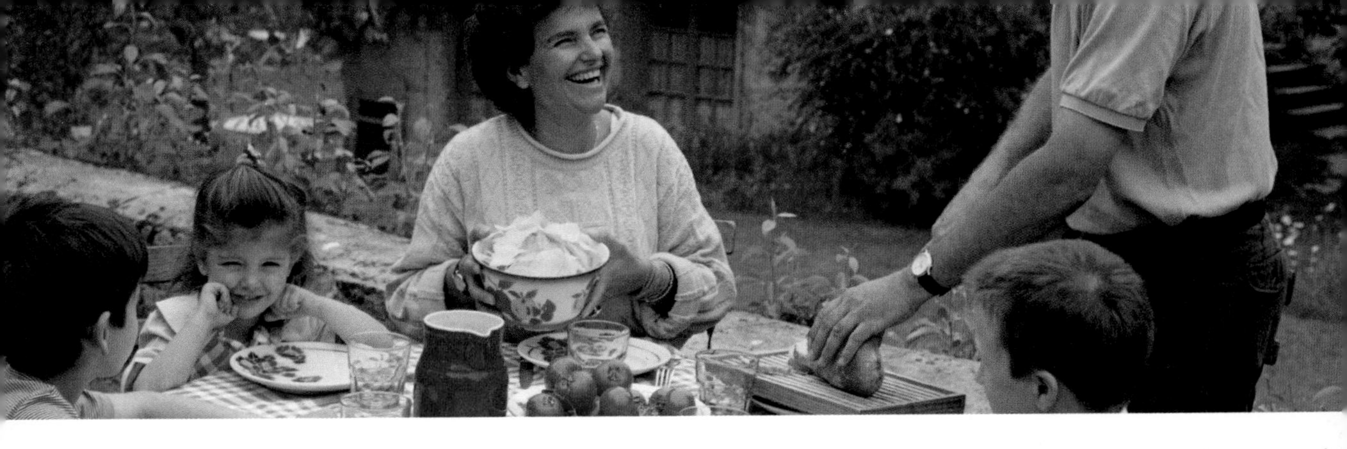

Then, in the early 1990s, carb counting received a lot of attention in the Diabetes Control and Complications Trial (DCCT) [also check out *Chapter 2*, page 23]. Over the years, carb counting has become a common approach to meal planning. Carb counting can be taught as a basic method of meal planning where the focus is to eat a prescribed number of grams of carbohydrate or carbohydrate choices (1 choice equals 15 g of carb) at meals and snacks. It can also be taught as advanced carb counting, which is used by many people with diabetes who take insulin several times a day or wear an insulin pump. People who use advanced carb counting take a specified amount of insulin based on the amount of carbohydrate they eat at meals and snacks. The book *Complete Guide to Carbohydrate Counting* (ADA, 2004) provides extensive information on this meal-planning approach.

The Plate Method

The Plate Method was adapted by several dietitians in Idaho in the 1990s from a meal-planning model first described in 1970 in Sweden. This method is designed to help you assemble healthy meals in the correct proportions and to spread the carbohydrate content of the meal evenly within each meal.

The central feature of this method is a plate that is divided into quarters. For both lunch and dinner, a person is encouraged to fill:

- 1/2 of the plate with vegetables
- 1/4 of the plate with starches
- 1/4 of the plate with meat
- one serving (cup) of milk
- one serving (small- to medium-size piece) of fruit

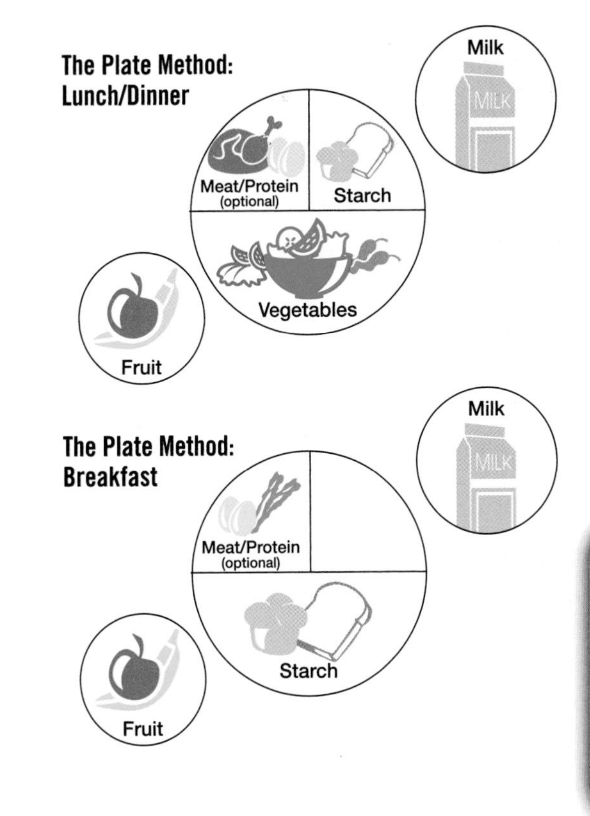

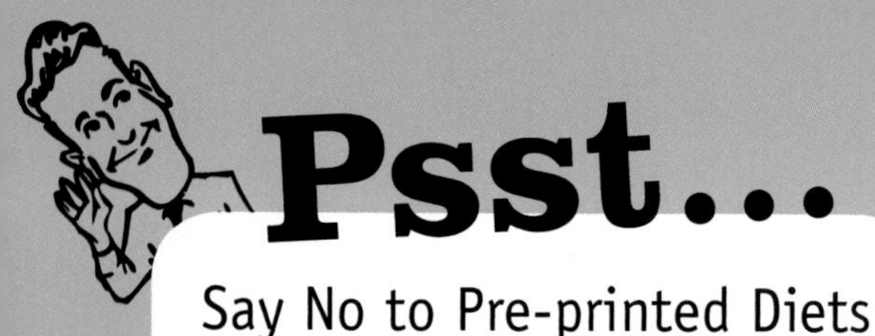

Psst...

Say No to Pre-printed Diets

For years, health care providers handed out pre-printed meals plans for different calorie levels—1,200, 1,500, 1,800, and so on. It has been shown over and over that it is difficult to follow a set meal plan, because it simply doesn't mesh with real life. You may find that you want or need a meal plan to help provide you with a framework for what to eat, how much to eat, and when. If you feel this will help, work with a dietitian to get this, but don't fall into the trap of looking for a rigid diet to follow long-term, because these diets rarely lead to long-term success. Becoming a healthier eater is a matter of making slow and steady behavior changes over time.

Myth

People with diabetes must eat 3 meals and 3 snacks each day

Fact

Years ago, health care providers would advise people with diabetes to eat three meals a day and three snacks to keep blood glucose levels in a safe range if they were on blood glucose–lowering medication. In those days, there was one type of blood glucose–lowering pills—sulfonylureas—or intermediate and regular types. Today, there are several groups of blood-glucose-lowering medications that don't cause hypoglycemia, along with insulin which causes fewer problems with low blood glucose. Today's advice is to include snacks in your eating plan if you want them, if your blood glucose still tends to drop below normal, or if you need snacks to get the calories or nutrients you require.

Wonder?

Why is the timing of meals so important?

To help manage your blood glucose levels, you'll want to:

1) Spread out your three meals throughout the day so you have about 4 to 5 hours between them.
2) Eat your meals at similar times from day to day.
3) Distribute the amount of carbohydrate at your meals as evenly throughout the day as you can, realizing that evening meals tend to be heavier than breakfast meals.

These three actions allow time between meals for blood glucose levels to come back down to your target zone before you eat again. These actions can also keep you from being too hungry between meals. Research shows that it can take longer after eating (in excess of 4 hours) for blood glucose to come back down to ideal pre-meal levels (70–130 mg/dl) in people with diabetes, especially in pre-diabetes and type 2.

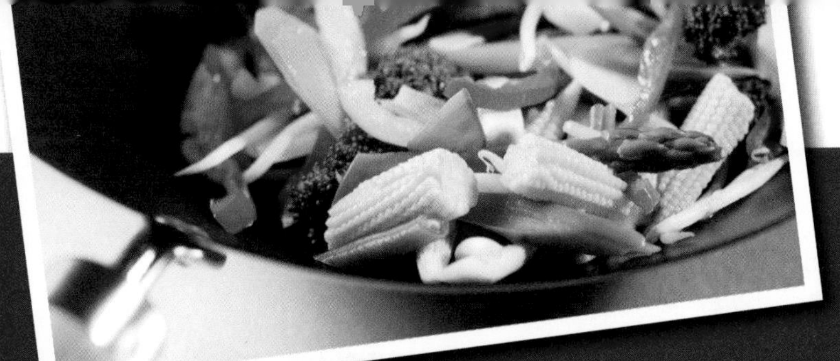

CHAPTER 6

Eat Healthy—Real Life Challenges and Solutions

Eating healthy was a challenge even years ago when people mainly ate meals cooked at home. Those days are gone. Today in our time-crunched, fast food driven world, it's even harder to abide by the healthy-eating guidelines. Food has become a part of nearly every life event and activity—from holiday and religious celebrations to business meetings or school-related fundraising events. It can be a challenge to put together healthy meals at these functions, in restaurants, and at other pit stops along the path of life.

This chapter offers you realistic solutions to the daily challenges of trying to eat healthy and manage diabetes in our challenging food environment. Try to slowly and steadily make positive changes in your eating habits to move in the direction of your nutrition and diabetes goals. Though we're surrounded by food at every turn, evidence suggests that healthy and convenient options are becoming more readily available in supermarkets, convenience stores, and restaurants.

What You'll Learn:

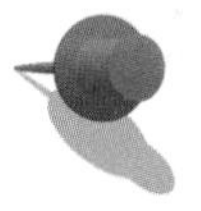

- The importance of planning to eat healthy and manage diabetes
- Food-shopping strategies
- What's on the Nutrition Facts label and how to let the label guide your food purchases
- All about sugar substitutes and sugar-free foods
- Portion-control tips, tactics, and tricks when eating at home and away
- Resources for cooking and baking with diabetes
- How to choose healthier restaurant foods, from American to ethnic fare

Planning—A Key to Healthy Eating

Though taking time to plan what you are going to eat for a week sounds arduous, you'll want to spend time to plan what you'll eat. If you are like most people, you buy the same foods week after week and then prepare and serve the same meals repeatedly. This is actually a good thing, because it makes your planning process easier.

Once you get into a groove that includes planning, you'll find that this approach actually saves you time and money and helps you become healthier. Think about how you can fit these planning steps into your life. Develop an inventory list for the foods you always want to have in your pantry, refrigerator, and freezer. Take stock of what you have and what you need to buy to keep your inventory as you want it. (Tip: Keep your inventory list in the kitchen, and add items as you run out of them.) And, spend a few minutes planning meals you'll prepare and eat during the next week. Add additional items you'll need to your shopping list.

Wonder?

How can I make meal planning easier?

If your goal is to get out of the convenience-food lifestyle that you know isn't healthy for you or your family, take advantage of what supermarkets have to offer. Supermarkets have become a cross between a supermarket and a restaurant with the amount of ready-to-eat foods they sell. You can choose from reasonably portioned healthy frozen meals or ready-to-eat main courses, sides, soups, and salads. If you're time-crunched, and cutting up greens for a salad just isn't going to happen, choose from ready-to-eat vegetables like carrots, tomatoes, celery, broccoli, and more. Grab a bag of pre-washed greens in your preferred variety [also check out *Chapter 5*, page 59]; ready-to-eat fruit like apple slices, pineapple chunks, sliced berries, and pieces of melon; and even whole-grain products like cereals, pasta, and breads. All of these options make it easier and faster to enjoy meals at home with less fuss.

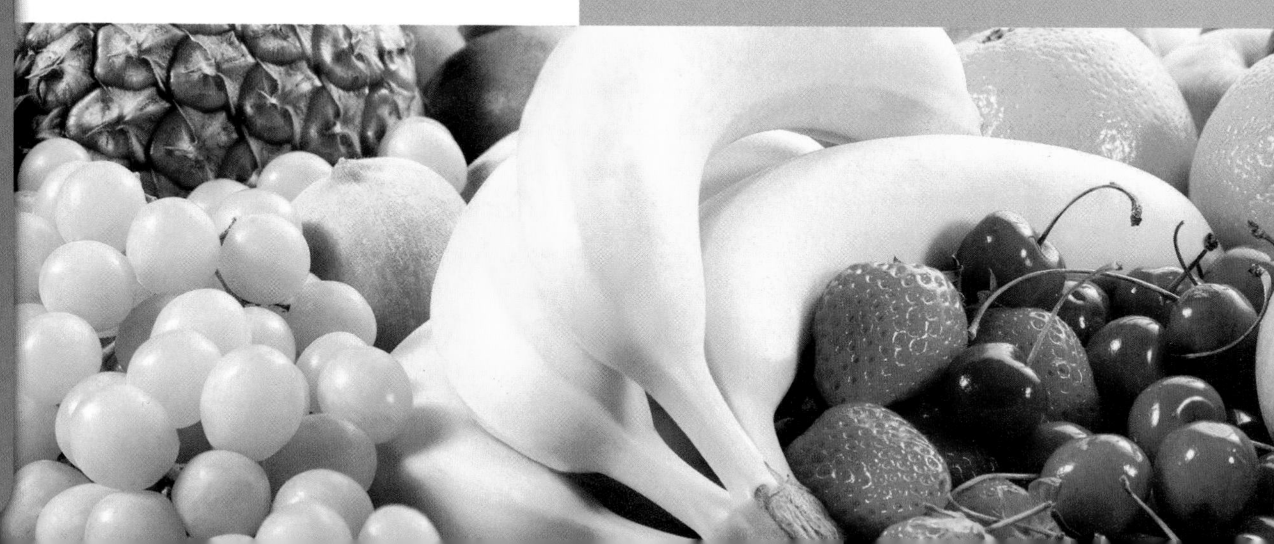

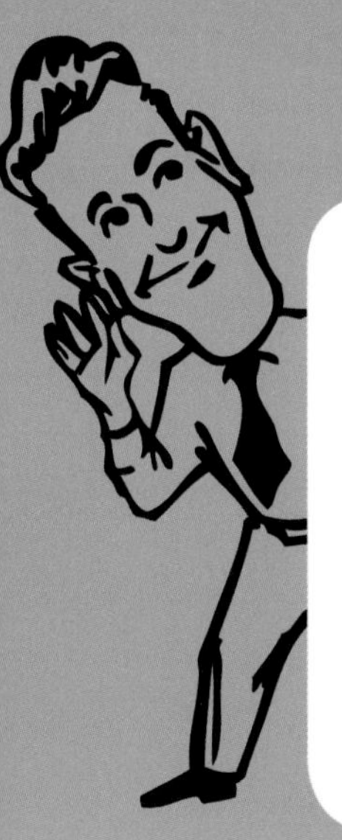

Psst...

Investigate Home Food- and Meal-delivery Services

The computer age, competition, and the time and energy crunch have given rise to services that can remove the drudgery of shopping, and save time and money. Check out supermarket-operated shopping services. You complete your order online, and foods are delivered to your home. You'll also find services that deliver meals (fresh, frozen, etc.) to your doorstep, customized for your nutrition needs and food preferences. You can even find cooks for hire who will prepare healthy meals for you and prepare them in, or deliver them to, your home. The possibilities are expanding, making it easier to help you save time and money.

TIPS + TACTICS

Ways to Shop Smart

- *Shop infrequently. The more organized you are, and the more storage space you have, the less frequently you have to shop.*
- *Shop at the same market, and choose one where you find most of what you need. Because you know where things are, you'll shop faster.*
- *Shop when the market is less crowded. Avoid the market between 5 and 7 p.m.*
- *Don't shop when you're hungry, to avoid temptation and a fuller shopping cart.*
- *Let your shopping list be your guide. Avoid dropping in impulse items.*
- *Don't feel compelled to walk every aisle. The healthiest foods are usually around the edges—fruits and vegetables on one wall, meats and poultry down another, and dairy foods along another wall.*
- *Read Nutrition Facts labels and ingredient lists to make sure that you know what you're buying and that the food fits into your meal plan.*

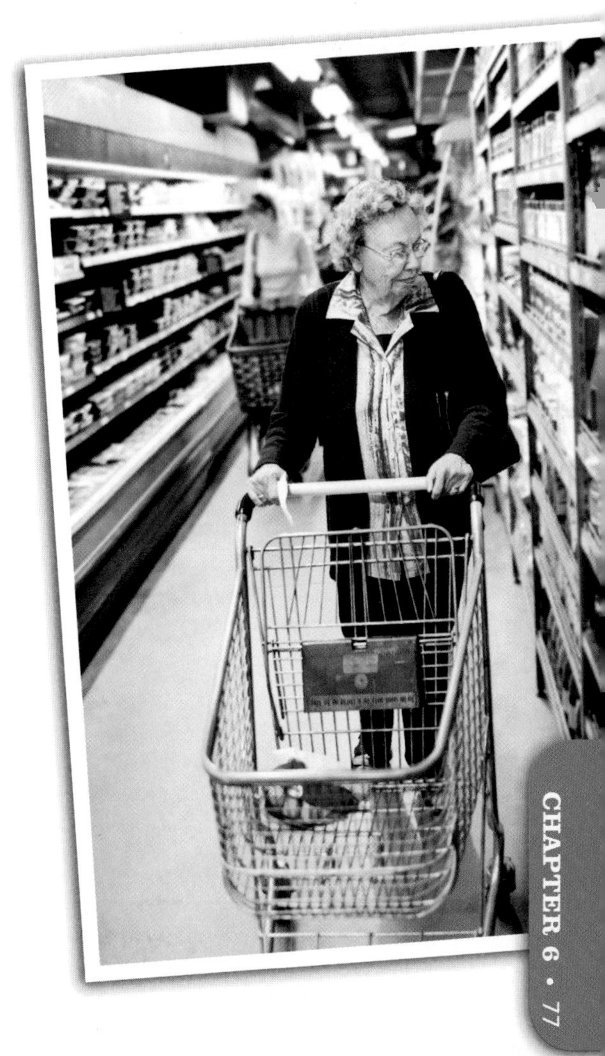

The Food Label's Nutrition Facts

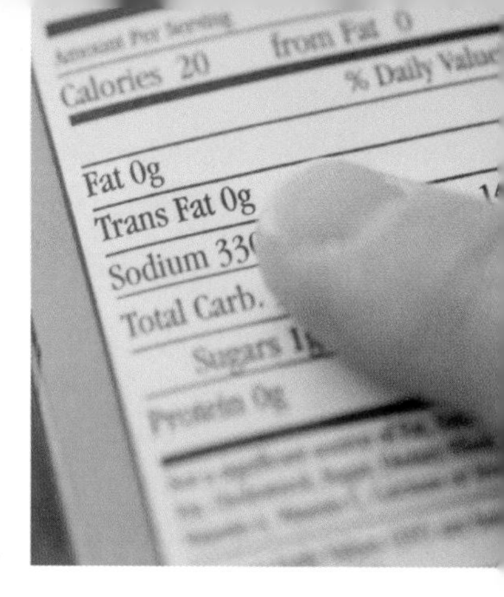

The Nutrition Facts label required on most packaged and processed foods is one of your best sources for nutrition information. The contents required on the Nutrition Facts reflect the federal laws and regulations from the Food and Drug Administration (FDA) and the U.S. Department of Agriculture (USDA). The Nutrition Facts label was changed significantly in 1994. The only major change since then occurred in 2006, when trans fat and information about certain food allergens began to be required by law.

Nutrition Facts

Serving Size 1 cup (228g)
Servings Per Container 2

Amount Per Serving

Calories 260 **Calories from Fat** 120

	% Daily Value*
Total Fat 13g	**20%**
Saturated Fat 5g	**25%**
Trans Fat 2g	
Cholesterol 30mg	**10%**
Sodium 660mg	**28%**
Total Carbohydrate 31g	**10%**
Dietary Fiber 0g	**0%**
Sugars 5g	
Protein 5g	

Vitamin A 4% • Vitamin C 2%
Calcium 15% • Iron 4%

*Percent Daily Values are based on a 2,000 calorie diet. Your Daily Values may be higher or lower depending on your calorie needs.

	Calories:	2,000	2,500
Total Fat	Less than	65g	80g
Sat Fat	Less than	20g	25g
Cholesterol	Less than	300mg	300mg
Sodium	Less than	2,400mg	2,400mg
Total Carbohydrate		300g	375g
Dietary Fiber		25g	30g

Calories per gram:
Fat 9 • Carbohydrate 4 • Protein 4

1. SERVING SIZE
2. SERVINGS PER CONTAINER
3. TOTAL FAT: The two types of fat that must be listed are saturated fat and trans fat. Manufacturers may also choose to list monounsaturated and polyunsaturated fat; however, if a nutrition or health claim is made, they must provide this information.
4. CHOLESTEROL
5. SODIUM
6. TOTAL CARBOHYDRATE: Two types of carbohydrates—dietary fiber and sugars—must be listed under Total Carbohydrate. Dietary fiber and sugars are the required sources of carbohydrate. Manufacturers may voluntarily list other sources, such as insoluble or soluble fiber, other carbohydrate, or sugar alcohols, but they must list them if they make health or nutrition claims.
7. PROTEIN
8. VITAMINS AND MINERALS: The percentage of the Recommended Daily Intake (RDI) in the food must be listed for vitamins A and C, calcium, and iron, must be listed. If a nutrition claim is made about another vitamin or mineral, the percentage of RDI in the food for that vitamin or mineral must be on the label.
9. PERCENT DAILY VALUES: The daily values are based on the amount of each nutrient needed by a person who eats 2,000 calories a day. Larger packages also must list the daily values for 2,500 calories a day. Percent Daily Values for total fat, saturated fat, cholesterol, sodium, total carbohydrate, and dietary fiber are listed to the right of each nutrient.
10. INGREDIENTS: (not shown) The FDA requires that ingredients be listed in descending order by how much of the ingredient is used, so the first ingredient is the one present in the greatest amount. The last ingredients are present in smaller amounts.

Wonder?

Why is "Sugars" on the Nutrition Facts label plural?

Sugars include all one-unit sugars (glucose and fructose) and two-unit sugars (sucrose, lactose, and high-fructose corn syrup). Foods may contain two types of sugars.

- Naturally occurring sugars: These sugars provide healthy sources of energy, vitamins, carbohydrate, and minerals. (Examples: fructose in fruit and lactose in milk.)
- Added sugars: These sugars are added to foods during food processing, in food preparation, or at the table. Food processing is now the greatest contributor of added sugars. Often, the added ingredient is high-fructose corn syrup.

All sugars—from natural sources or added—contain 4 calories per gram. They are 100 percent carbohydrate. The current use of the word "sugars" doesn't allow you to decipher between the two types of sugars; however, you can determine the sources of sugars by reading through the ingredients.

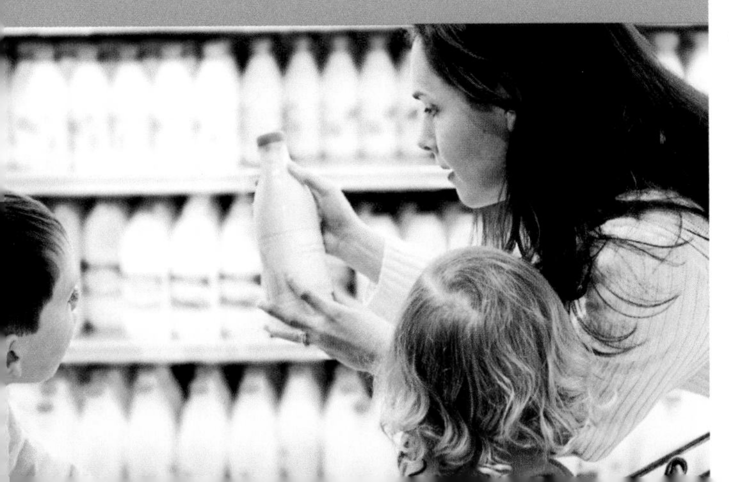

Sizes of Servings

The serving sizes on food labels for nearly 140 categories of foods are standardized and regulated by the FDA. The standard servings are intended to be a typical serving, but they tend, for many people, to be on the small side. The serving size must also be provided in household measures, such as cups or table-spoons, and it must list the number of items, so you can get a good sense of the quantity. For example, the serving size on a cracker label might read 15 crackers (28 g/1 oz).

The nutrition information provided on Nutrition Facts is for one serving on most foods. Some foods packaged for individual use that contain more than one serving, such as a 20-ounce bottle of soda, must provide nutrition information for the total amount of food in the serving. The FDA has hinted that it may decide to require companies to abide by this practice for more foods.

Reduced-Sugar, No-Sugar Added, and Sugar-Free Foods

If there is one thing people think they know about diabetes, it's that people with diabetes need to avoid foods that contain sugar. Hopefully, you know that's no longer true [also check out *Chapter 5*, page 59]. You probably have discovered lots of reduced-sugar and so-called sugar-free foods on supermarket shelves. Foods labeled sugar-free or no sugar added aren't necessarily carbohydrate- or calorie-free. The calorie count depends on which sweeteners have been used in the food, along with the other ingredients in the food. Learn the categories of the ingredients used to manufacture these foods, and their names, then decide whether you want to include them in your meal plans.

NO-CALORIE SWEETENERS (SUGAR SUBSTITUTES)

Today, there are five FDA-approved no-calorie sweeteners, acesulfame potassium (common brand name Sunette), aspartame (NutraSweet), neotame, saccharin (Sweet 'n Low), and sucralose (Splenda). These sweeteners have all undergone rigorous research (through the FDA food additive approval process) and have been shown to be safe for all Americans to use, including people with diabetes and women who are pregnant.

The main no-calorie sweeteners used today are aspartame and sucralose. They are found in many foods and beverages, including diet sodas, fruit drinks, syrups, yogurts, ice cream, jams, and other products. They are also available in packets or as granular products to use like sugar for sweetening foods or for cooking and baking. These sugar substitutes contain almost no calories or carbohydrate and don't raise blood glucose. As long as you don't use more than ten packets or teaspoons a day, you don't need to be concerned with these few calories and grams of carbohydrate. Sugar substitutes can help you greatly lower the carbohydrate and calories you eat.

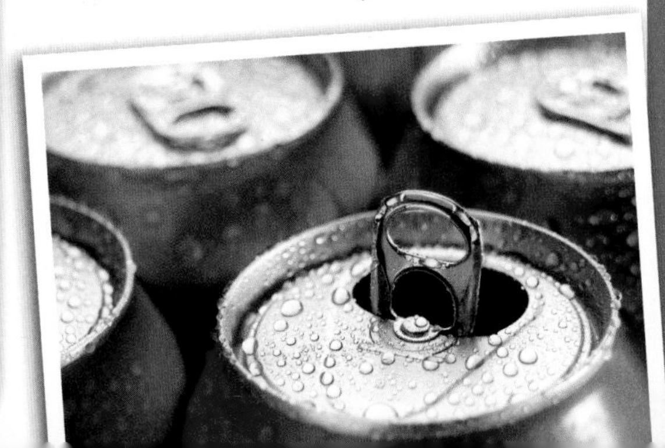

Wonder?

What about the dietary supplement stevia?

Stevia is currently categorized as a dietary supplement. Dietary supplements are not required to go through the same intensive research and FDA approval as some sugar substitutes. Two stevia producers are partnering with large beverage manufacturers to research stevia and bring it to the market. Cargill is working with Coca-Cola on Truvia (a form of stevia call rebiana), while the manufacturers of Equal (Merisant Company) and PepsiCo are partnering to bring Purevia (a form of stevia called Rebaudioside-A) to the market. Stevia has gone through the FDA's Generally Recognized as Safe (GRAS) process.

By the Numbers

Regular Sugar vs. No-Calorie Sweetener

Here is a comparison between a regularly sweetened fruit drink and a fruit drink sweetened with a no-calorie sweetener.

Type of drink	Regularly sweetened fruit drink	No-calorie fruit drink
Serving Size	8 ounces	8 ounces
Calories	110	10
Carbohydrate (g)	30	2
Sugars (g)	29	0

By the Numbers

Regular Sugar vs. Sugar Alcohol

Here is a comparison of regular ice cream and ice cream sweetened with a sugar alcohol.

Type of ice cream	Regular	No-sugar-added, light
Serving Size	1/2 cup	1/2 cup
Calories	140	100
Total Fat (g)	8	5
Carbohydrate (g)	15	15
Sugars (g)	15	4
Sugar Alcohol (g)	0	3

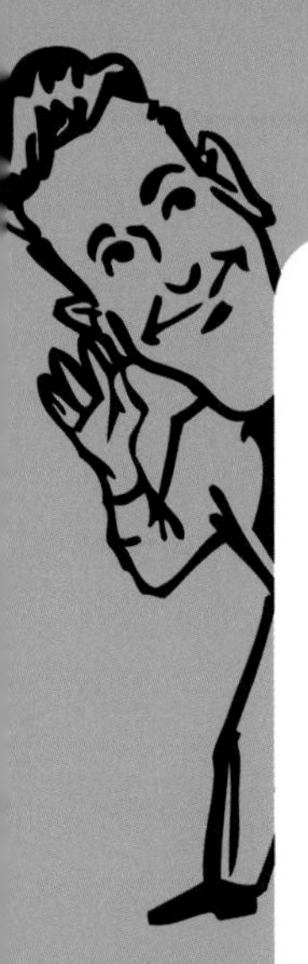

Psst...

Choosing to Use Sugar-Free Foods or Not

Deciding whether to use sugar-free foods and which foods to eat is up to you, your taste buds, and your nutrition and diabetes goals. Many sugar-free foods—especially those sweetened with no-calorie sweeteners, such as diet carbonated and noncarbonated drinks, hot cocoa, yogurt, and syrups—can satisfy your sweet tooth, reduce your waistline, lower your blood glucose, and may improve your blood lipids due to less saturated fat intake. Find a few sugar-free foods that truly offer you a calorie savings and help you stay on track with your nutrition and diabetes goals.

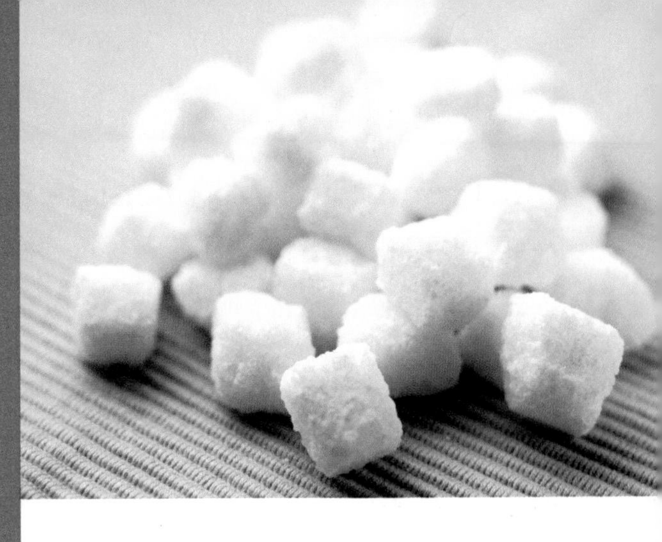

REDUCED-CALORIE SWEETENERS: POLYOLS (SUGAR ALCOHOLS)

Sugar alcohols are a group of ingredients commonly used in sugar-free foods. Interestingly, they're not sugar or alcohol. They are carbohydrate-based ingredients that contain half the calories of sugar on average (2 calories vs. 4 calories per gram). Polyols can replace sugar in foods like candy, cookies, and ice creams. Polyols contain about half the calories of sugar because they aren't completely digested. A downside of polyols is that they can cause gas, cramps, and/or diarrhea in some people or in large amounts. According to the FDA, foods with large amounts of polyols must provide an information statement that notes: "Excess consumption may have a laxative effect."

Replacing sugars with polyols can cause a lower rise in blood glucose than with regularly sweetened foods; however, people don't tend to use these foods frequently enough to result in a significant lowering of calorie or carbohydrate intake or blood glucose. The calories and grams of carbohydrate per serving of sugar-free foods sweetened with polyols often are only minimally reduced.

Wonder?

If I count carbs to calculate my insulin doses to cover food, do I need to subtract the grams of fiber or not?

It depends! Bearing in mind that most people don't eat more than 2–5 grams of carbs per meal, this small amount of fiber isn't going to impact your insulin doses and blood glucose much. However, if you use carb counting to estimate your meal time rapid-acting insulin doses and eat certain foods and/or meals that are in excess of 5 grams of fiber, and you feel your carb counting is precise, then subtract these grams of fiber from the total carbs for the meal. Calculate your insulin dose from this reduced carb total.

Resources for Nutrition Information

At times, you will come across foods you want to eat that don't come with a label or nutrition information (such as some restaurant foods), as well as times that you don't have nutrition facts by your side. Many resources are available both online and off.

ONLINE:

- *www.diabetes.org/myfoodadvisor*
- *www.ars.usda.gov/nutrientdata*
  This is the USDA's National Nutrient Database for Standard Reference. This database, updated annually, contains nutrition information for about 7,000 commonly eaten foods. It is downloadable to a PC and searchable online or downloadable to a PDA.
- *www.mypyramidtracker.gov*
  This government online dietary assessment, part of the mypyramid website, provides information on diet quality, related nutrition messages, and links to nutrient information.
- *www.calorieking.com*
- *www.nutritiondata.com*
- www.dietfacts.com

OFFLINE:

- *The Doctor's Pocket Calorie, Fat and Carbohydrates Counter*, by Allan Borushek. Family Health Publisher. 2007 (www.calorieking.com).
- *The Ultimate Calorie, Carb, & Fat Gram Counter,* by Lea Ann Holzmeister. ADA, 2006.
- *Guide to Healthy Restaurant Eating, 4th edition*, by Hope Warshaw. ADA, 2009

Portion-Control Tools

There is no doubt that the portions of foods served in America are a BIG reason for our expanding waistlines, along with the epidemics of pre-diabetes and type 2 diabetes [also check out *By the Numbers: How Portions Have Grown*, page 85]. Therefore, a key to healthier eating is portion control—a tall task when you are served large portions in restaurants.

The critical reason to weigh and measure your foods is to reacquaint your eyes (and stomach) with reasonable portions. When you first start to follow a healthy eating plan, weigh and measure your foods frequently. Get your portions in line with the amounts you should eat, and then you can weigh and measure your foods less frequently. The more you weigh and measure, the more precise your portions will be, and the better you'll estimate portions with your eyes and hands when you eat out [also check out *Portion Control Tools on the Road*, page 84]. Controlling portions of the less healthy foods you eat is a relatively easy and powerful way for you to achieve your diabetes and nutrition goals. So, gear up to start weighing and measuring your foods.

Portion-Control Tools for the Home

Have these measuring tools handy. You may have them stored away. Dig them out, dust them off, and find them some counter space. Keeping them in view increases their use.

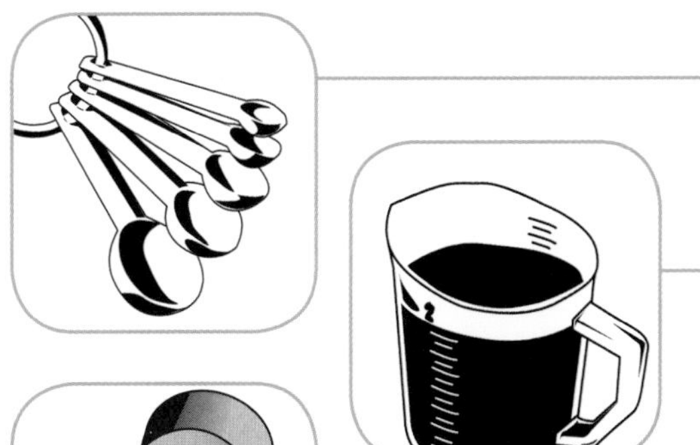

Have a set of measuring spoons that includes 1/2 teaspoon, 1 teaspoon, 1/2 tablespoon, and 1 tablespoon.

Have a 1-cup measuring cup with lines showing 1/4, 1/3, 1/2, 2/3, and 3/4 cup measures. A liquid measuring cup should be clear (glass or plastic). To measure liquids correctly, set the cup down and bend down at eye level to make sure the liquid reaches the proper line.

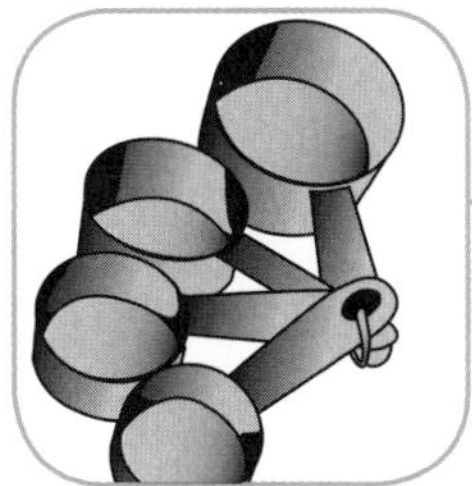

Have a set of measuring cups that includes 1/4-cup, 1/3-cup, 1/2-cup, and 1-cup measures. Choose the correct size for your serving, and fill it to the top. Level it with the flat edge of a knife.

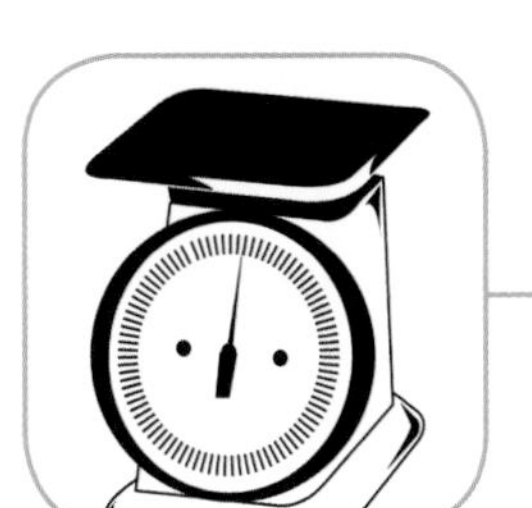

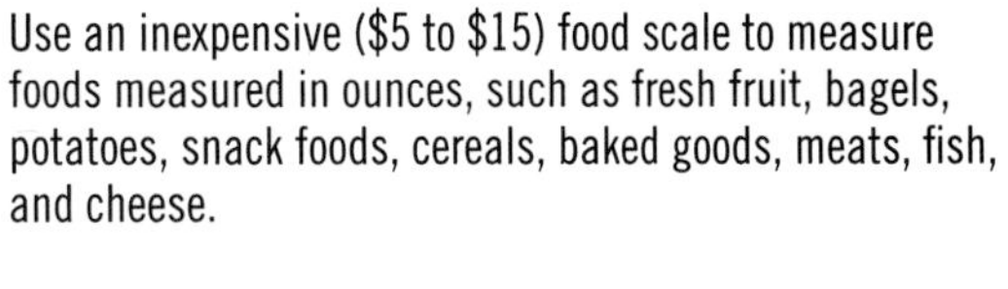

Use an inexpensive ($5 to $15) food scale to measure foods measured in ounces, such as fresh fruit, bagels, potatoes, snack foods, cereals, baked goods, meats, fish, and cheese.

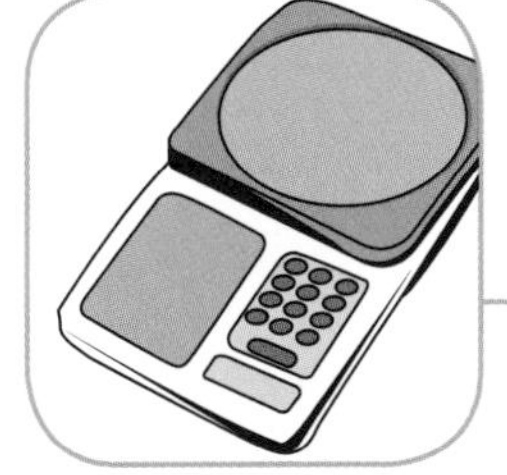

More expensive scales ($25 to $190) are available. They measure more precisely in ounces, pounds, grams, or kilograms and may provide the gram weight and grams of carbohydrate based on an internal database, which certainly helps with carb counting (*www.diabetesnet.com* is a good resource for these scales).

TIPS + TACTICS

Control Portions at Home

- *Use measuring equipment to get and keep your eyes in line with proper portions. Always keep measuring spoons, cups, and a scale on the counter.*
- *Use smaller plates and bowls. Less food looks like more food on smaller plates.*
- *Don't serve family style. Avoid putting bowls, pots, or casserole pans on the table.*
- *Don't leave the extras out when you sit down to eat if you don't want to eat them. When you buy produce—fruits, vegetables, and starches—buy the smallest pieces. Look for small apples, bananas, and potatoes.*
- *When you buy meat, fish, or poultry, buy what you need for the meal, rather than too much, to limit overeating.*

Control Portions on the Road

- *Steer clear of items with portion descriptors that are large (unless you split them), such as:* giant, grande, supreme, extra large, jumbo, double, triple, double-decker, king size, *and* super.
- *Don't fall for deals in which the "value" is to serve you more food so that you can save money. That's not a value to you.*
- *Avoid all-you-can-eat restaurants or buffets. They simply encourage overeating.*
- *Split, share, and mix and match menu items to get what you want to eat in the portion you want to eat it.*
- *Use your well-trained eyes and hands to estimate proper portions.*
- *If you know that the portion you'll be served will be too large, ask for a take-home container when you place your order. Put away the second serving before you dig in.*

Portion-Control Tools on the Road

It is one thing to have measuring equipment at home, but like most Americans, you probably eat many meals away from home. Have no fear! When you're on the road, your eyes and hands become your portion-control tools. They work well at home, too, once you have correct portions nailed down.

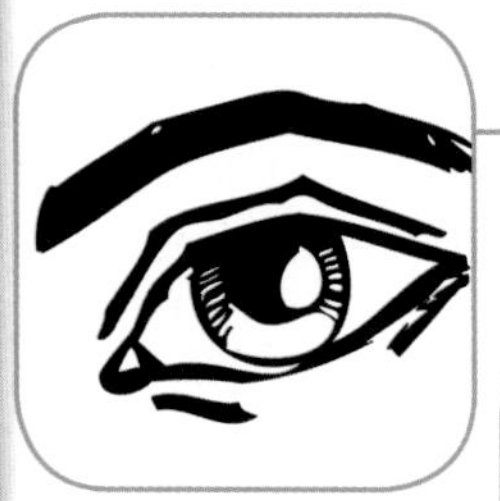

Don't underestimate a well-trained set of eyes. Your eyes are an invaluable measuring tool because they travel with you. Just make sure they are honest!

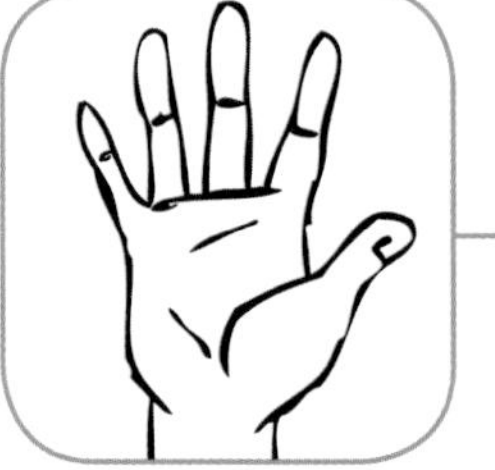

- Thumb tip (from tip of finger to first knuckle) = 1 teaspoon
- Thumb (from tip of finger to second knuckle) = 1 tablespoon
- Two fingers lengthwise = 1 ounce
- Palm of hand = 3 ounces (A regular-sized deck of cards is 3 ounces)
- Tight fist = 1/2 cup
- Loose fist or cupped hand = 1 cup

Note: These guidelines hold true for most women's hands, but some men's hands are much larger. Check out the size of your hands in relation to various portions.

By the Numbers How Portions Have Grown

To see how portions have grown over 20 years, look at these comparisons.

Food	Portion 20 Years Ago	Portion Today
Bagel	3-inch diameter, 140 calories	6-inch diameter, 350 calories
Cheeseburger	330 calories	590 calories
Spaghetti and Meatballs	1 cup pasta, 3 meatballs, 500 calories	2 cups pasta, 3 large meatballs, 1,000 calories
French Fries	2 1/2 ounces, 210 calories (today's small order at a fast-food restaurant)	7 ounces, 610 calories (today's large order at a fast-food restaurant)
Turkey Sandwich	1 sandwich on 2 slices bread, 320 calories	1 sandwich on large roll, 820 calories

Source: National Heart, Lung, and Blood Institute (www.nhlbi.nih.gov).

If I Only Knew . . .

Measuring foods at home would help me assess restaurant portions . . .

The two most important items in my kitchen are my mother's old measuring cups and an inexpensive ($10) food scale. At home, these measuring tools keep me honest and have helped train my eyes to accurately estimate portions in restaurants. For example, at a Chinese restaurant, I can look at the rice bowl and scoop out just about 2/3 cup of rice because I use a 1/3-cup measuring cup at home to measure a portion of rice. At my favorite Italian restaurant, I visualize one cup of pasta on my plate at home, and when the bread comes, I can guess how much Italian bread equals the size of a piece of commercial bread. Measuring foods at home helps me eat in restaurants with less stress and anxiety about getting off track. I can relax and enjoy eating out. Thanks, Mom!

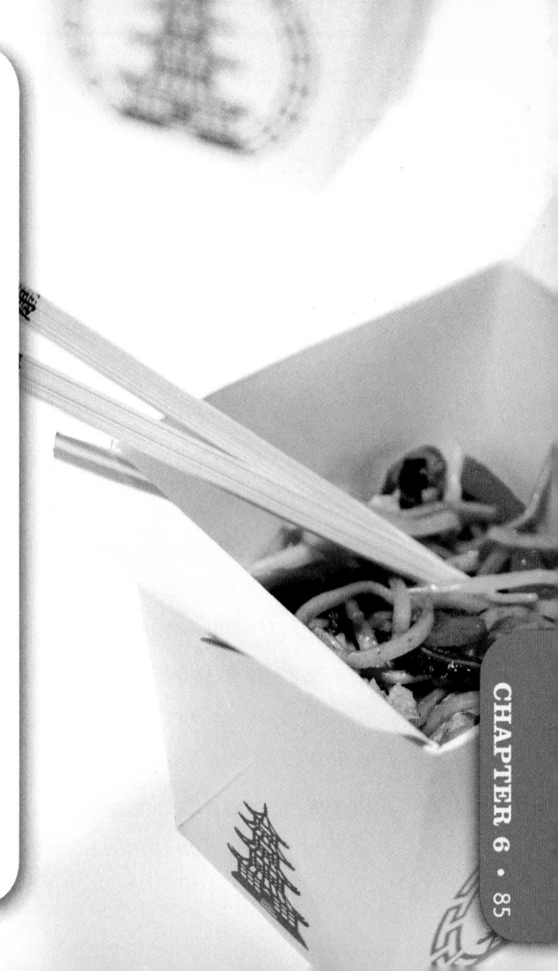

Healthier Restaurant Eating—Taking Out or Eating In

In today's fast-paced world, restaurant eating has become a part of our daily lives, and Americans are eating more meals out each week than ever before. Dining out has become a social activity, where family and friends gather to spend time together or relax after a long day of work. Don't feel that having diabetes prevents you from eating and enjoying restaurant meals. Yes, restaurant foods have some pitfalls, but if you arm yourself with a few critical skills and strategies, there's no reason you can't enjoy restaurant foods healthfully [also check out *Tips and Tactics: Healthier Restaurant Eating*, below].

Four pitfalls lead to the big challenges to healthy restaurant eating.

1. Foods are often high in fat and high in calories from oils or shortening; butter and cream; salad dressing; sour cream; cheese or cheese sauce; and butter, cream, and eggs.
2. Foods are often high in sodium from salt; ingredients like soy sauce, meat tenderizers, broth, ham, or bacon; sauces and gravies; use of prepared canned food, such as soups and vegetables; and salad dressings.
3. Meals may focus on the large portion of protein (meat, poultry, or seafood) particularly in American-style restaurants—steak houses, delicatessens, sandwich shops, and family restaurants.
4. Portions are often oversized. This encourages overeating.

TIPS + TACTICS

Healthier Restaurant Eating

- *Move away from thinking that every restaurant meal is a special occasion. You can have a restaurant meal that is both healthy and enjoyable.*
- *Don't enter a restaurant that serves no healthy foods.*
- *Have your order in mind when you call, drive up, or enter the restaurant. Don't even open the menu. It may tempt you to go off track.*
- *Learn to spot foods high in fats and calories, cooking methods that add fat, and the names of high-fat dishes.*
- *Be creative and practice portion control with the menu. Don't automatically order a main course. Opt for a soup and salad, an appetizer and soup, or a half portion. Or eat family style—share a few items with your dining partners. This is easy to do in Asian restaurants and is getting easier in other restaurants with the movement toward smaller plates.*
- *Make reasonable requests, such as asking for your sandwich on healthier bread or asking for mustard instead of mayonnaise.*
- *If you know that the portion you'll be served will be too large, ask for a take-home container when you place your order. Put away the second serving before you dig in. Double your pleasure by enjoying the leftovers when you are truly hungry again.*

If I Only Knew...

Special orders don't upset them...

I love to eat out... always have and always will! It's social and relaxing. But having diabetes has certainly thrown a few wrenches into my carefree way of ordering. I had to get over being shy or the notion that I was being a difficult customer when asking about the ingredients in a dish or for a substitution. As I've become more comfortable making special requests, I have also realized that special orders don't generally upset wait staff as long as I'm reasonable and pleasant. Many diners have special needs and wants, from vegetarians, to gluten-free diners, people with allergies, and those watching their calories.

By the Numbers

Restaurant Eating

Statistics show that Americans:

- eat more meals out now than ever before (an average of 6 meals per week).
- eat one quarter of their restaurant meals from fast-food restaurants.
- spend nearly 1/2 their food dollars purchasing foods to eat away from home.
- eat nearly 1/3 of their calories away from home and, they aren't the healthiest calories with added sugars, unhealthy fat, and too much sodium leading the way. Fruits and vegetables are often missing in action.

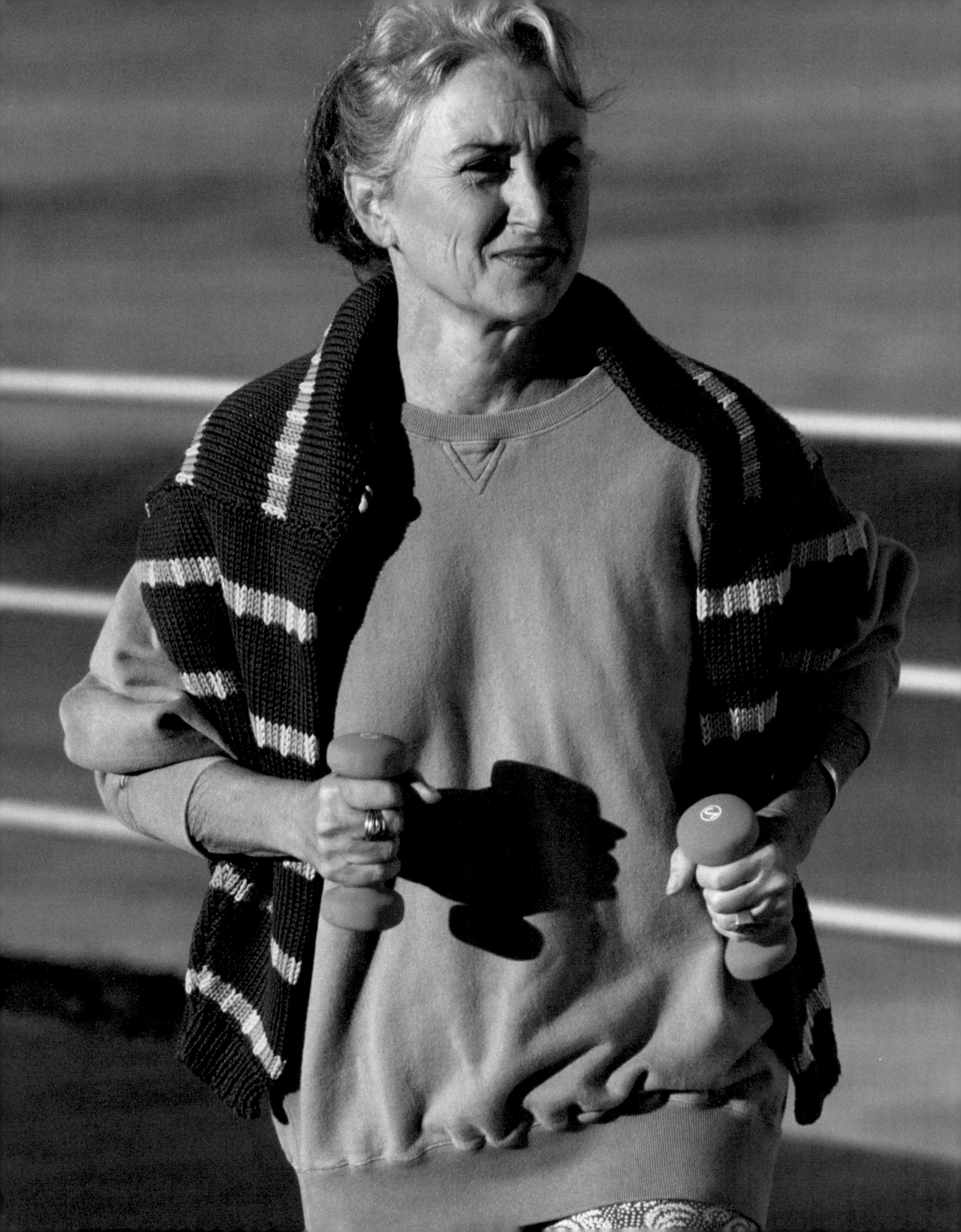

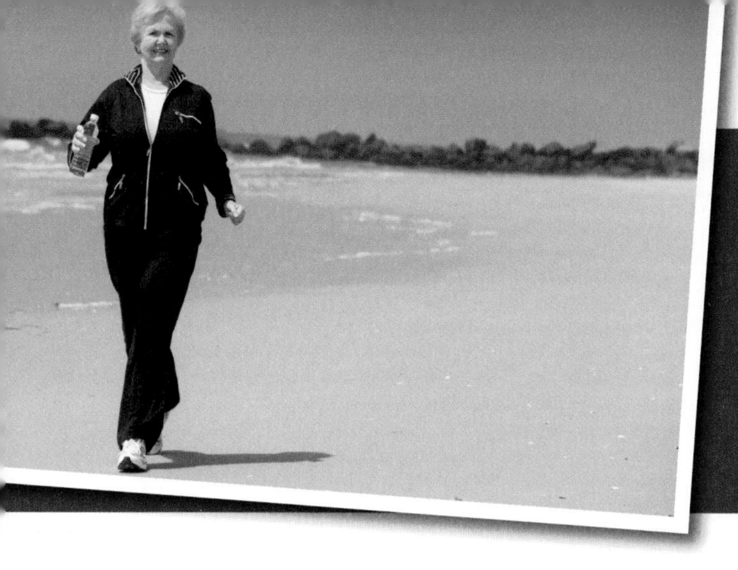

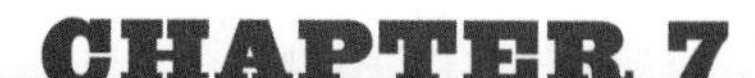

CHAPTER 7

Get Up, Get Active

Being more active can help you prevent or delay getting type 2 diabetes, and it is also a powerful treatment to help manage your diabetes. You may already know this, but when it comes to physical activity, knowing doesn't always translate into doing. When you're ready to get moving, there are some things you need to be careful about. Learn what they are, follow the tips, and reap the benefits. You may love to be active, or you may be one of those people who have barriers that keep you from being more active; either way, you will learn that you don't have to spend hours at a gym or run three miles to get measurable results. A moderate amount of physical activity provides a significant return on your time investment almost immediately. Invest wisely.

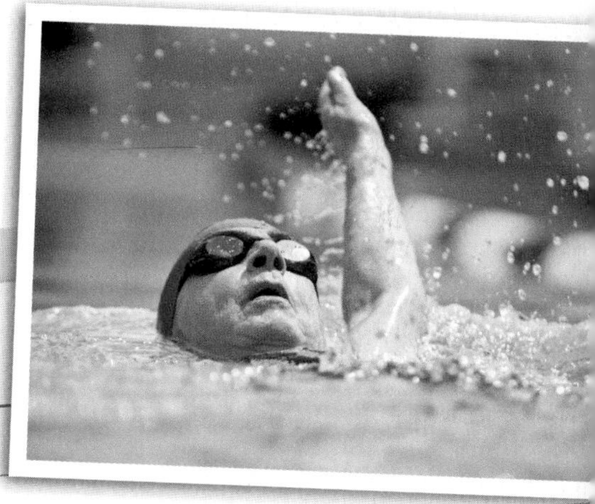

What You'll Learn:

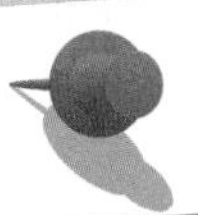

- The benefits of being physically active
- How to fit physical activity into your life
- Knowing the different types of exercise and how to implement an exercise plan
- The recommendations for physical activity for people with diabetes
- Your heart rate range and how to exercise in that range
- How to identify and get over your barriers to being physically active
- How using a pedometer can motivate you to exercise more

Benefits of Physical Activity

Exercise and physical activity do more than help you lose weight; they strengthen your lungs, heart, and muscles. Physical activity is important for everyone at every age and fitness level. Physical activity benefits you not only medically but psychologically as well. It's been shown to help reduce stress, improve sleep, and even improve your moods, and that's just a start. It can also help you reach your weight-loss goals and reduce the risk factors for heart disease and stroke.

When it comes to managing diabetes, the benefits of physical activity are even more significant. Physical activity can improve insulin actions, lower your blood glucose levels, and even improve A1C levels in people with type 2 diabetes. When health care professionals recommend a treatment, be it medication, surgery, a meal plan, or an exercise program, they weigh the benefits and risks. When it comes to diabetes and physical activity, the benefits outweigh the risks, especially if you know the risks and take a few extra steps to prevent them.

If you are aware of the benefits of physical activity but have difficulty incorporating exercise in your life, you are not alone. Many people have barriers to being physically active. Once you identify your obstacles and come up with solutions, you can learn how to incorporate physical activity into your everyday life. Just remember, don't try to do too much at one time [also check out *Chapter 4*, page 49].

By the Numbers

How Active Are Americans?

The Centers for Disease Control and Prevention reports these findings, despite the proven benefits of physical activity.

- More than 50% of American adults do not get enough physical activity to provide health benefits.
- 25% of adults are not active at all in their leisure time. Activity decreases with age and is less common among women than men and among those with lower income and less education.
- More than 1/3 of young people in grades 9–12 do not regularly engage in vigorous physical activity.
- Daily participation in high-school physical education classes dropped from 42% in 1991 to 33% in 2005.
- In 2005, 10% of high school students did not participate in any moderate or vigorous physical activity.

Benefits of Physical Activity

- Prevents or delays the onset of type 2 diabetes
- Improves insulin action
- Lowers blood glucose levels
- Improves A1C levels in type 2 diabetes
- Lowers blood pressure
- Improves lipids (cholesterol)
- Improves body composition
- Reduces several risk factors for heart disease and stroke
- Improves sleep
- Reduces stress

Exercise vs. Physical Activity

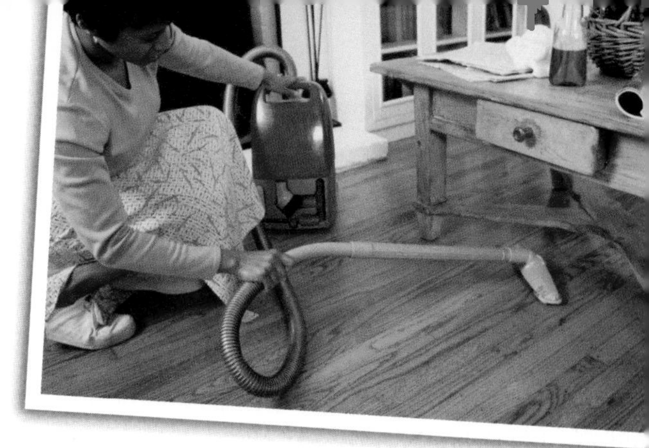

It is a common misconception that exercise and physical activity are the same thing. Although the words are used interchangeably, there is a difference. Exercise is generally broken down into three categories: aerobic, anaerobic, and stretching. Physical activity can include anything that gets you moving or doing more than you would by just sitting at home. Some people don't like the word exercise. For them, exercise means things like running, swimming, or going to a gym. These thoughts keep people from doing much of anything, but we have found that you can get health benefits from just being more active. Taking a walk, gardening, and vacuuming are considered physical activity and can help you manage your diabetes. So get out there and get moving.

There are many reasons to start a physical activity program. You might be trying to lose weight, maintain your current weight, improve your heart health, or lower your blood glucose. Whatever the reason, it's important to understand what your goals are and make a plan for achieving them. If you are trying to lose weight, the first rule of thumb is that you need to burn more calories than you consume. Bottom line? If you take in fewer calories than you use, you will most likely lose weight. Maintaining that weight loss is very important. Most of the National Weight Control Registry's members report that they keep their weight off by maintaining a low-calorie, low-fat diet and doing high levels of activity. Ninety percent of these members exercise, on average, about one hour per day [also check out *Chapter 16*, page 207]. So now that you know how important it is to get up and get moving, let's talk about the types of exercise and what they can do for you.

Wonder?

What are the best beverages to drink when you exercise?

Exercise should make you sweat. When you sweat, you lose fluids. To replace them, drink fluids during and after exercise if your activity is intense. Water is your best choice, but if you are exercising for a long time, you may want a drink that contains carbohydrate. If so, make sure you look at the Nutrition Facts. You may need to prepare by diluting some fruit juices or sports drinks beforehand to prevent you from drinking too much, and your blood glucose level going too high [also check out *Chapter 6*, page 75].

Aerobic Exercise

The most effective type of exercise for achieving weight-loss goals is aerobic exercise (also known as cardio) because it works out your heart, lungs, arms, and legs and increases your heart rate and burns calories. Aerobic means "with oxygen." Aerobic physical activity is rapid physical activity that improves, or is intended to improve, the efficiency of your body's cardiovascular system in absorbing and transporting oxygen. To get the best results from aerobic exercise, it is important to keep up a consistent pace over an extended period of time. The more strenuous the activity, and the longer the time you do it, the more benefits you will reap. Some of the most common examples of aerobic exercise are dancing, brisk walking, jogging, running, swimming, and bicycling, but they can include many other activities that require constant motion. Along with burning calories and fat, aerobic exercise can help you improve insulin sensitivity.

Anaerobic Exercise

Anaerobic means "without air" or "without oxygen." Anaerobic physical activity is short-lasting, high-intensity activity where the demand for oxygen from the exercise exceeds the oxygen supply. Anaerobic activity is more commonly known as strength training or resistance training. This type of activity relies on energy from sources that are stored in the muscles. Examples of strength training include weight lifting, pushups, jumping rope, and many more [also check out *Examples of Anaerobic Activities*, page 93]. Strength training benefits you because it builds more muscle, which means you will burn more calories while at rest. Scientific research has shown that increasing your muscle mass can reduce insulin resistance and lower blood glucose levels. Be sure to also allow 48 hours between sessions so your muscles have the opportunity to recovery, and you have less chance of an injury.

By the Numbers

Calories Burned During Aerobic Exercise

These calculations are based on a 5'10" man weighing 154 pounds. If you weigh more, you will burn more calories. On the other hand, if you weigh less, you will burn fewer calories.

Type of Exercise	Calories burned in 30 minutes
Dancing	165
Walking (3 1/2 miles/hour)	140
Swimming	255
Running/Jogging (5 miles/hour)	295
Golf (Walking)	165

Source: Dr. Buynak's 1-2-3 Diabetes Diet *(ADA, 2006).*

DEFINITION:

resistance training: physical training that utilizes isometric, isotonic, or isokinetic exercise to strengthen or develop the muscles.

Examples of Anaerobic Activities

- Weight lifting
- Push-ups
- Pull-ups
- Squats
- Lunges
- Sprints (e.g., running, biking)
- Jumping rope
- Hill climbing
- Isometrics (when one part of the body is used to resist the movement of another part of the body)
- Any rapid burst of hard exercise

Myth

When you exercise, you gain weight because fat turns to muscle, and muscle weighs more than fat.

Fact

A pound of muscle weighs the same as a pound of fat, but muscle is denser; therefore, it takes up less space than fat. Fat does not turn to muscle, but when you start to be more active and build muscle, you usually decrease your body fat. As you become more physically active, you may not see a change in the scale right away, but you may see that you are going down in size and that your clothes fit better.

Stretching

Stretching is another important part of your exercise regimen because it helps you increase your flexibility. Stretching should be a part of your everyday activity and should be included before and after your exercise sessions. Yoga, martial arts, and Pilates are all considered stretching or flexibility exercises, but you need to find an instructor to properly learn the exercises. If you have diabetes, be sure to check with your health care provider about any complications that could arise when trying these exercises. When stretching, it is important to remember that you should stretch slowly and smoothly, don't bounce, remember to breathe, and only go as far as you can without pain. Try to do each stretch for 15–20 seconds at a time to gain the most flexibility benefits.

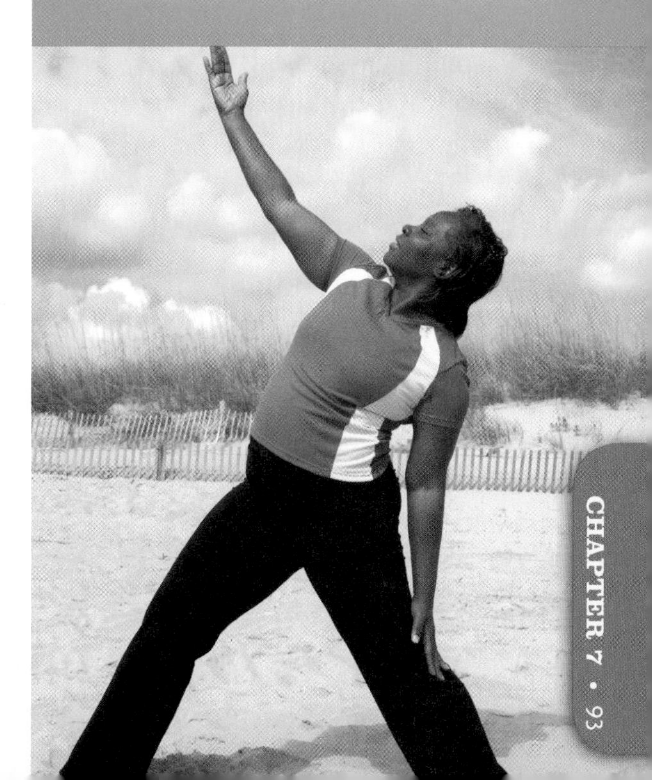

Research Brief

Other Benefits of Physical Activity

Scientists from the Peninsula Medical School in Exeter, U.K., found a direct link between levels of physical activity in middle age and physical ability during the latter part of life, regardless of weight. Dr. Iain Lang, who headed the research team, found that middle-aged people who maintained a reasonable level of physical activity were less likely to become unable to walk distances, climb stairs, maintain their sense of balance, stand from a seated position with their arms folded, or sustain their grip as they got older. The study found the rate of decreased physical ability later in life was twice as high among those less physically active. The study also revealed that being overweight or obese was associated with an overall increased risk of physical impairment but that, regardless of weight, people who engaged in heavy housework or gardening, played a sport, or had a physically active job were more likely to remain mobile later in life.

Researchers found that physical activity of about 30 minutes three or more times a week resulted in fewer than 13 % of people developing some sort of physical disability, while this rate increased to 24 % where subjects were less active.

Dr. Lang said the findings were similar in the U.S. and the U.K., which suggests they are universal and that exercise in middle age does more than benefit people in terms of weight loss. It also helps them remain physically healthy and active later in life. And, as far as results from activity are concerned, weight does not seem to be an issue.

If I Only Knew . . .

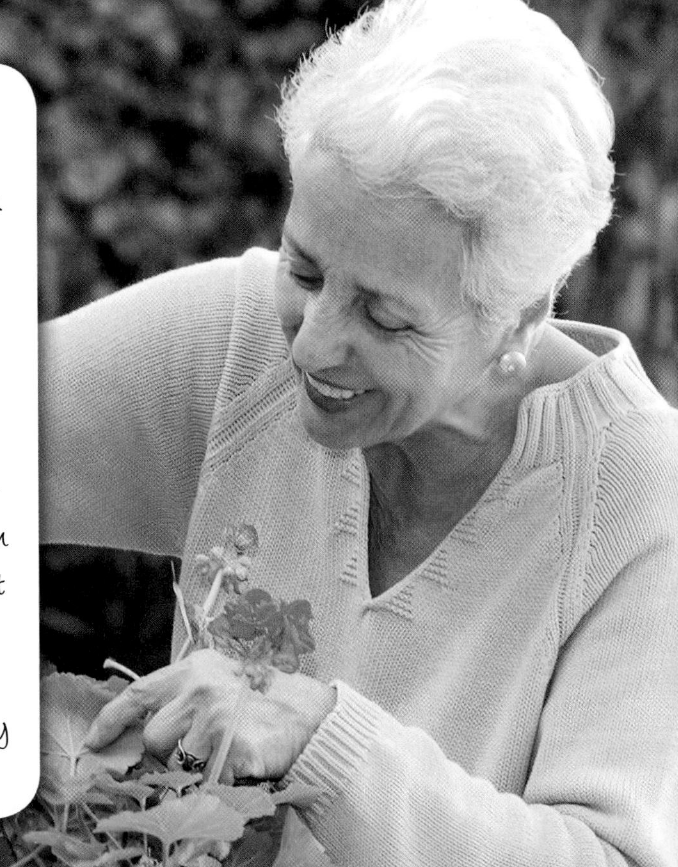

Gardening is exercise, too!

Exercise is such a dull word. It makes me think of treadmills and jumping jacks. This does not motivate me. So, I move more instead of exercise. Some days, I might take a walk for 30 minutes or do weights at the gym, but many days I walk in short spurts to get a cup of coffee, or to go to the bank or post office—any errands I can do on my feet, rather than in my car. I find excuses to organize the basement or straighten up the house. When the weather is nice, I try to get out into my garden to do a little raking, digging, or watering, or I walk my dog. This is what works for me.

Working Physical Activity Into Your Life

Two of the biggest questions when talking about exercise are: how long do I need to exercise for, and how often should I do it? If you don't currently exercise regularly, it's best to ease into an exercise program. Talk to your health care provider for tips on how to get started and where to begin. As a rule, aim to get your heart rate up for at least 30 minutes a day, 5 or more days a week to obtain maximum health benefits. If you don't have 30 minutes, you can break it down into three 10-minute intervals or two 15-minute intervals. If you're goal is weight loss, you may need to increase those numbers.

The ADA recommends that people with diabetes should perform at least 150 minutes of moderate-intensity aerobic activity a week. People with type 2 diabetes should also perform resistance training three times per week. Don't forget to stretch before and after every activity.

By the Numbers

ADA's Recommendations for Physical Activity

The ADA recommends that people with type 2 diabetes get the following amount of physical activity every week.

- At least 150 minutes of moderate-intensity aerobic activity per week
- Resistance training at least three times a week (on nonconsecutive days)

Tracking Your Heart Rate for Optimal Results

When starting an exercise program, it's important to know your resting heart rate and also to understand the range that your heart rate should be in when exercising, so you are working hard enough to receive health benefits, but not too hard to cause injury. Figuring out your resting heart rate is as easy as five simple steps.

1. Gently place the tips of your index and second finger on the palm side of your other wrist below the base of your thumb. Or gently place the tips of these fingers on your lower neck, on either side of your windpipe.
2. Lightly press with these fingers until you feel a pulse (the blood pulsing beneath your fingers). You may need to move your fingers around in the general area to feel your pulse.
3. Look at a watch or a clock with a second hand as you gently press on this area.
4. Count the beats you feel for 15 seconds, and multiply number by 4 to get your pulse.
5. Fill in the blanks to find your heart rate.
   ___ beats in 15 seconds ___ x 4 =
   ___ (your heart rate).

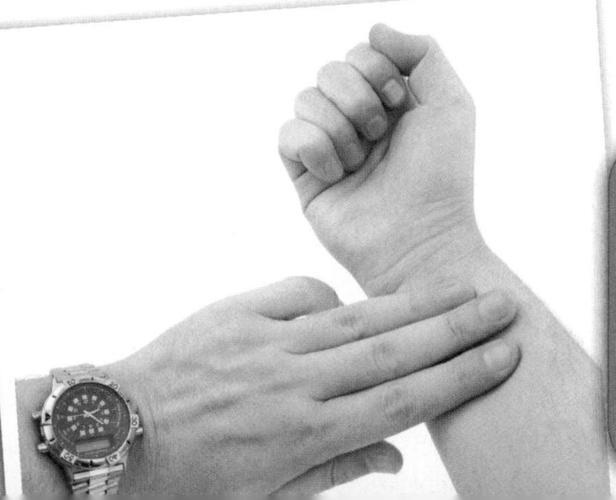

Now that you know what your resting heart rate is, use the formula below to calculate the target range for your heart rate during physical activity. This is the range where you're receiving the best health benefits, but you're not working your body too hard to cause injury. If you are 50 years old, try to get and keep your heart rate in the range of 94 to 117 beats per minute to ensure you are getting moderate-intensity aerobic physical activity.

Using the formula below, fill in the blanks:

1. 220 - ___ your age = your moderate heart rate (MHR)
2. Multiply your MHR X 0.55 = ___ bottom range of beats per minute
3. Multiply your MHR X 0.69 = ___ top range of beats per minute
4. Your Target heart range is ___–___ beats per minute

When you perform physical activity, check your pulse to see that you are within this range.

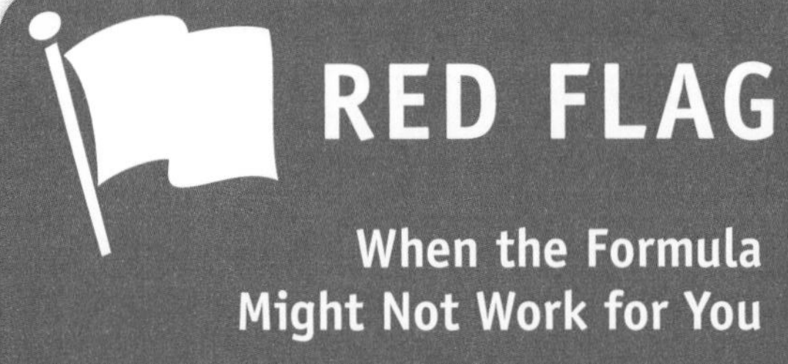

When the Formula Might Not Work for You

If you have nerve damage, or if you are taking certain heart and/or blood pressure medications, your heart may beat more slowly. Check with your health care provider about this. If this is true for you, your heart rate is not a good guide for how hard to exercise. Instead, exercise at what you feel is a moderate level of exertion. Moderate means not too hard and not too easy. You should be able to talk during your physical activity.

Wonder?

What should my heart rate be?

Normal heart rate/pulse

Age	Normal heart rate/ pulse at rest
Children (6–15 years old)	70–100 beats per minute
Adults (18 years and older)	60–100 beats per minute

Decreasing Risks of Physical Activity

Although being physically active should be a part of everyone's diabetes plan, there are some things you need to know and do before you add physical activity to your treatment plan. Although, for the most part, the benefits outweigh the risks, the risks can be dangerous, so you want to avoid them. The most common problems people with diabetes experience during physical activity are low blood glucose (hypoglycemia), high blood glucose (hyperglycemia), musculoskeletal system problems (bones, joints, tendons, and muscle problems), and other diabetes risks associated with complications.

Preventing Hypoglycemia During Exercise

Physical activity improves insulin action for people with type 2. This means it helps your body use the insulin you make or take more efficiently. Because of this, you are at risk for low blood glucose during and even up to 24 hours after you exercise, especially if you are taking medication(s) that have the side effect of low blood glucose [also check out *Chapter 8*, page 101, and *Chapter 15*, page 195]. Closely monitor your blood glucose numbers before and after exercise to see if you need to adjust your food or medications to keep your numbers up. If your numbers are lower than your target, you may need to have a snack before, during, and/or after your activity. Or you may need to change your medication dose. Although recommendations must be individualized to your needs, if you find you are getting low, a rule of thumb is for you to consume 10–20 grams of carbohydrate for every 30 minutes of moderate physical activity [also check out *Chapter 6*, page 75].

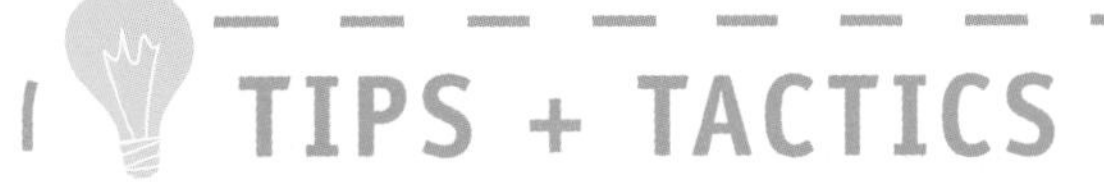

Help Prevent Hypoglycemia With Exercise

- *If you are taking diabetes medications with a side effect of low blood glucose, keep your blood glucose above 90mg/dl before exercising.*
- *If you take insulin, keep your blood glucose above 110mg/dl.*
- *If you have other complications or concerns about hypoglycemia, keep your blood glucose above 120mg/dl.*
- *If you are not taking medications that cause hypoglycemia, or are not taking any blood glucose–lowering medication, you will most likely not experience hypoglycemia.*
- *If your blood glucose is < 100mg/dl pre-exercise and you are taking a medication that can cause low blood glucose, the ADA recommends you have a pre-exercise carbohydrate snack to prevent hypoglycemia.*

Preventing Hyperglycemia During Exercise

Physical activity usually decreases blood glucose, but some people notice their blood glucose rises in response to exercise, which is usually due to lack of insulin. There are times when your blood glucose is high, and you should not exercise. In order to prevent hyperglycemia from occurring, it's important to check your blood glucose frequently when you start your physical activity. If you're able, check before, during, and after the activity to see how your glucose responds to physical activity. The only way to really know is to check. If your blood glucose starts at 110mg/dl before activity and rises to 150mg/dl after exercise, and your A1C is < 7%, then this is nothing to be concerned about. You will most likely see it go down after exercising. On the other hand, if your A1C is > 7%, you are on several medications that lower your blood glucose, you are trying to avoid taking insulin, and if your blood glucose starts out at 200mg/dl and goes up to 250mg/dl, this is something to be concerned about. Talk with your health care provider about this. You may need insulin.

Wonder?

How often should I check my blood glucose when I exercise?

- Check twice before you exercise. Check 30 minutes before, and again just before you begin. If your blood glucose is more than 250–300 mg/dl and rising, wait until it levels off. When it is > 100mg/dl and less than 250, begin your activity.
- Check during your exercise. You will want to check during your exercise if you are trying an exercise for the first time, when you feel or think your blood glucose might be getting too low, or when you will be exercising more than an hour (check every 30 minutes).
- Check after exercise. After exercise, your body restores glucose to your muscles and liver by removing it from your blood. This can go on for as long as 10 to 24 hours. During this time, your blood glucose levels may fall too low [also check out *Chapter 15*, page 195].

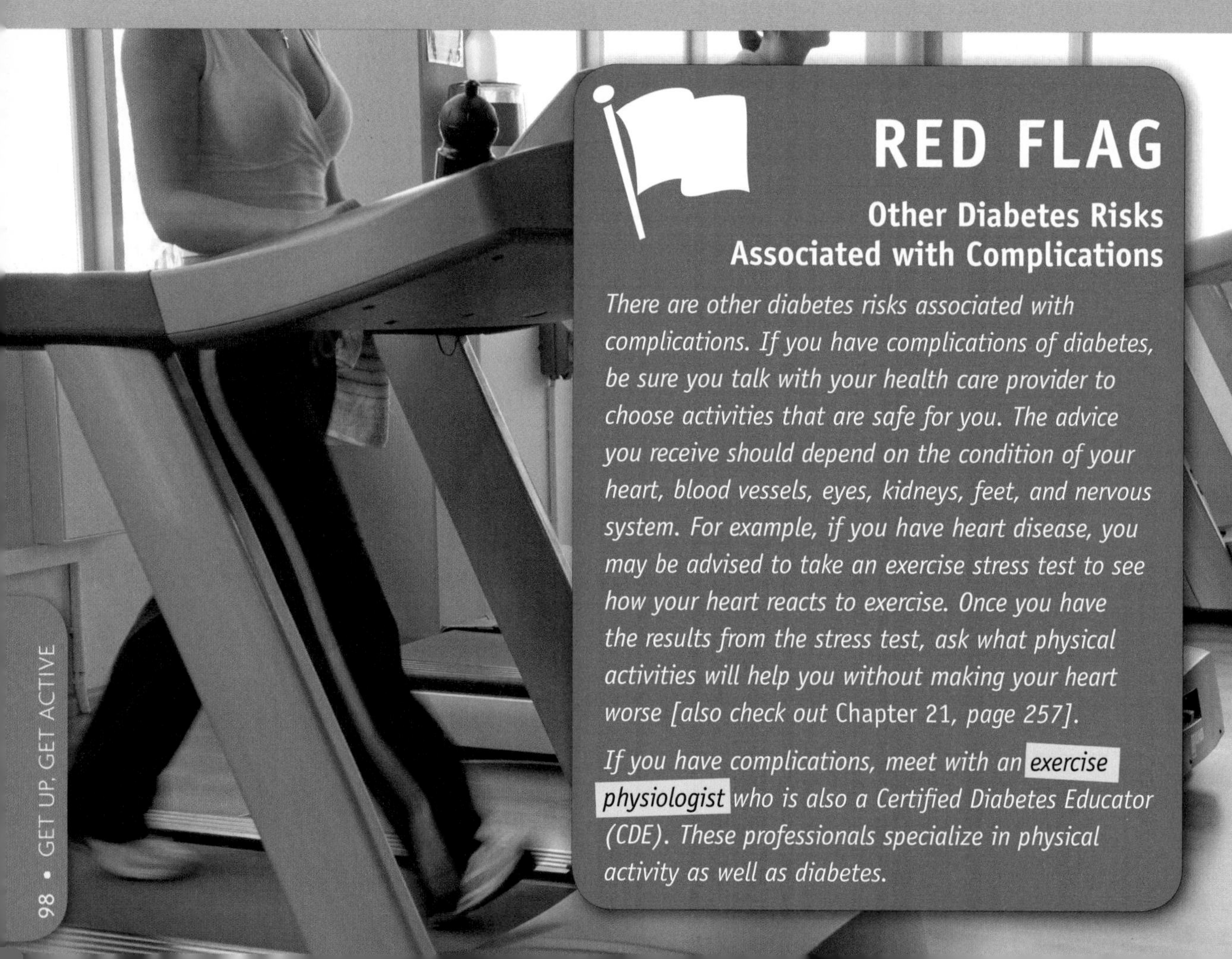

RED FLAG

Other Diabetes Risks Associated with Complications

There are other diabetes risks associated with complications. If you have complications of diabetes, be sure you talk with your health care provider to choose activities that are safe for you. The advice you receive should depend on the condition of your heart, blood vessels, eyes, kidneys, feet, and nervous system. For example, if you have heart disease, you may be advised to take an exercise stress test to see how your heart reacts to exercise. Once you have the results from the stress test, ask what physical activities will help you without making your heart worse [also check out Chapter 21, *page 257].*

If you have complications, meet with an exercise physiologist *who is also a Certified Diabetes Educator (CDE). These professionals specialize in physical activity as well as diabetes.*

Tracking Your Progress by Counting Your Steps

One of the easiest ways to get and stay motivated on your exercise regimen is to use a pedometer to track your daily step averages. A pedometer is a small, portable device that counts each step you take. Some just count steps, while some count the distance you travel. Pedometers are used to measure your physical activity and to motivate you to move more.

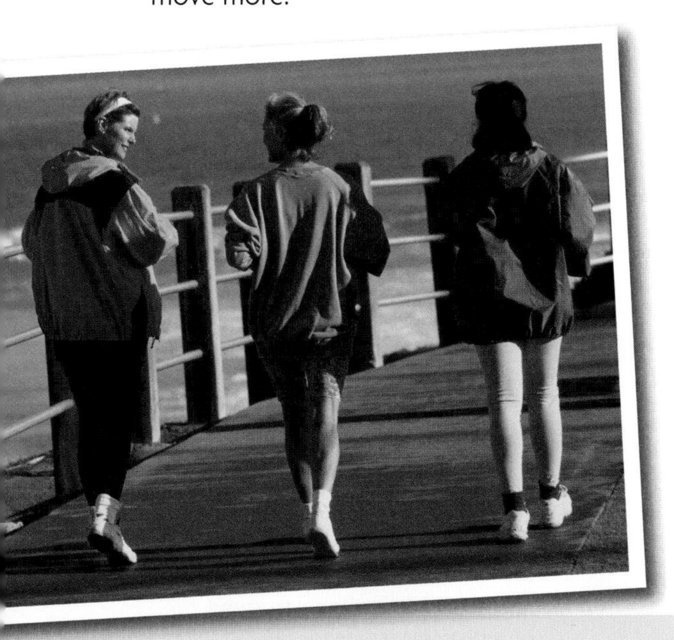

Wonder?

What's the best time of the day to exercise?

The time you **will** exercise is the best time to exercise. Many people have difficulty finding time for physical activity, so the busier your schedule, the harder it will be to meet your goals. Find the best time for you, and do it. If there are times of the day you know your blood glucose is usually low, that would not be the time to exercise. Remember, the recommendations are 30 minutes per day most days of the week.

There are many pedometers on the market, so purchase one that works. To see if yours works properly, wear it as directed in your user's manual. Take 100 steps, and see how the number on your pedometer matches your number of steps. Some pedometers count activities, such as bending, and give you credit for steps you aren't taking. These are considered interference, not steps. The more accurate ones count only steps.

Figure out your average daily step total by wearing it for three days and then dividing your total by three. Once you know your average step total, set a realistic goal to try and increase your steps every day. If you think you need to be more active, try to increase your daily steps by 500 (about five minutes of walking), and continue to increase your steps every week.

DEFINITION:

exercise physiologist: a specialist trained in the science of exercise and body conditioning who can help people plan a safe, effective exercise program.

Become More Active for the L-O-N-G Run, for Life

Before starting an exercise program, decide to make the changes you can and will make for the long run. Rather than getting all excited at first, overdoing it, and then burning out, make small, realistic goals. Start with one goal, and master that by doing it for at least three weeks before you think of adding another. For example, if you find your day is long, and there is a lot to do when you get home at the end of the day, set your alarm clock a half hour earlier. Wake up and work in some physical activity before you start your day.

Think about what you like and don't like to do. If you are a people person, you may want to join a gym. If you are a self-starter, you may just choose to take a walk or two every day by yourself.

Keep it simple, and keep it real. If you watch a lot of TV, get up and move during each commercial break. Instead of taking one big bag of garbage out, take out several smaller bags, so you'll go out more often. If you are cooking, instead of using a tray for dinner, walk each plate to the table. Make the effort to move a little more each day.

If I Only Knew . . .

Maintaining my weight could be so social . . .

I find, for me, that doing an activity with a friend is much more fun—and more motivating—than exercising alone. I have a friend who walks with me around the neighborhood. We gab, share stories, and before we know it, 30 minutes have passed. We don't have a specified time during the week, but we call each other at least once or twice a week, even if we only have 20 minutes to spare. I have another friend—a business colleague—with whom I arrange gym "dates." We work on our aerobic machines together and sometimes take a walk before entering the gym.

TIPS + TACTICS

Ways to Accumulate Pedometer Steps

- *Take a walk. Walk by yourself, with a friend, a family member, or a dog. Pick a destination to walk to, such as the grocery store, the cleaners, or the park.*
- *Step in place while you talk on the phone, or watch TV, or while waiting for your luggage, or a ride, or in the grocery line.*
- *Step or dance to music. Dance around the house while you do your household chores, mop the kitchen, clean the bathroom, dust, and vacuum.*
- *Take the stairs. If you are able to walk steps, take the stairs instead of the elevator. If taking the stairs seems to be too many steps, take the elevator, then get off a floor or two away from your destination and walk the rest of the way.*
- *Get up and get it yourself. Instead of asking someone else to get something for you, get up and get it yourself.*

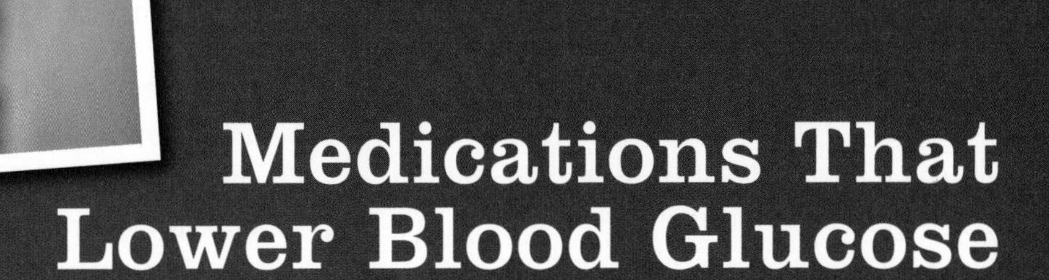

CHAPTER 8

Medications That Lower Blood Glucose

Prior to 1995, there were only two types of medications available to lower blood glucose—insulin and one class (category) of pills called sulfonylureas. Today, there are more types of insulin on the market, over a half dozen categories of pills, and even two injectable medications besides insulin.

Insulin was first used in a human being in 1922, while pills to lower blood glucose didn't exist until the 1950s. A biguanide, the second class of oral blood glucose–lowering medications, was approved for use in the U.S. in 1995. Metformin is still the only biguanide approved in the U.S. Since the early 2000s, several more new classes of blood glucose–lowering medications have been approved by the Food and Drug Administration (FDA).

As research continues to reveal more about the underlying physiological causes of rising blood glucose levels over the years, medications are being developed to go directly to the cause. If you don't currently take a blood glucose–lowering medication and are not reaching your target blood glucose levels before and/or after meals in spite of eating healthy and being physically active, you may need to use one or more medications to lower your blood glucose level.

What You'll Learn:

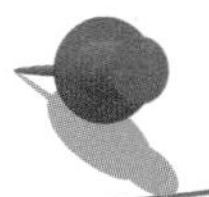

- Blood glucose–lowering medications can help you achieve your blood glucose goals
- More medications to lower your blood glucose are available today than ever before
- Common progression in the use of blood glucose–lowering medicines in type 2 diabetes
- How to take your medications correctly
- Helpful tips about taking your blood glucose–lowering medications

Progression of Type 2 Diabetes Over Time

Type 2 diabetes doesn't happen overnight. It starts with inflammation, which causes insulin resistance. Insulin resistance increases the demand for more insulin to keep your blood glucose normal. Although you are not aware of this at the time, several different things are happening in your body during this time. Your blood glucose may be normal, but your high insulin levels can cause high blood pressure, an increase in triglycerides, a decrease in HDL, and even weight gain, especially in your abdominal area. In time, you lose many of your beta cells, and your blood glucose rises because you have a relative deficiency of insulin being made in your pancreas, and you also have insulin resistance, which makes it harder for your body to use the insulin you do make.

Myth

Taking insulin makes diabetes complications worse

Fact

The reason why people often develop complications after they start to take insulin is that they keep putting it off and wait too long to start taking it. It's the high blood glucose levels over time that causes complications, not taking insulin.

Wonder?

I have type 2 diabetes; will I ever need to take insulin shots?

You may. Because experts now know that good blood glucose control from the day you are diagnosed with diabetes is critical to your long-term health, your health care provider may feel you need one or more blood glucose–lowering medications right away. Experts also know that type 2 diabetes progresses with time. They estimate that you have already lost at least half of your beta cells when you are diagnosed. Your ability to make your own insulin will continue to dwindle over time. This is the reason that you may need to continue to progress your blood glucose medications—either increased doses and/or adding new classes of medications over time.

If you live a number of years with type 2 diabetes, you will probably eventually need some insulin. In fact, many experts agree that people with type 2 diabetes should be started on insulin earlier than they generally are. When you are first diagnosed with diabetes, you may be able to manage your diabetes with a healthy lifestyle and the medication metformin. As time goes on, you may need to add more medication to reach your blood glucose target levels both before and after meals. The great news is that taking insulin or other injectables has never been easier. The needles on syringes are now shorter, thinner, and sharper. Insulin pens are readily available and are convenient to use. So, while insulin or other injectables might be in your future, know that using them will be easier than you imagine.

Progression From Normal Blood Glucose to Pre-Diabetes and Type 2

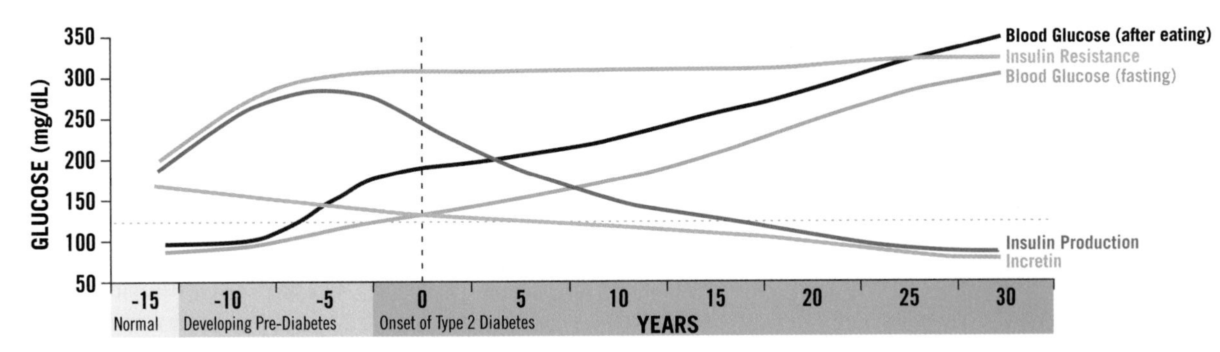

By the time pre-diabetes progresses to type 2 diabetes, your pancreas has already lost 50% or more of your beta cells—your body's insulin-making capability. The process from pre-diabetes to diabetes can take several years, and you may experience very few or no symptoms at that time. Your insulin-producing capacity will continue to decline even further after you are diagnosed with diabetes, which is the reason you may eventually need to add insulin or another injectable to your medications.

It's important to understand what is happening within your body during this time, so you can fully understand how the blood glucose–lowering medications can help. The four main reasons your blood glucose is high are because your:

- pancreas isn't making enough insulin to manage your blood glucose
- liver isn't releasing glucose as it should
- muscle cells aren't taking in glucose like they should
- incretin production from your intestine is on a decline.

Understanding what is going on in your body to keep your blood glucose levels high will help you understand how the medicine you take can help you to manage your blood glucose. The graphic on the next page illustrates how oral and injectable medications work within your body to lower blood glucose levels.

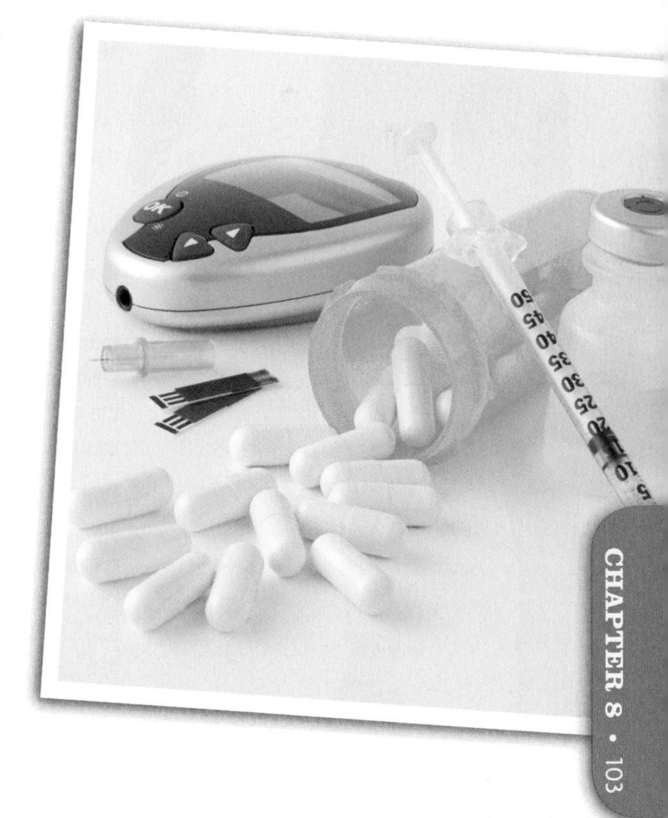

How Blood Glucose–Lowering Medications Work in the Body

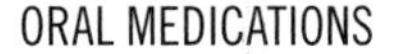

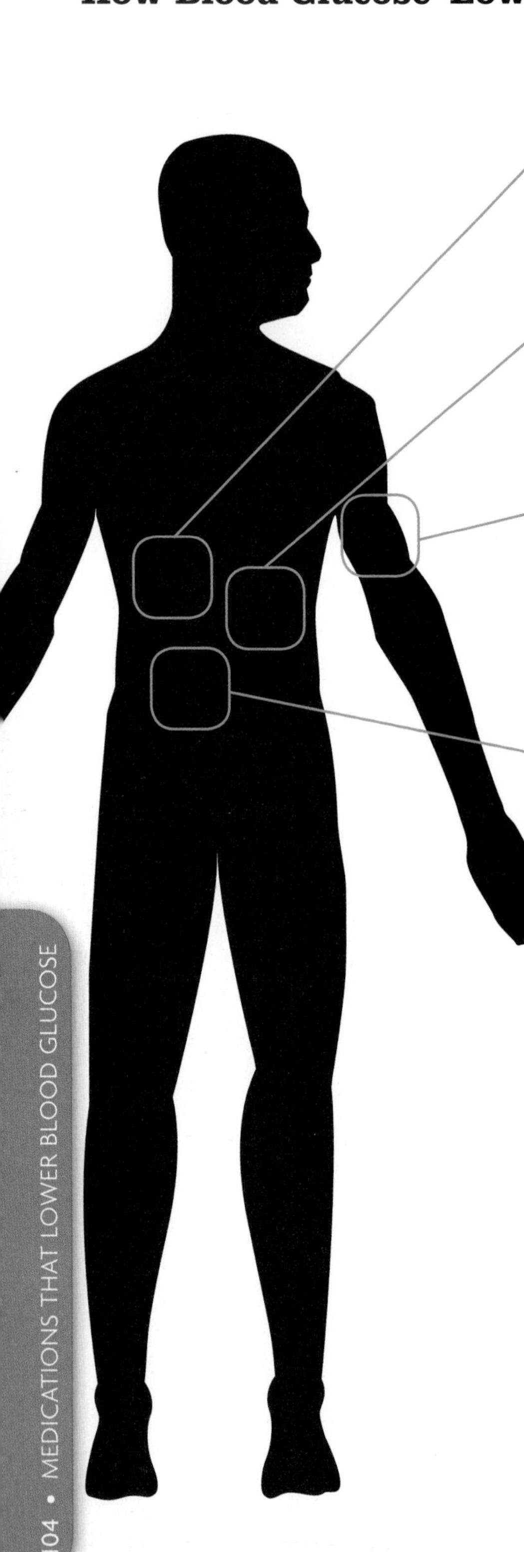

ORAL MEDICATIONS

Biguanides (metformin is the only one) work mainly on your liver to decrease the amount of glucose it produces, and also work on your muscles and fat cells to increase the amount of glucose they use to decrease insulin resistance.

Sulfonylureas work on your pancreas to stimulate the beta cells of your pancreas to produce more insulin. For sulfonylureas to work, your beta cells must still have the ability to produce insulin.

Meglitinides (nateglinide, repaglinide) work on your pancreas much like sulfonylureas, except they are faster acting and work to lower blood glucose for just a few hours.

Thiazolidinediones, glitazones for short (pioglitazone, rosiglitazone), work mainly on your muscles to increase your cell's insulin sensitivity. They also work on your liver to decrease the amount of glucose it produces.

Dipeptidyl peptidase IV Inhibitors, DPP-4 Inhibitors for short (sitagliptin) work in your intestines by inhibiting the enzyme dipeptidyl peptidase-4 (DPP-4), which breaks down hormones normally released in response to a meal to regulate your blood glucose after eating. By inhibiting this enzyme, the hormones can work to lower your blood glucose after eating. These medications are oral incretin mimetics.

Alpha-glucosidase inhibitors (acarbose, miglitol) work on your intestines to inhibit alpha-glucosidase, an enzyme that is needed to break down carbohydrate for digestion. By inhibiting this enzyme, carbohydrate are not broken down as efficiently, and carbohydrate absorption is delayed.

INJECTABLE MEDICATIONS

Exenatide (brand name Byetta) is an incretin mimetic that is taken by injection. It mimics the effects of naturally occurring hormones and can help your body make more insulin. Exenatide is the synthetic version of a protein discovered in the saliva of the Gila monster, a large lizard that is native to the southwestern U.S. There are other medications in this class that are in various stages of the drug-approval process.

Pramlintide (brand name Symlin) is a synthetic (man-made) form of the hormone amylin. In the 1980s, scientists began to understand that people who have type 1 diabetes not only make no insulin but also make no amylin. People with type 2 diabetes have a dwindling supply of both insulin and amylin. Amylin is a hormone formed in, and put out by, the beta cells of your pancreas. It regulates the timing of glucose release in your bloodstream after eating by slowing the emptying of your stomach.

Blood Glucose Lowering Medications for Type 2

Oral glucose–lowering medications do not benefit people with type 1 diabetes. These pills work best in tandem with a healthy eating plan and regular physical activity. This way, you have three therapies working together to lower your blood glucose levels. Although you may find that your blood glucose levels go down when you begin taking pills, your blood glucose levels may not get to your target range. Or, if they do, they may not stay there for long. Remember, type 2 diabetes is a progressive disease; in time, you will most likely need to take more medication or different medications, including insulin, to manage your diabetes.

If you were diagnosed with diabetes recently, and your blood glucose is pretty easy to control, you will likely be able to use one or more of the blood glucose–lowering medications other than insulin to keep your blood glucose levels near normal; however, if you have had diabetes for more than 10 years or if you already take more than 20 units of insulin each day, the variety of oral medications probably won't control your glucose.

Even if blood glucose–lowering medications do bring your blood glucose levels near the normal range, you may still need to take insulin for a short time if you have a severe infection, need surgery, are hospitalized, or are under great stress. All of these tend to raise blood glucose levels, and oral medications may not be able to control blood glucose levels during these stressful times.

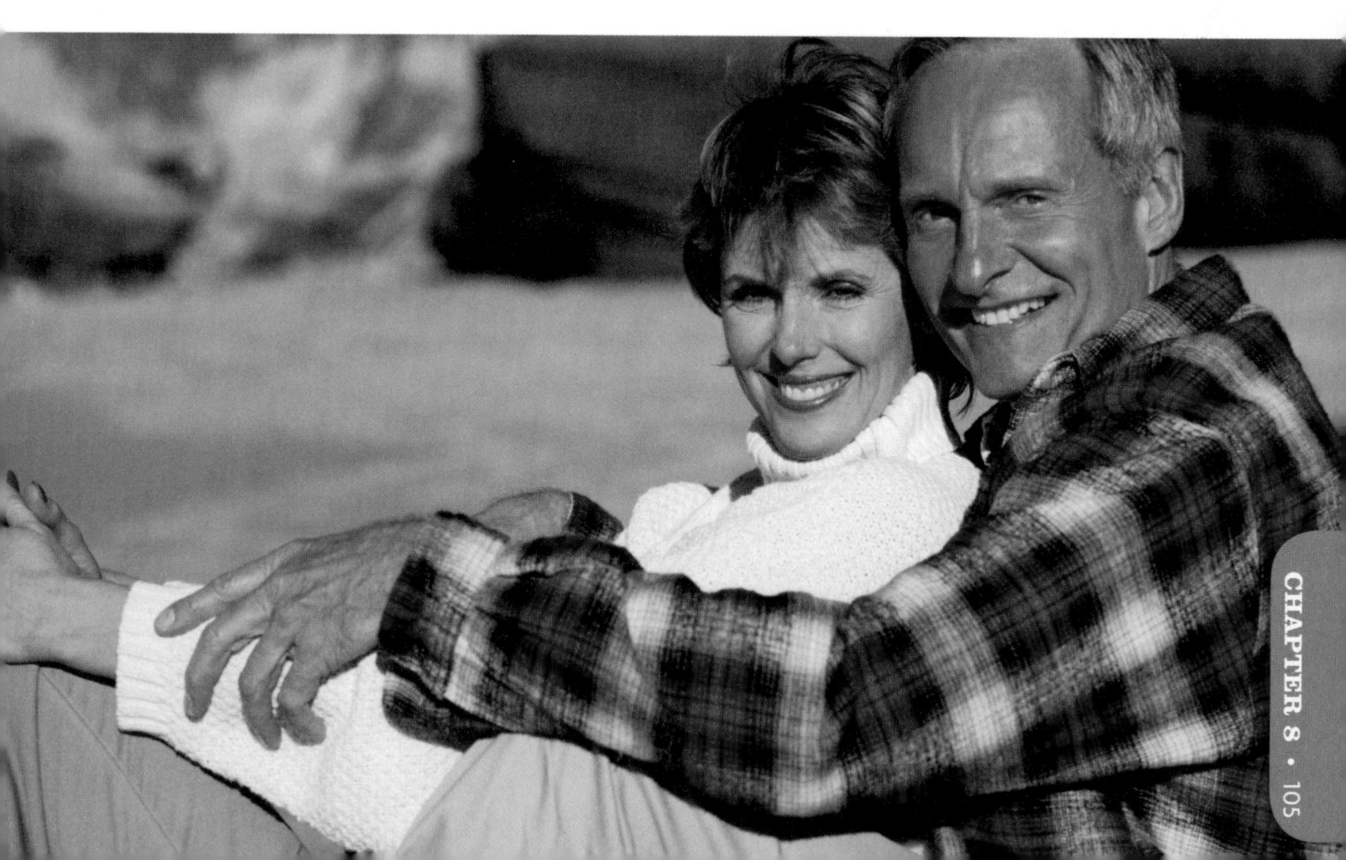

Oral Blood Glucose–Lowering Medications for Type 2

Target Organ	Class	Brand Name	Generic Name	Generic?
Intestines	alpha-Glucosidase inhibitors	Precose	acarbose	No
		Glyset	miglitol	No
	DPP-4 Inhibitors	Januvia	sitagliptin	No
	Bile-sequestering agent (can cause low blood glucose when taken with other medications that lower blood glucose)	WelChol	colesevatam hydrochloride	No
Liver, muscles, and fat cells	Biguanides	Glucophage	metformin	Yes
		Glucophage XR, Glumetza, others	metformin (long-acting)	Yes
		Riomet	metformin (liquid)	No
	Thiazolidinediones (TZDs)	Actos	pioglitazone	No
		Avandia	rosiglitazone	No
Pancreas	Meglitinides (can cause low blood glucose, but risks lower than with sulfonylureas)	Starlix	nateglinide	No
		Prandin	repaglinide	No
	Sulfonylureas (can cause low blood glucose) Note: Drugs followed by an asterisk are older sulfonylureas. They tend to cause more hypoglycemia and are seldom used today.	Amaryl	glimepiride	Yes
		Glucotrol	glipizide	Yes
		Glucotrol XL	glipizide (long-acting)	Yes
		DiaBeta, Micronase	glyburide	Yes
		Glynase PresTab	glyburide (miconized)	Yes
		Diabinese	chlorpropamide*	Yes
		generic only	tolazamide*	Yes
		generic only	tolbutamide*	Yes

Comments/Precautions
Take with the first bite of each meal. ADVANTAGES: Acarbose and miglitol normally do not cause weight gain. SIDE EFFECTS: Gas, bloating, and diarrhea. To minimize side effects, ask your doctor about starting with a low dose and building up slowly. WHO SHOULDN'T TAKE: People with inflammatory bowel disease, other intestinal diseases, or obstructions. HYPOGLYCEMIA: Acarbose and miglitol don't cause hypoglycemia when used alone. When used with certain other diabetes medications, low blood glucose can occur. In these cases, treat hypoglycemia with glucose tablets, glucose gels, or fruit juice.
ADVANTAGES: Does not cause weight gain. SIDE EFFECTS: May occasionally cause stomach discomfort and diarrhea. CAUTIONS: If you have kidney problems, your doctor may prescribe lower doses and may do blood tests to see how well your kidneys are working.
This is a new medication that received its indication to be used for people with type 2 diabetes in January 2008. Colesevelam hydrochloride is a non-absorbed, lipid-lowering polymer that binds bile acids in the intestines, impeding their reabsorption. SIDE EFFECTS: Common side effects are constipation, nasopharyngitis (inflammation of your nasal passages and upper part of your pharynx), indigestion, hypoglycemia when taken with other medications that lower your blood glucose, nausea, and high blood pressure. WHO SHOULDN'T TAKE: People who have or have had an intestinal blockage, blood triglyceride levels of greater than 500 mg/dL, or a history of pancreatitis (inflammation of the pancreas). DRUG INTERACTIONS: Interferes with thyroid medications, glyburide, oral contraceptives. Tell your health care provider if you have a Vitamin A, D, E, or K deficiency, or if you are pregnant, planning to become pregnant, or breastfeeding.
ADVANTAGES: Metformin does not cause weight gain and may improve cholesterol levels. It does not cause low blood glucose (hypoglycemia) when used alone. SIDE EFFECTS: Nausea, diarrhea, or loss of appetite (these should subside within a few weeks). To minimize side effects, take with meals. In some cases, the dose may need to be reduced and then gradually increased as the body gets used to the medicine. Lactic acidosis is a rare but serious side effect. WHO SHOULDN'T TAKE: Metformin may not be right for you if you have kidney problems or severe respiratory problems, are 80 or older, are taking medication for heart failure, have a history of liver disease, drink alcohol excessively, or are hospitalized.
It typically takes 4 to 6 weeks to see an effect on your blood glucose. SIDE EFFECTS: Can cause weight gain, fluid retention, and heart failure. Call your doctor right away if you have any signs of heart failure, such as rapid weight gain, shortness of breath, edema (fluid retention in ankles, legs, or hands), or fatigue. LIVER TESTS: Your doctor should check your liver function prior to starting these medications and periodically throughout your treatment. Call your doctor right away if you have any symptoms of liver damage, such as nausea, vomiting, abdominal pain, fatigue, loss of appetite, or dark urine. WOMEN: These medications may cause women who are not ovulating and haven't gone through menopause to begin ovulating again, enabling them to conceive. Also, oral contraceptives may be less effective when taking these medications. AVANDIA: Carries a potential increased risk of heart attack.
Take at start of meals. Skip the dose if you skip a meal.
Probably safe in people with kidney disease, but people who have kidney disease or who are elderly should be started on a lower-than-usual dose.
Most effective when taken with a meal, and may be more effective when taken 30 minutes before a meal.
Should be taken with a meal.
Effects may last entire day. May not be suitable for people with kidney disease.
More readily absorbed than regular glyburide, so the strengths of the tablets are different.
Longest-acting drug in this class, so it has a higher potential to cause low blood glucose. Not recommended for elderly people and those with kidney disease. May cause low blood sodium levels, jaundice, and possibly skin rashes.
People with kidney disease may need smaller doses. Used infrequently.
An older agent; used infrequently for diabetes.

Adapted from American Diabetes Association 2008 Resource Guide

Two Medications in One Pill

You may need to take more than one class of medication to effectively lower your blood glucose. For example, you may take a biguanide (metformin) and a sulfonylurea (glimiperide). Because it may be easier and less expensive for you to take one pill rather than several, pharmaceutical companies often combine two medications in one. At the time of this writing, these are the combination pills available. See the chart below for examples of combination pills.

Injectable Medications Other Than Insulin

There are also two classes of injectable medications on the market to help lower blood glucose: exenatide (Byetta) and pramlintide (Symlin).

Exenatide is the synthetic (man-made) version of the hormone exenatide, which slows down the rate at which your body absorbs food, helps you feel full more quickly, decreases the amount of glucose that your liver produces, and helps some people lose weight. Exenatide is approved by the FDA for use with metformin, a sulfonylurea, or a combination of the two. Your health care provider may consider exenatide for you if you have not achieved adequate glycemic control with metformin or a sulfonylurea.

Pramlintide (Symlin) is an analog of amylin, a hormone found in your body, and is released by the same cells that produce insulin. It works by helping to control your blood glucose after meals and signals the brain's satiety center, to provide a feeling of fullness earlier. Symlin helps suppress your appetite and lowers high blood glucose levels after meals. Symlin should be taken before a meal that has at least 250 calories or 30 g of carbohydrates. It cannot be mixed with insulin, so it must be taken as a separate injection. When starting on Symlin, you should work with your health care provider to reduce your mealtime insulin and follow the Symlin dose instructions. Nausea and insulin-induced hypoglycemia are the only two known side effects.

Examples of Combination Pills

Class	Brand Name	Generic Name	Generic?
Combination Pills *See cautions for each drug in the combination, listed separately on the previous page.*	Glucovance	metformin + glyburide	Yes
	Avandamet	metformin + rosiglitazone	No
	Metaglip	metformin + glipizide	Yes
	Actoplus Met	metformin + pioglitazone	No
	Janumet	metformin + sitagliptin	No
	Duetact	pioglitazone + glimepiride	No
	Avandaryl	rosiglitazone + glimepriride	No

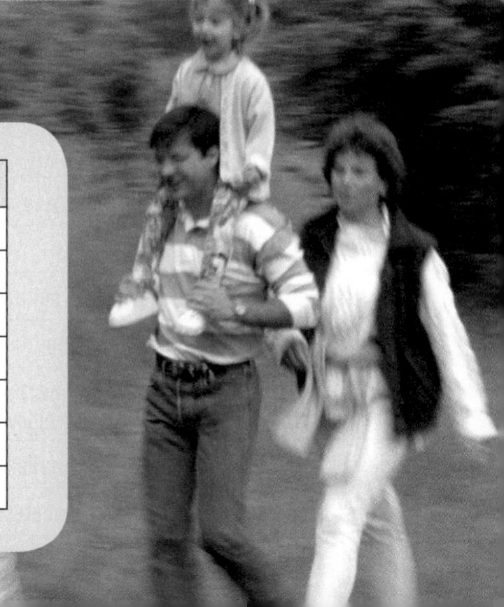

DEFINITION:

analog: a genetically engineered form of insulin that is derived from the human insulin molecule. An analog acts in the same basic way as the body's native insulin.

Wonder?

I've heard that checking my blood glucose is more painful than giving myself an injection. Is this true?

Everybody is different, but for many people it's true that checking blood glucose can be more painful. Think of people who are blind. They use their fingertips to touch and decipher things because there is an abundance of nerves in fingertips. These nerves protect you. If you touch something hot, you know to stay away. But if you need to take shots, you will, for the most part, give yourself a shot in your abdomen, your arm, or your leg. There is less concentration of nerves in those areas, so you usually don't feel it as much.

Road Maps to Progress Blood Glucose Medications

Over time, type 2 diabetes progresses, and you have a dwindling supply of insulin being produced by your beta cells; you also have continuing insulin resistance. There's an expanding choice of medications that treat the different problems of type 2 diabetes, and your provider can combine medications in myriad ways based on your individual needs and tolerance to specific medications. Your blood glucose–lowering medications should be increased and/or added over time to control your blood glucose levels. To stay healthy, you need to get and keep your A1C at 7% or less (eAG of 154 or less) as quickly as possible and keep it there over time.

So, what path should you and your health care provider follow to achieve this goal? Experts from the ADA provide an algorithm, or roadmap, for health care providers (and you) to follow. To develop this, they consider the medications' effectiveness, safety, how well they are tolerated, ease of use, and cost.

Experts now suggest that at diagnosis of type 2, people be started on metformin along with healthy lifestyle changes. Metformin should be initiated slowly because of potential side effects and then slowly increased to the maximum effective dose if needed to control blood glucose levels.

If metformin alone doesn't achieve target goals at this point or in the future, either an intermediate- or long-acting insulin or a sulfonylurea can be added and increased as needed. As blood glucose increases over time, more insulin and/or other medications should be added. To achieve your goals, be aware of your blood glucose targets, and monitor your blood glucose before and after meals [also check out *Chapter 13*, page 163]. Know when you should call or send in your blood glucose results and discuss how and when to make changes in your medications.

You shouldn't wait for three to six months between visits to make necessary changes in your medications. Also, don't keep putting off progressing your diabetes treatment by telling your provider that you will try harder on your eating plan or by being more active regardless of whether you need to start an oral medication or an injectable one. You'll want to continue to work on living a healthier lifestyle and getting to a healthy weight because it's good for your diabetes and overall health, but research shows that weight loss at this point is unlikely to improve your blood glucose enough. Keep in mind that *you* have not failed, it's *your pancreas* that's failing.

Insulin and Blood Glucose Control

Today, there are insulins that work much like the insulin your body makes. The needles on syringes and pens are thinner, shorter, and sharper than ever; some are even called mini needles. Most people are relieved to find out that they can hardly feel the needle when they give themselves a shot. It's a whole new world when it comes to giving yourself insulin. If you need insulin, don't fight it. After their first injection, most people look back and wonder why they made such a big deal out of going on insulin. They wonder why they didn't start sooner, because they could have felt better so much sooner.

There are many benefits to taking insulin. The first, and probably most important, is that you can take as much as you need to achieve blood glucose control. (This isn't so with any other blood glucose–lowering medication.) Go slow and only make changes advised by your health care provider. Unlike other types of medications that may stop working over time, if you use the right amount, insulin will continue to keep your blood glucose under control. Insulin is a very safe drug with a limited number of side effects. Potential hypoglycemia and possible weight gain are common side effects.

DEFINITIONS:

basal: the insulin needed to manage blood glucose levels between meals and overnight. This may be provided by long-acting insulin or rapid-acting insulin in a pump.

bolus: the insulin needed to control the rise of blood glucose after food intake or to help lower a high blood glucose level. Bolus insulin is usually provided by a rapid-acting insulin.

TIPS + TACTICS

Insulin Injection Tips

- *Select a site that has no scar tissue. Make sure your site is one to two inches from scars, bruises, or your belly button.*
- *Use the same part of your body for selected injections. i.e., all morning shots in the abdomen, evening injection in the arm, and bedtime injection in the thigh.*
- *Use insulin that is at room temperature. You can use insulin that has been refrigerated but it will absorb slower and it may sting.*
- *Make sure no air bubbles remain in the syringe before injection. (These small air bubbles are not dangerous, but if you don't get rid of them you won't get the amount of insulin you need.)*
- *Keep muscles relaxed when injecting.*
- *Penetrate the skin quickly.*

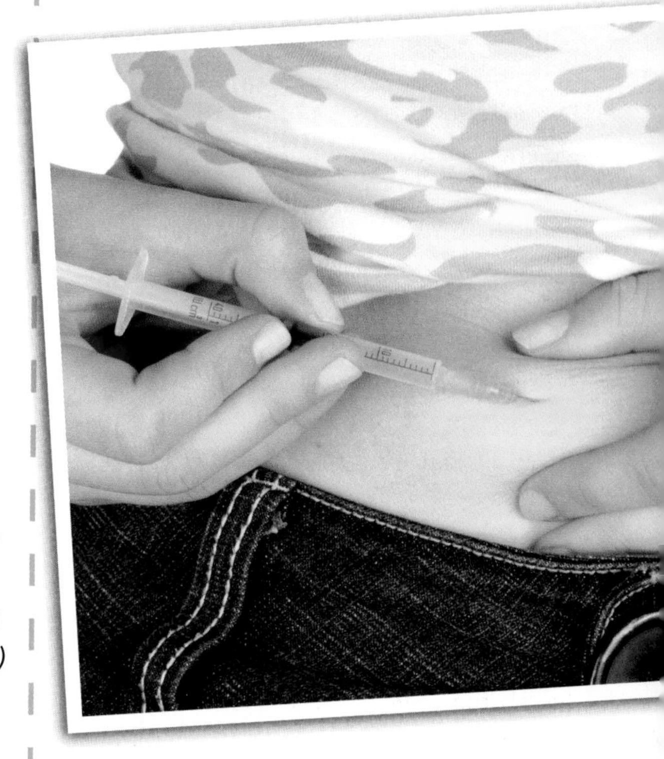

If you have type 1 diabetes, you will need to take insulin, because your pancreas no longer makes insulin on its own. Typically, you will need to take insulin three to four times a day to keep your blood glucose under control, or if you wear an insulin pump, it will deliver a small amount of insulin all day (basal insulin), and you can program it to give you specific amounts of insulin when you eat or if your blood glucose is too high (bolus insulin).

If you have type 2 diabetes, and you are not able to hit your blood glucose goals consistently with oral medications, you will probably need to take insulin. As the disease progresses, your body may stop making insulin altogether, at which time you will need to take insulin [also check out *Progression From Normal Blood Glucose to Pre-Diabetes and Type 2*, page 103].

Nearly all insulin in use today is called human insulin. It is not obtained from humans but is manufactured through recombinant DNA technology. It is made to look almost identical to human insulin [also check out *Chapter 1*, page 5]. There is a lot to learn about insulin, so start with the things you need to know to get started. There is more to know, but as you learn, the best way to manage your diabetes is to do a little at a time and build on that.

Starting Insulin

When you start an insulin regime, it's important to first understand what insulin is and how it performs in your body. Insulin is a hormone that helps your body use glucose for energy and regulates your blood glucose. Now you're ready to start learning about the mechanics. Your health care provider should teach you how to give yourself an injection, probably having you practice with normal saline (salt water) the first time.

Next, your provider should discuss with you how often you should take your insulin. You will also need to know the times you need to take it, such as before meals and before bed. If you have type 2, your health care provider may first have you start with one injection of long- or intermediate-acting insulin before bed, along with your other blood glucose–lowering medications. If your blood glucose is not where it should be, your health care provider will raise the dose and/or add more injections, a pre-mixed insulin, or rapid-acting

Are you insulin resistant or resistant to taking insulin?

There are really two types of insulin resistance. One is when your body is resistant to your insulin [also check out *Chapter 1*, page 5]. The other is psychological insulin resistance. This is when health care providers or people who have diabetes put off starting insulin because either the health care professional is not comfortable with it or because the person who needs it isn't comfortable with taking insulin. Once you know how important insulin is for you, it's easier to get over your resistance to taking insulin. If you or your health care professional has insulin resistance, this can delay you getting the insulin you need early on to manage your blood glucose levels. If you take medications, and your blood glucose is not in your targets both before and after meals, talk with your health care provider about adding insulin. Don't put it off.

Psst...

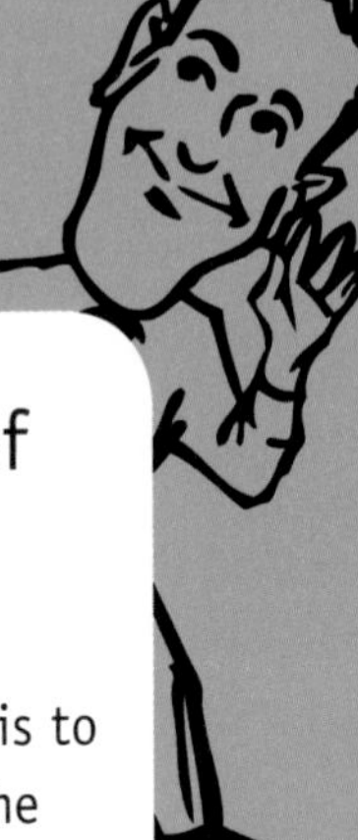

Three main characteristics of the insulin you take

The easiest way to understand how to manage your blood glucose with insulin is to know the three main characteristics of the insulin you take.

- Onset: the length of time before your insulin reaches your bloodstream and begins lowering blood glucose.
- Peak Time: the time during which your insulin is at its maximum strength in terms of lowering your blood glucose. (Note: long-acting insulins have no peak.)
- Duration: how long your insulin continues to lower your blood glucose.

If I Only Knew . . .

Insulin shots don't hurt much . . .

I worked hard to avoid insulin shots. At first, I was on one pill, and then I had to progress to two. My blood glucose continued to rise, and I continued to feel tired. The first time I tried to give myself a shot, I was glad to see a thin, short needle. Filling the syringe was easy, but it took me 15 minutes to find the nerve to stick it into my stomach. When I did, I jammed it so hard that I bruised myself. I added a third pill to my regimen to try and keep from having to inject myself again. When it was clear that oral medications still weren't working, another provider showed me a trick: pinch the skin area with my free hand, and use one gentle motion to inject the needle. No pain! What a relief! My blood glucose improved immediately with insulin.

insulin before meals. There are several different ways to hit your blood glucose target, so work with your health care provider to find out what will work for you.

If you have type 1 and are just starting on insulin, your health care provider will probably start you on four injections per day—one a long-acting insulin and then an injection of rapid-acting before meals. Because your blood glucose may be high when you start on insulin, you may need more insulin to start and less once your body adjusts.

TIPS + TACTICS

How to Dispose of Needles

- *If you can do it safely, clip the needles off the syringes so no one can use them. It's best to buy a device that clips, catches, and contains the needle. Do not use scissors to clip off needles. The flying needle could hurt someone or become lost.*
- *If you don't destroy your needles, recap them yourself.*
- *Place the needle or entire syringe in an opaque (not clear) heavy-duty plastic bottle, like a bleach or detergent bottle with a screw cap or a plastic or metal box that closes firmly. Do not use a container that will allow the needle to break through, such as a plastic milk container.*
- *Do not recycle your syringe container. Throw it out in the regular trash.*
- *Your area may have rules for getting rid of medical waste like used syringes. Ask your refuse company or city or county waste authority what method meets their rules.*
- *When traveling, take your used syringes home. Pack them in a heavy-duty, puncture-proof holder, such as a hard plastic pencil box, for transport.*

For more information on needle disposal, visit www.safeneedledisposal.org.

It's also important to learn how to store insulin and dispose of needles. Whether you use an insulin pen, insulin syringe, or insulin pump, there are needles that need to be disposed of as well.

Types of Insulin

There are four different types of insulin: rapid-acting, short-acting, intermediate-acting, and long-acting. Each type has different onsets, peaks, and durations. Remember that everyone has a unique response to insulin, so the times mentioned here are approximate. You will learn by experience how long the insulin takes to work for you.

Rapid-acting insulin enters and leaves your bloodstream quickly, so if you are taking it before you eat, you should start taking it about 15–20 minutes before you sit down to eat. The only exception is if you are taking it to correct high blood glucose levels or if your blood glucose is too low [also check out *Chapter 15*, page 195]. Because these insulins leave the bloodstream within about three to four hours, there is less chance of hypoglycemia several hours after the meal than with short-acting insulin.

Regular or short-acting insulins usually reach the bloodstream within 30 minutes after injection. If you take them before meals, you should wait about 30 minutes after taking your insulin to eat. Typically, the higher the dose of regular insulin, the longer its duration of action. This insulin is not used as much as the rapid-acting insulins today.

Intermediate-acting insulin is called N or NPH, which stands for Neutral Protamine Hagedorn. NPH is the only intermediate-acting insulin currently marketed, and it is often used in combination with regular insulin. In people with type 2 diabetes, it is also sometimes used at bedtime along with other medications that lower type 2 diabetes. NPH

By the Numbers

Insulin Action

Insulin	Onset	Peak	Duration
Rapid-Acting: lispro, aspart, glulisine	10–20 min	1–3 hrs	3–5 hrs
Short-Acting: regular, R	30 min–1 hr	2 1/2–5 hrs	3–5 hrs
Intermediate-Acting: NPH, N	1–2 hrs	4–8 hrs	10–20 hrs
Long-Acting: detemer, glargine	1–2 hrs	relatively flat, no pronounced peak	Up to 24 hrs

Psst...

Recent observations suggest that rapid-acting insulin doesn't get absorbed and lower blood glucose as quickly as practitioners first thought when the first one was approved in 1995. Most experts agree that the maximum blood glucose–lowering effect of rapid-acting insulin occurs closer to 90 to 120 minutes after it is injected. If this is what you experience, the optimal time to take rapid-acting insulin is 15–20 minutes or more before you eat, rather than just before or after you start to eat. The best way to know is to check your blood glucose at various times after you have taken your insulin, or with the use of a continuous glucose monitor (CGM). If your after-meal glucose levels are still too high, you may want to try taking your insulin earlier. If that doesn't work, you may need to increase your before-meal insulin doses.

insulin is not used as much as the long-acting insulins today.

Long-acting insulins have continuous, relatively "peakless" action that mimics natural basal (background) insulin secretion. These must not be mixed with any other type of insulin. They can be injected any time during the day as long as they are taken around the same time each day. They should not be administered intravenously. Some people take long-acting insulins every 12 hours rather than every 24 hours but this depends, in part, on which long-acting insulin you take.

Wonder?

Why can't you take insulin orally?

Insulin is a protein drug that is degraded in your stomach and prevents pure insulin from doing its job to maintain your blood glucose.

Combining or Mixing Insulins

You may use either rapid- or short-acting insulins with a long-acting insulin or NPH insulin in an effort to mimic the body's natural insulin secretion. Because long-acting insulins do not provide a peak to cover meals, most people need to take a bolus dose of rapid- or short-acting insulin before they eat, to provide coverage for the rise of blood glucose from food intake.

If you are taking regular or rapid-acting insulin and long-acting insulin, note that both types of insulin are clear in appearance. If you take both of these insulins, it is very important that you choose the correct insulin from the correct vial. Companies are now making the vials or the labels look different to help prevent you from taking the wrong insulin.

When combining insulin, there are some important things you need to remember. First, NPH insulin mixes easily with short-acting regular insulins. Mixtures containing the rapid-acting insulins should be injected immediately after mixing them and should only be mixed with NPH under the guidance of your health care provider. The long-acting insulins can't be mixed in the same syringe with other insulins and should be injected separately in a syringe or pen alone.

Premixed Insulins

Premixed insulins may be convenient for you if you take two types of insulin at one time and if the types of insulins you take can be mixed. They come with a certain percentage of one type of insulin and a percentage of the other type of insulin. For example, some mixtures are called 70/30, which means it's 70% of an intermediate insulin and 30% of a regular- or short-acting insulin. These come pre-mixed either in vials or insulin pens. Premixed insulins don't allow you to be as flexible with the timing of your meals but can be helpful if you have poor eyesight or dexterity. Insulin pens may also be useful for you if you have either of these issues.

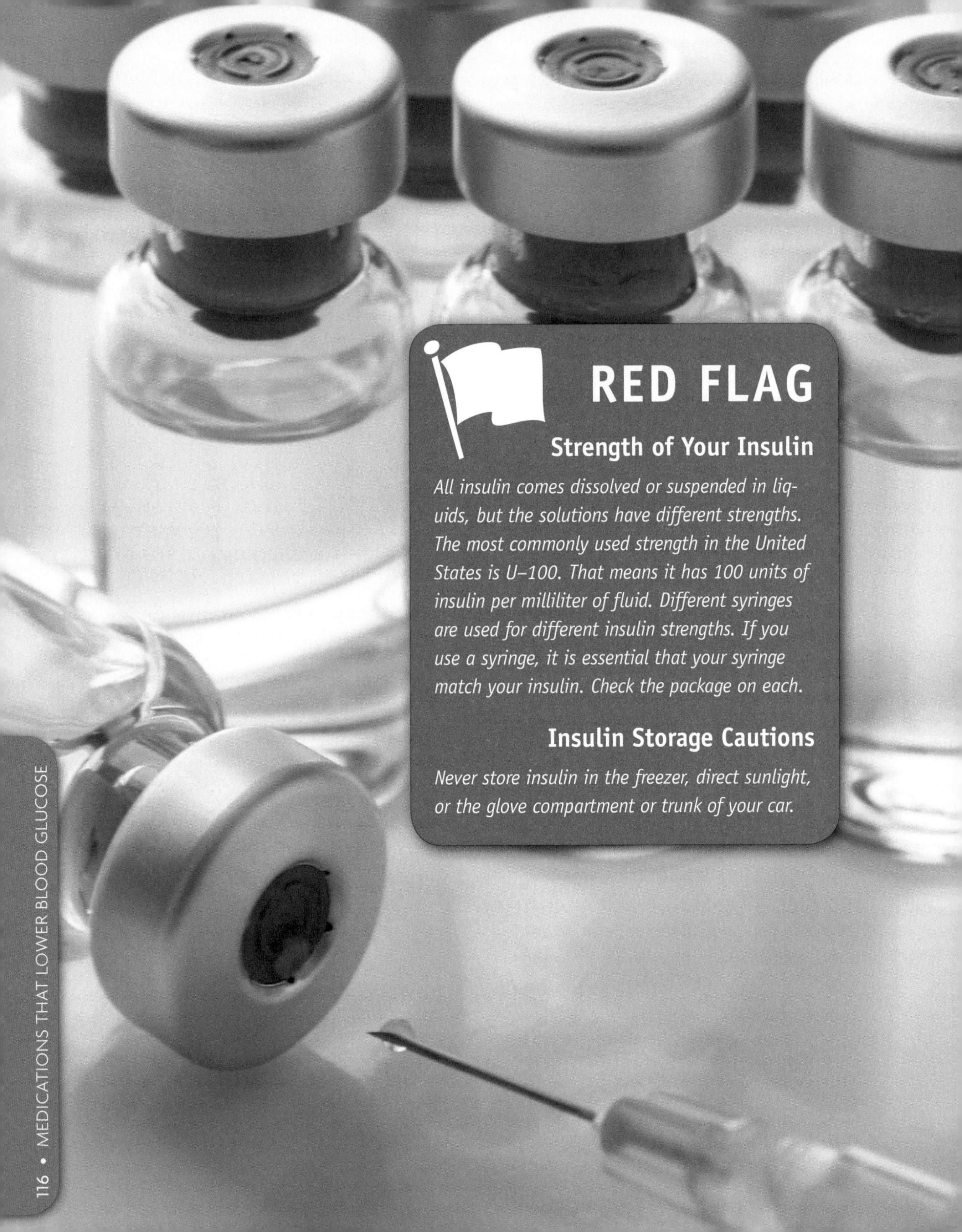

RED FLAG

Strength of Your Insulin

All insulin comes dissolved or suspended in liquids, but the solutions have different strengths. The most commonly used strength in the United States is U–100. That means it has 100 units of insulin per milliliter of fluid. Different syringes are used for different insulin strengths. If you use a syringe, it is essential that your syringe match your insulin. Check the package on each.

Insulin Storage Cautions

Never store insulin in the freezer, direct sunlight, or the glove compartment or trunk of your car.

Ways to Administer Insulin

At this time, there are several ways to take insulin: syringe, insulin pen, insulin pump, and other injection aids and alternatives. You can work with your health care provider to find out what method works best for you.

A syringe is a device used to inject medications or other liquids into your body tissues. The syringe for insulin has a hollow plastic tube with a plunger inside and a needle on the end. Today's syringes are smaller and have thinner needles and special coatings that work to make injecting as easy and painless as possible. Syringes come in different sizes and have different size needles. Talk to your health care provider about whether you need a prescription or not (some states require them, but others don't) and which syringe is right for you.

Insulin pens are becoming more available and more popular today. An insulin pen looks like a writing pen, only instead of a writing point, there's a needle, and instead of an ink cartridge, there's an insulin cartridge. These devices are convenient, accurate, and often used by people on a multi-dose regimen. These pens are particularly useful for people whose coordination or vision is impaired, people who have a fear of needles, and people who are on the go. Insulin pens come with one kind of insulin or a pre-mix. If you use a pre-mixed insulin, you'll need to follow package instructions to ensure the insulin is well mixed. If you are interested in trying an insulin pen, talk to your health care provider.

An insulin pump is a small, computerized insulin-delivering device, about the size of a small cell phone, that you wear all the time.

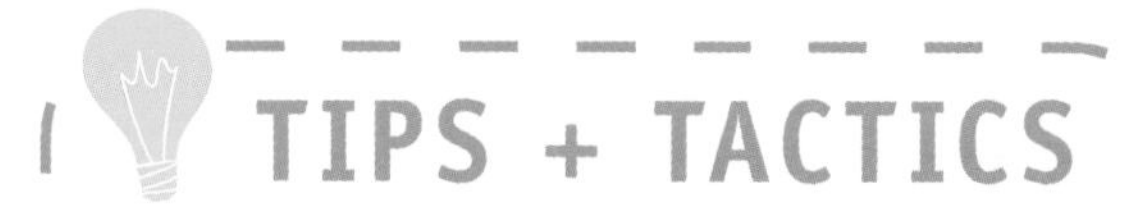

Insulin Safety and Storage

There are several things to keep in mind when considering how to store your insulin. Use the tips below to keep your insulin working to its full effectiveness.

- *TEMPERATURE. Manufacturers recommend you keep the insulin you are presently using at room temperature as long as you will use the amount in the vial or pen within 30 days. If you don't use the vial or pen within 30 days you should discard the remaining insulin. Store your extra unopened vials and insulin pens in your refrigerator until you are ready to use it.*
- *EXPIRATION DATE. Don't use insulin beyond its expiration date. There is no guarantee you will be getting the intended strength of your insulin past that date. The expiration date can be found on your insulin vial, insulin pen cartridge, or pen.*
- *APPEARANCE. If you notice particles, clumps, or discoloration on any of your insulin, do not use it. Return the unopened bottle to the pharmacy for an exchange or refund. If it is an opened bottle, discard it.*

An insulin pump delivers a basal dose of insulin constantly and the user decides how much rapid-acting insulin to deliver before meals. An insulin pump doesn't manage your blood glucose automatically but, if used properly, has the capability of improving glucose management.

Injection Aids and Alternatives

Injection aids and alternatives can make it even easier to give yourself an injection, as well as give you an alternative if you are still having difficulty with injections.

Visual aides like magnifiers are available if you have difficulty seeing to draw up your insulin properly. Insulin pens work well if you are visually impaired, because you can hear and count how much insulin you draw up.

Infusers create "portals" into which you inject insulin. With an infuser, a needle or catheter is inserted into subcutaneous tissue and remains taped in place, usually on the abdomen, for 48–72 hours. The insulin is injected into it rather than directly through the skin into the fatty tissue. Some people are prone to infections with this type of product, so be sure to discuss the necessary cleaning procedures with your health care provider.

Jet injectors release a tiny jet stream of insulin, that is forced through your skin with pressure. These devices have no needles, so they can be a good option for people with needle phobias. They are not pain-free and can sometimes cause bruising. These devices can be expensive, so find out whether your health plan will pay for it up front. Insulin delivery with these devices is not always stable, so you will need to work closely with your health care provider to ensure good blood glucose management while you adjust to one of these devices.

Often manufacturers will make sample products available to you before you make a purchase. Talk with your health care provider about these kinds of products because they can sometimes get you samples. Look for items that are easy to use and durable. Some items require more skill and dexterity on the part of the user than others, so try several before you buy. Make sure that the injection aid you purchase works with the supplies you use and works well for you.

Psst...

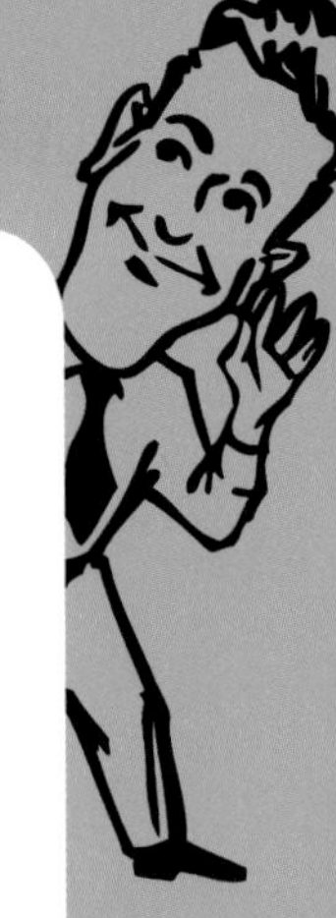

Online Resources About Taking Insulin

The following websites are excellent resources for learning more about the different ways to administer insulin. A diabetes educator is also an excellent resource for learning everything you want to know about insulin.

www.bddiabetes.com/us/

www.changingdiabetes-us.com/

www.goinsulin.com/

www.medtronicminimed.com

www.myomnipod.com

www.animascorp.com

www.disetronic-usa.com/dstrnc_us/

www.childrenwithdiabetes.com/pumps

www.lillydiabetes.com

DEFINITION:

subcutaneous: under the skin.

Insulin injection areas

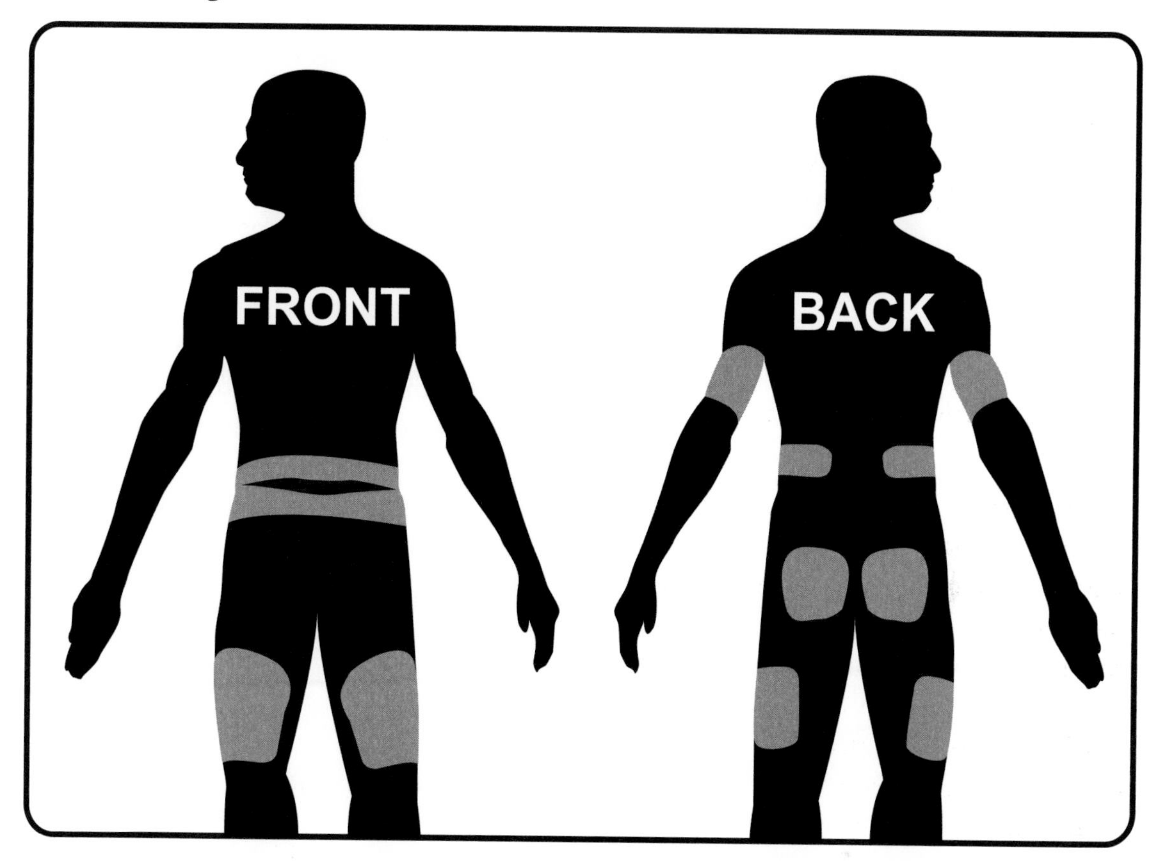

Site Rotation

The place on your body where you inject insulin can affect your blood glucose level. Insulin enters the blood at slightly different speeds when injected at different sites. Insulin shots work fastest when given in the abdomen (but just slightly faster). Insulin arrives in the blood a little more slowly from the upper arms and even more slowly from the thighs and buttocks. Injecting insulin in the same general area (for example, your abdomen) will give you the most consistent results from your insulin.

Don't inject the insulin in exactly the same place each time; move around in the same general area. For example, giving your before-breakfast insulin injection in the abdomen and your before-supper insulin injection in the leg each day gives more consistent blood glucose results. If you inject insulin near the same place each time, hard lumps, extra fatty deposits, or scar tissue may develop. The new insulins cause less scar tissue than the older insulins, but it's still good to change sites. Scar tissue can be uncomfortable and unsightly, and can make your insulin action less reliable. Work with your health care provider to choose the best sites for your insulin injections. Make a site-rotation plan to help you avoid inconsistent insulin absorption and fluctuating blood glucose levels.

Insulin In the Future

Scientists have been searching for new ways to administer insulin for many years. They thought they had found success in 2006, when Exubera, the first inhaled insulin, was approved by the FDA; however, Exubera did not sell well and was taken off the market in 2008. The exact reason for Exubera's failure is not fully known, although there are theories out there. Some believe that the inhaler was too bulky, or the insulin was too expensive. There were also concerns about the dangers of exposing the lungs to insulin, or the possibility that people just weren't happy with their blood glucose levels while on it. In the end, maybe it just turned out that taking insulin by injection wasn't as hard as it seemed.

So, what's to come almost 100 years after insulin was created and changed the lives of so many people? Pharmaceutical companies and researchers are looking into smaller inhalers for inhaled insulin, insulin that you spray in your mouth, insulin pills, and insulin skin patches. Stay tuned to ADA resources for updates. If these work well, they will definitely be welcomed. Until then, be glad there is something that can save, prolong, and improve your life...good-old insulin by injection.

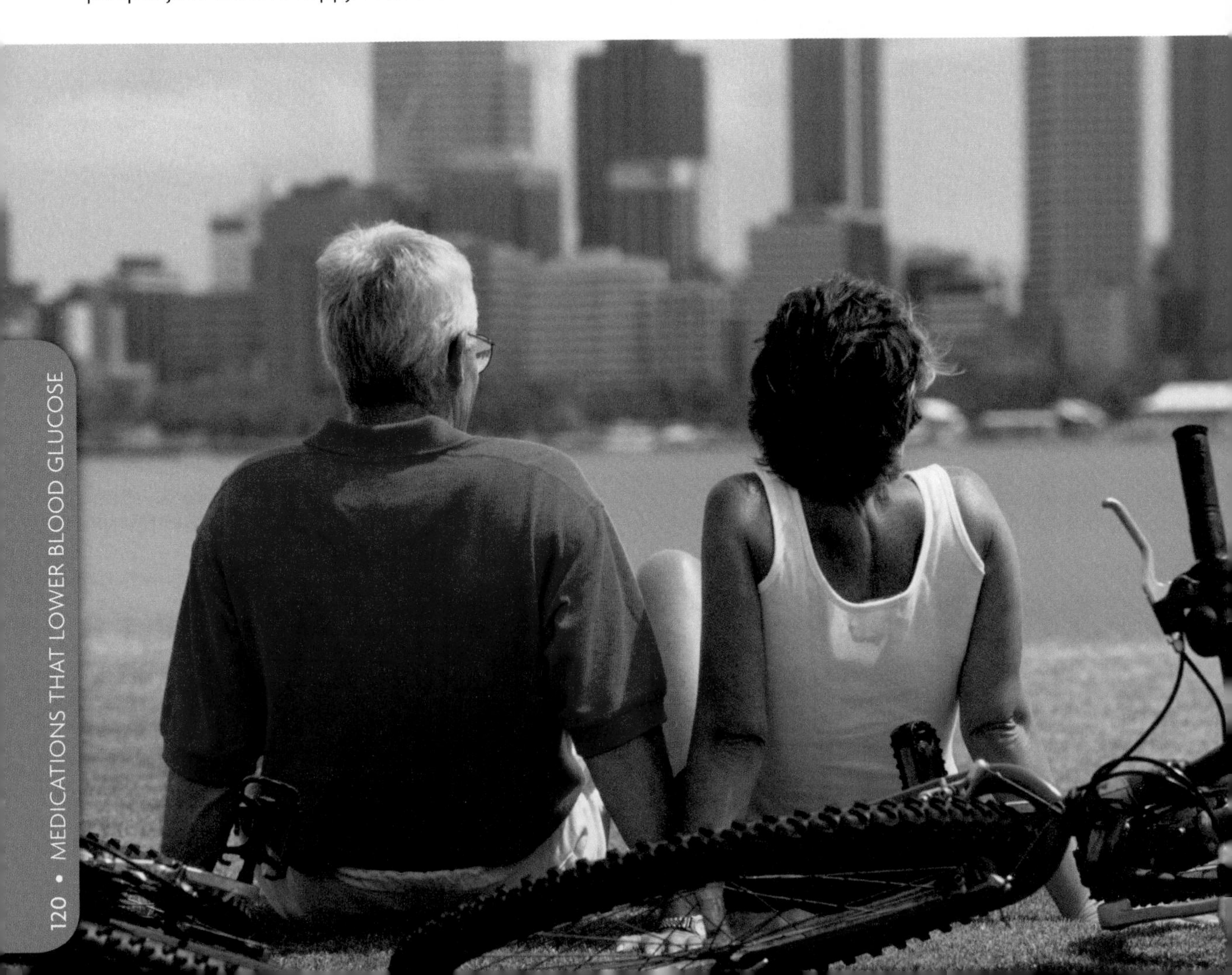

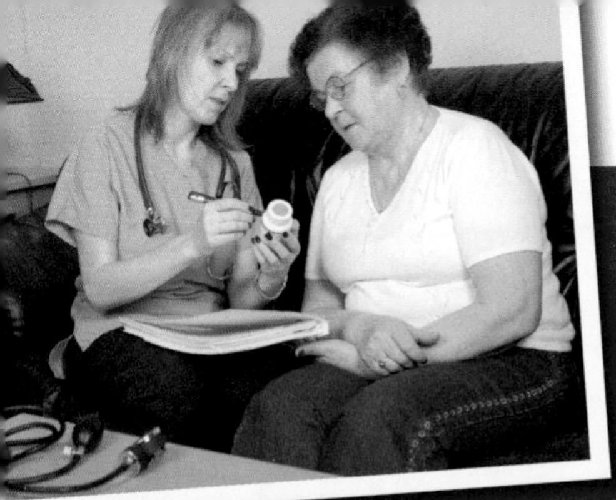

CHAPTER 9

Other Medications to Manage Diabetes

Today, experts agree that if you control your ABCs over the years, you can prevent or delay the common complications of diabetes—such as heart disease, heart attacks, and strokes. Blood glucose control is not the only measurement you need to be concerned about when you have diabetes. You also need to control your blood pressure and cholesterol. Your health care provider may recommend medications to achieve your targets. As you have learned, there are recommended numbers—or targets—for managing your ABCs. Many health care professionals use the term treat to target, meaning to use whatever it takes to help you reach and maintain your targets [also check out *Chapter 2*, page 23]. In this chapter, you will be reminded of recommended target goals and recommendations about how to reach those goals, as well as a bit about other medications that are often prescribed for people who have diabetes.

What You'll Learn:

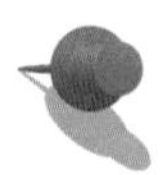

- To stay healthy and prevent/delay diabetes complications, it's also important to control your blood pressure and blood lipids
- Many people with diabetes need to take medications in addition to making lifestyle changes to manage high blood pressure and blood lipids
- Common medications in use to prevent or manage high blood pressure and heart disease
- Common side effects and warnings about blood pressure and heart disease medications
- How medications for other health problems can affect your diabetes

B Stands for Blood Pressure

Two out of three people who have diabetes also have high blood pressure. Because most of the complications of diabetes are related to both elevated blood glucose and elevated blood pressure, it is important you make managing your blood pressure a priority. Blood pressure is the force of blood exerted on the inside walls of your blood vessels. It is expressed as a ratio in millimeters of mercury (e.g., 130/80mmHg, read as 130/80). The first—or top number—is the systolic pressure, which indicates the arterial pressure occurring during contraction of the left ventricle of the heart. This is the measurement of your heart when it beats. The second—or bottom—numberis the diastolic pressure, which is the arterial pressure during the interval between heartbeats. This is the measurement when your heart is at rest.

If your blood pressure is above the recommended target goal, it can cause problems. It is important that you try to get your blood pressure to < 130/80mmHg at all times of the day. It varies just like your blood glucose.

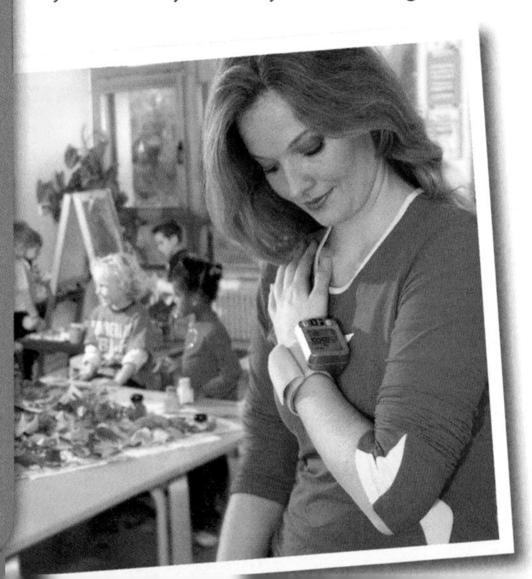

By the Numbers

ADA Recommendations for Blood Pressure

- If you have a systolic blood pressure of 130–139 mmHg or a diastolic blood pressure of 80–89 mmHg, you should be encouraged to make lifestyle changes for a maximum of three months. If your targets of < 130/80mmHg are not achieved in that time, you should be treated with the addition of one or more medicine that lowers your blood pressure.
- If you have more severe high blood pressure (systolic blood pressure ≥ 140 or diastolic blood pressure ≥ 90 mmHg) when you are diagnosed or when you follow up, you should receive medication in addition to lifestyle therapy.
- The medications you receive should include one of two classes of medications: an angiotensin converting enzyme (ACE inhibitor) or an angiotensin receptor blocker (ARB). If you are not able to tolerate one class of these medications, your health care provider should recommend the other class for you. If these medications don't lower your blood pressure to your target range, your health care provider should recommend that you add another class of medication called a thiazide diuretic or a loop diuretic.
- It is not unusual for you to need two or more types of medications to lower your blood pressure to your target range.
- If you are pregnant and have diabetes and chronic high blood pressure, your blood pressure target goals should be 110–129/65–79 mmHg for your health as well as your baby's health.

DEFINITIONS:

angiotensin converting enzyme (ACE inhibitor): an oral medication that lowers blood pressure. For people with diabetes, especially those who have protein (albumin) in their urine, it also slows down, prevents, and can reverse kidney damage.

angiotensin receptor blocker (ARB): an oral medicine that is used to treat high blood pressure and can slow down, prevent, or reverse kidney damage.

diuretic: any substance that increases the production and elimination of urine.

Treatment Strategies for High Blood Pressure

If your blood pressure is high, drug treatment is not the only option. Although there are no well-controlled studies of healthy eating and physical activity in the treatment of high blood pressure in people with diabetes, studies in people who do not have diabetes have shown blood pressure–lowering effects similar to using one kind of blood pressure medication. This has been done by:

- Reducing your sodium intake and excess body weight
- Increasing your consumption of fruits, vegetables, and low-fat dairy products [also check out *Chapter 5*, page 59]
- Avoiding excessive alcohol consumption [also check out *Chapter 15*, page 195, and *Chapter 18*, page 229]
- Increasing activity levels [also check out *Chapter 7*, page 89]
- Losing about 10 pounds

These strategies not only help your blood pressure, but also your blood glucose and lipids.

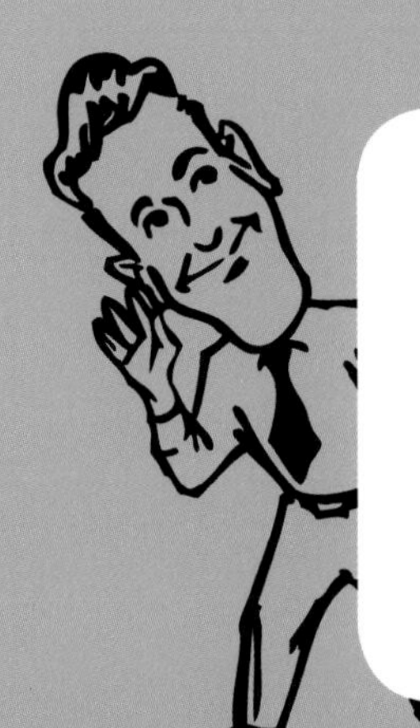

Psst...

Blood Pressure Medications

If you take blood pressure medications, check your blood pressure at home to see how you are adjusting to your medication. If you should experience side effects and need to contact your health care provider, this information will help your health care provider make an informed assessment [also check out *Chapter 13*, page 163, and *Chapter 21*, page 257].

ACE Inhibitors and Angiotensin Receptor Blocker (ARBs)

ACE inhibitors are oral medications that lower your blood pressure by blocking an enzyme that narrows your blood vessels. ACE stands for angiotensin (an-gee-oh-TEN-sin) converting enzyme. By opening your blood vessels, it lowers your blood pressure. This allows your blood to flow more freely through your vessels and delivers blood and oxygen to your heart and other parts of your body. For people with diabetes, especially those who have protein (albumin) in the urine, it also helps slow kidney damage. Some health care providers recommend ACE inhibitors to prevent kidney damage even if you don't have high blood pressure. Angiotensin (an-gee-oh-TEN-sin) receptor blockers (ARBs) are a class of oral medicines that lower blood pressure, much like ACE inhibitors, except they block certain chemical receptors that cause your blood vessels to narrow.

As with any medication, there is always the possibility of mild to severe side effects. Talk with your health care provider if you experience any of these side effects of ACE inhibitors and ARBs:

- Dizziness, faintness, or lightheadedness when you change from a lying or sitting position to a standing position. This may be the strongest when you first start taking this medication and it may go away.
- Symptoms of high potassium: Confusion, weakness, irregular heartbeat, shortness of breath, and numbness or tingling in hands, feet, or lips.

ACE Inhibitors

Generic	Brand	Generic Available?
captopril	Capoten	Yes
enalapril	Vasotec	Yes
lisinopril	Prinivil, Zestril	Yes
ramipril	Altace	Yes
quinapril	Accupril	Yes

ARBs

Generic	Brand	Generic Available?
losartan	Cozaar	No
olmesartan	Benicar	No
valsartan	Diovan	No

Thiazide-like Diuretics

Generic	Brand	Generic Available?
hydrochlorothiazide or HCTZ	Diuril, Esidrex	Yes
methyclothiazide	Enduron	Yes
indapamide	Lozol	Yes
metolazone	Zaroxolyn	Yes

Loop Diuretics

Generic	Brand	Generic Available?
furosemide	Lasix	Yes
bumetanide	Bumex	Yes
ethacrynic acid	Edecrin	Yes

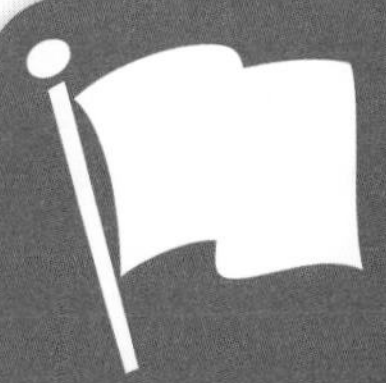

RED FLAG

ACE Inhibitors and ARBs Warnings

- *ACE inhibitors or ARBs are not recommended during pregnancy. These medications may harm your unborn baby. Use an effective means of birth control while taking these medications. If you become pregnant while on these medications, speak with your health care provider as soon as you find out you are pregnant.*
- *Tell your health care provider if you are breastfeeding or have diabetes, heart disease, kidney disease, liver disease, or lupus. This includes telling your dentist you are on these medications.*
- *This medicine may make you dizzy or drowsy. Avoid driving, using machines, or doing anything else that could be dangerous if you are not alert.*
- *Your blood pressure may go up if you stop using this medicine. High blood pressure usually has no symptoms. Even if you feel well, do not stop using the medicine without asking your health care provider.*
- *Most ACE inhitors and ARBs are not recommended for children. Children should not take these medications unless they are prescribed by a licensed pediatrician.*

- Problems with urination, pain in the side or lower back, dry mouth, increased thirst, muscle cramps, nausea or vomiting, a sore throat, fever, headache, stuffy or runny nose, mouth sores, unusual bruising, chest pain, a fast or irregular heartbeat, and/or swelling of your lower legs, ankles, and feet. Contact your health care provider.
- Allergic reactions. If you notice a red, itchy skin rash, don' treat the rash; this can be a reaction to the medication. If you have swelling of your neck, face, and tongue, this is a medical emergency. In both cases, contact your health care provider.
- Cough. This is usually a dry hacking cough. Tell your health care provider. You may need a cough medicine, or you may need to be switched to another medication.
- Change in taste. You may notice a salty or metallic taste in your mouth or notice a decrease in your sense of taste. This usually goes away in time.

Diuretics

Diuretics, also known as water pills, help lower your blood pressure by getting rid of excess water and salt. There are several classes of diuretics. They each increase the amount of urine you excrete, but each does so in its own unique way. The two classes are thiazide-like diuretics and loop diuretics. Thiazide-like diuretics lower your blood pressure more than loop diuretics, cause moderate increases in sodium excretion, and are appropriate for long-term use. Loop diuretics are more powerful than thiazide-like diuretics and are often used for people who have congestive heart failure symptoms in emergency situations.

Side effects of thiazide-like and loop diuretics are related to increased urination. You not only get rid of unneeded water, but also electrolytes like sodium and potassium. If you lose too much water or electrolytes, you can get dehydrated and have electrolyte imbalances. Many of the side effects are related to losing too much fluid or electrolyte imbalances.

- Increased urination. Either an increase in frequency or amount. This can last several hours after taking your medication.
- Dehydration caused by losing too much fluid. Signs include extreme thirst, extremely dry mouth, dark-colored and/or decreased urine output, constipation, and dizziness.
- Electrolyte imbalances. Have your electrolytes checked before and during treatment. Taking these kinds of diuretics puts you at risk for low potassium and sodium. Symptoms include irregular heart rhythm, confusion, muscle weakness, muscle cramps or weakness, extreme tiredness, loss of appetite, nausea, and vomiting. If you have any of these symptoms, contact your health care provider right away.
- Dizziness, faintness, or lightheadedness when you change from a lying or sitting position to a standing position. Change positions slowly. Contact your health care provider if this does not go away.
- Sore throat, fever, cough, ringing in your ears, unusual bruising or bleeding, and rapid weight loss. These are serious side effects. Stop taking this medication, and contact your health care provider right away.

DEFINITION:

electrolytes: electrolytes are minerals in your blood and other body fluids that carry an electric charge. It is important that your electrolytes are in a certain balance, because they affect the amount of fluid in your body, the acidity (pH) of your blood, muscle action (your heart is a muscle), and other important processes.

- Itchy red skin or rash. This can indicate an allergy to your medication. Stop taking it, and contact your health care provider.
- Diuretics may cause an increased blood glucose in some people. If you notice this, do not stop taking this medication, but talk with your health care provider about this.

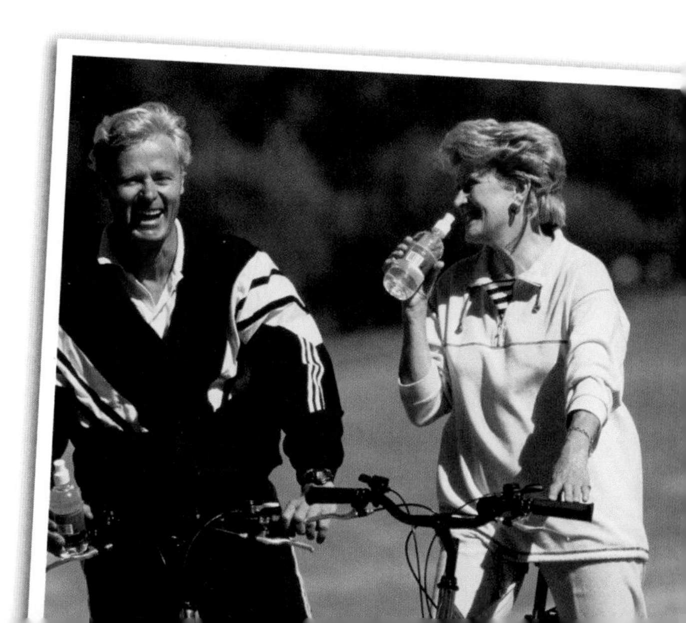

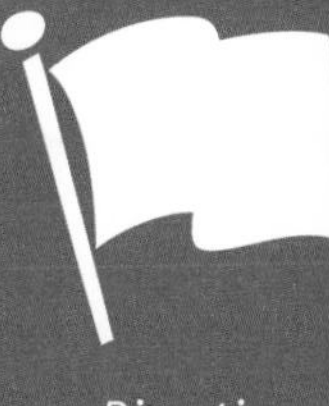

RED FLAG

Diuretic Warnings

- *Diuretics are not recommended during pregnancy. These medications may harm your unborn baby. Use an effective means of birth control while taking these medications. If you become pregnant while on diuretics, speak with your health care provider as soon as you find out you are pregnant.*
- *Tell your health care provider if you are breastfeeding or have diabetes, heart disease, kidney disease, or liver disease. This includes telling your dentist you are on these medications.*
- *If you stop using this medicine, your blood pressure may go up. High blood pressure usually has no symptoms. Even if you feel well, do not stop using the medicine without asking your health care provider.*
- *Most diuretics are not recommended for children. Children should not take these medications unless they are prescribed by a pediatrician.*

Wonder?

When is the best time to take my blood pressure medication?

That depends on you, your medication, and your blood pressure. If you can only remember to take it a certain time of the day, let your health care provider know that. Hopefully, your health care provider will recommend something you can take only once a day. Since early morning high blood pressure is serious and often seen in people who have diabetes, you want to make sure your early-morning numbers are within your target range. If you are taking your medications in the morning, and your blood pressure is above your target, talk with your health care provider to see if you should take your pills in the evening instead, so it will be working to cover your early-morning rise [also check out *Chapter 13*, page 163].

Combinations of Blood Pressure Medicines

Because many people who have high blood pressure need to take two or more classes of blood pressure–lowering medications, many times two classes of these medications are in one pill. For example, you may be taking an ACE inhibitor and a thiazide-like diuretic in one pill rather than two separate pills. You may not be able to tell by the name, but one way to know is if your pills have two numbers on them. For example, if you are taking Capozide, it would say Capozide 25/15, which means there are 25mg of captopril and 15mg of hydrochlorothiazide in your pill. Ask your health care provider whether you are taking any combination pills. If so, you need to be aware of the effects and side effects of both.

C Stands for Cholesterol (Lipids)

People with type 2 diabetes have an increased prevalence of lipid (or cholesterol) abnormalities, which contribute to their high risk of heart disease. Because of the high incidence of heart disease in people who have diabetes, it is important for you to be aware of your lipid levels so you can prevent and treat heart disease. As with blood pressure, drug treatment is not the only prevention and treatment for lipid abnormalities; however, because medications called statins can prevent and treat heart disease, they are recommended along with lifestyle modification for most people over 40 years old who have diabetes. Statins (or HMG-CoA reductase inhibitors) are a class of drugs used to lower lipid levels in people who have or are at risk for heart disease.

How Statins Work

Statins lower cholesterol by inhibiting the enzyme HMG-CoA reductase in your liver, resulting in an increased clearance of low-density lipoprotein (LDL) from the bloodstream and a decrease in LDL cholesterol levels. The first results can be seen after one week of use, and the effect is maximal after four to six weeks. If statins help you reach your target lipid goals, it does not mean you should stop taking your medication. It means your medication is working, and you should continue to take it.

Side Effects of Statins

Most people tolerate statins well, but there are side effects. Some of these side effects

Statin Medications Available in the U.S.

Generic	Brand	Generic Available?
rosuvastatin	Crestor	No
atorvastin	Lipitor	No
lovastatin	Mevacor, Altoprev	Yes
fluvastatin	Lescol	No
pravastatin	Pravachol	Yes
simvastatin	Zocor	Yes

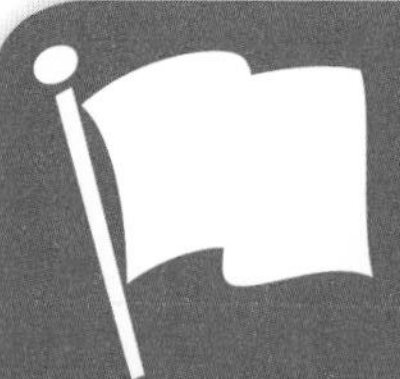

RED FLAG

Statin Warnings

- *Statins are not recommended during pregnancy. These medications may harm your unborn baby. Use an effective means of birth control while taking these medications. If you become pregnant while on these medications, speak with your health care provider as soon as you find out you are pregnant.*
- *Tell your health care provider if you are breast-feeding or have diabetes, heart disease, kidney disease, or liver disease. This includes telling your dentist you are on these medications.*
- *If you stop using this medicine, your lipids may go up. Elevated lipids have no symptoms. Even if you feel well, do not stop taking your medicine without asking your health care provider.*
- *Statins should only be used in children when recommended and under the care of a pediatrician.*

Wonder?

What is hs-CRP, and what does it have to do with my risk for heart and blood vessel diseases?

High-sensitive C-Reactive Protein (hs-CRP) is a protein found in your blood that can detect the level of inflammation in your body. There are currently no recommendations by the ADA or the American Heart Association (AHA) as to when the test should be ordered and who should have the test. Most people have their hs-CRP tested when they have their lipids tested, but you can choose to test more often if your health care provider thinks it's necessary.

AHA and the Centers for Disease Control and Prevention (CDC) define risk groups as:

- Low risk: less than 1.0 mg/L
- Average risk: 1.0 to 3.0 mg/L
- High risk: above 3.0 mg/L

Although inflammation is your body's normal response to infections, injury, and fever, researchers now believe that chronic inflammation can lead to the progression of heart and blood vessel diseases, which can eventually lead to heart attacks and strokes. Recent research suggests that people who have an hs-CRP result in the high-risk group in spite of a normal LDL cholesterol level should take a statin medication to lower their hs-CRP and LDL cholesterol levels even further. Because diabetes already puts you at high risk of heart and blood vessel diseases, your health care provider may already have you on a statin medication. If not, ask whether you should be on one [also check out *Chapter 2*, page 23]. Recent infections, injuries, and general inflammation, such as rheumatoid arthritis, can increase your hs-CRP and give you a falsely elevated estimate of risk.

go away as your body adjusts to your medication. These are:

- Muscle and joint pain. Many times, this goes away; however, if this persists, talk with your health care provider about switching to a different statin.
- Gastrointestinal (GI) problems. You may experience nausea, diarrhea, and/or constipation. If these symptoms persist, ask your health care provider about switching to a different statin.

While most side effects will go away in time, there are a few side effects that can be potentially serious in the long run. The most dangerous is the increase in liver enzymes, which can lead to liver damage. You may not experience any symptoms related to this, so it's especially important to have your liver enzymes checked prior to starting a statin and periodically throughout taking the medication. If there is only a mild increase, discuss with your health care provider whether you should continue, decrease the dose, or stop treatment completely. If the increase is severe, you will most likely be instructed to stop taking it, which will bring your liver enzymes back to normal.

With high doses of statins, you are also at an increased risk of muscle pain and tenderness, otherwise known as statin myopathy. There is also the possibility that you could develop rhabdomyolysis, a rare but serious disorder that causes the muscle cells to break down and release a protein into the blood that can cause kidney damage. If you notice any muscle aches or pains, report them to your health care provider immediately.

Combination Therapy

Sometimes lifestyle strategies and statins will not be able to get you to your target levels. With statins, you will most likely see a decrease in your total cholesterol and your LDL, but not always your triglycerides and your HDL [also check out *Chapter 2*, page 23]. If this is the case, your health care provider may recommend combination therapy using statins and other lipid-lowering agents.

As with some of the medications that lower your blood glucose, as well as some to decrease your blood pressure, there are combination lipid-lowering pills that have more than one agent in them. Some of them even have one agent to lower your blood pressure and one agent to lower your lipids. There are also pills that have combination agents for your cholesterol. Make sure you know what medication you are taking. You may be taking a combination pill and not even know it.

Aspirin

Aspirin has been demonstrated to prevent cardiovascular problems, such as strokes and heart attacks. Since diabetes and heart disease are so closely related, the ADA recommends you take a baby aspirin (81 mg) or a regular aspirin (325 mg) daily if you:

- have a history of heart disease
- are more than 40 years old
- have other risk factors, such as a family history of heart disease or high blood pressure
- smoke
- have high lipid levels

Psst…

Other benefits to taking statins

- Decreased inflammation. Decreasing inflammation can stabilize the lining of the blood vessels throughout your body.
- Relaxation of blood vessels. This can decrease blood pressure.
- Blood-thinning properties. This can help reduce your risk of blood clots.
- Kidney protection. This is thought to be due to the anti-inflammatory, lipid-lowering, and blood pressure–lowering effects of statins.
- Prevention of cancer. The studies on this effect have been mixed.
- Prevention of arthritis and bone fractures. More research needs to be done in this relationship.
- Decreased risk for, and possible treatment of, Alzheimer's and dementia. Although more research is needed, this could be because of the anti-inflammatory effects of statins.

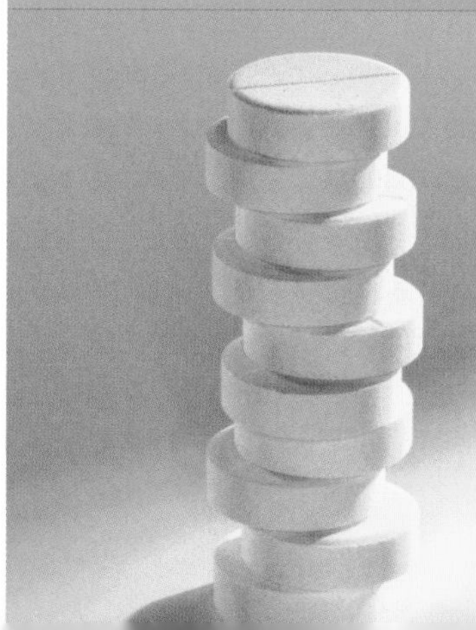

- have protein in your urine

Exactly how aspirin works is not completely understood, but it may be because it helps keep your red blood cells from clumping together. These cells seem to clump more readily in people with diabetes. It may also be related to its anti-inflammatory action.

Taking aspirin is not without risk; it can cause stomach and intestinal bleeding, which is why people with bleeding ulcers shouldn't take aspirin. This risk can be reduced by taking an enteric coated aspirin, and avoiding taking aspirin on an empty stomach. Aspirin is not recommended in people under 30 years old and is contraindicated in people under 21 years old because of an associated risk of Reye's syndrome.

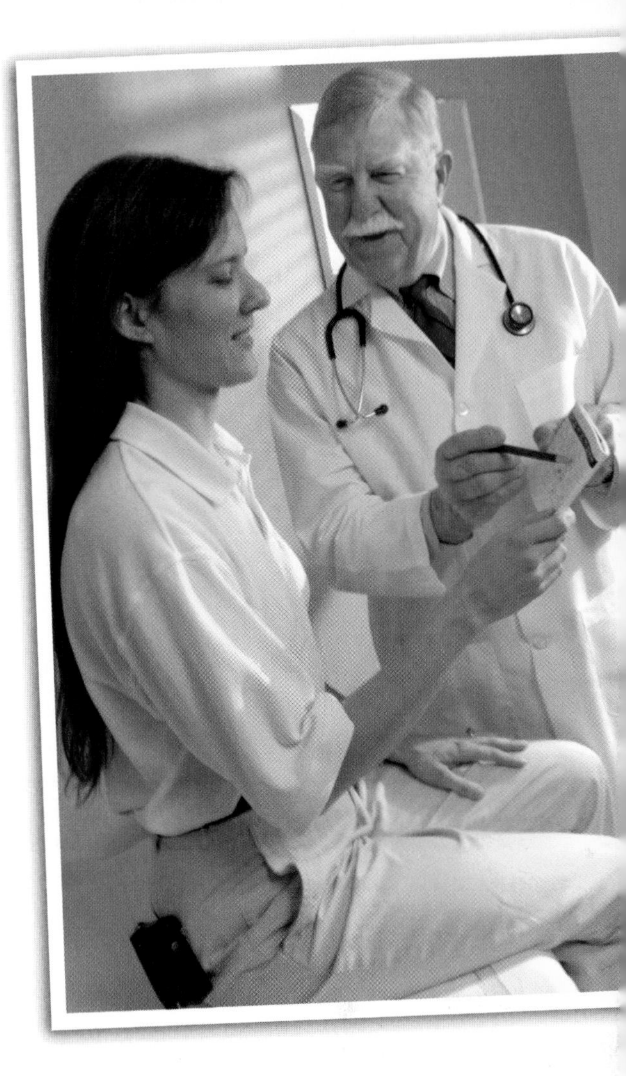

Other Medications

Diabetes may not be the only health issue you have. You may be taking other medications for your other diseases or health problems. If so, it's important that you learn about how the medications you take to manage your diabetes interact with other medications. Sometimes one medication will increase or decrease the effectiveness of another medication. This is very important for you to know, so you can get the most benefit from all your medications with the smallest amount of negative side effects.

Thyroid Medications

There is a high incidence of thyroid problems in people with diabetes. If your thyroid is not functioning correctly, this can affect your blood glucose, blood pressure, and cholesterol, among other things. If you are taking any type of thyroid medications, know that an elevated thyroid hormone may increase your blood glucose and blood pressure. Monitor your blood glucose, blood pressure, and lipids with the understanding that if you notice changes in these numbers, it could be related to your thyroid. Work with your health care provider to have your thyroid levels checked on a regular basis and to have your medications adjusted as needed.

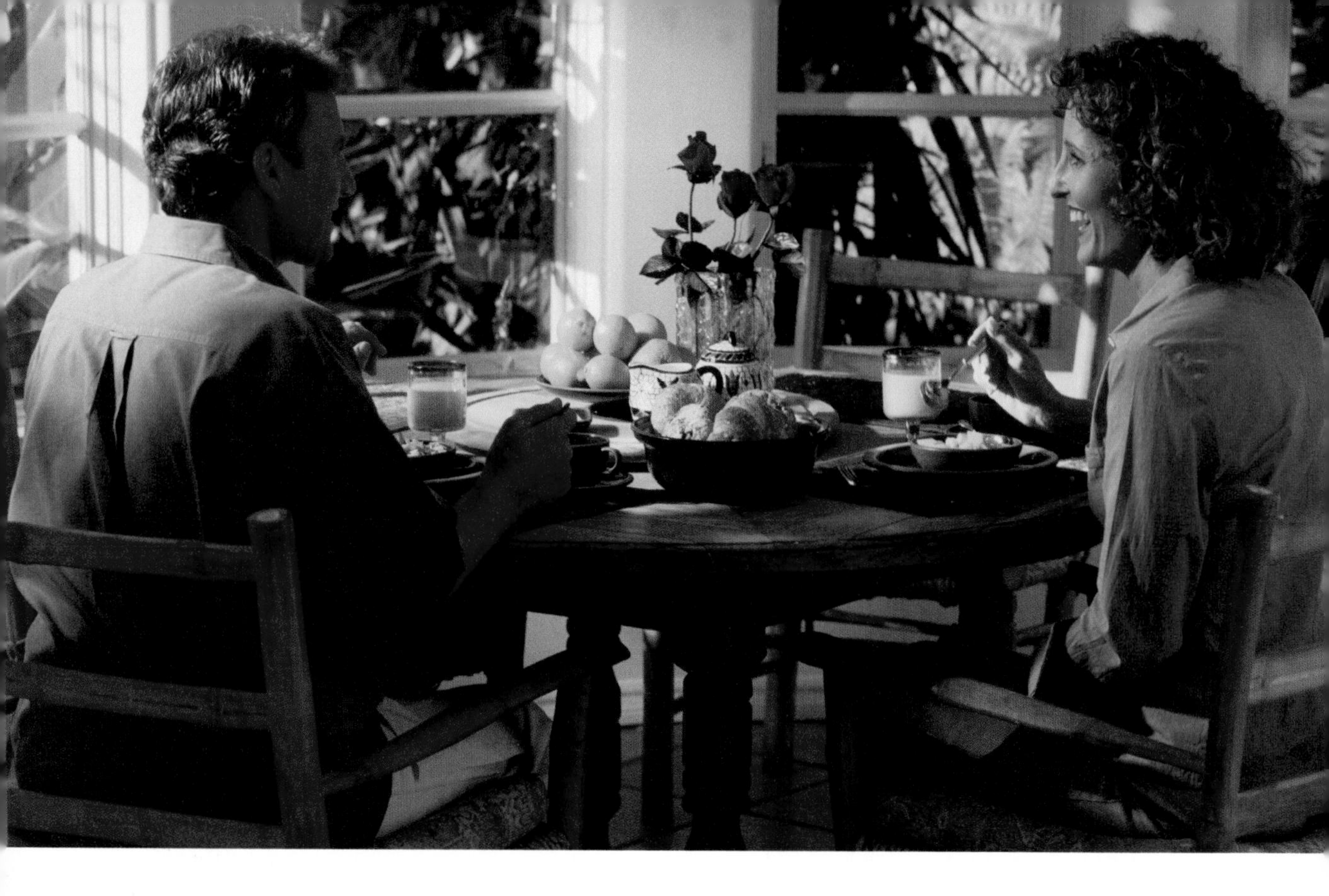

Steroids

Steroids are the shortened term for corticosteroids. Corticosteroids are man-made drugs that closely resemble cortisol, a hormone your adrenal glands produce naturally. Corticosteroids are different from the male hormone–related steroid compounds that some athletes abuse. Steroids work by decreasing inflammation and reducing the activity of your immune system. Corticosteroid medications include cortisone, prednisone, and methylprednisolone. Steroids are used to treat a variety of conditions in which your body's defense system malfunctions and causes tissue damage, such as allergic reactions, asthma, rheumatoid arthritis, and severe pain. Taking steroids to manage an inflammatory condition can induce the onset of type 2 diabetes in people at risk.

The occurrence of side effects depends on the dose, type of steroid, and length of treatment. For people with diabetes, it is not unusual to experience an increase in blood glucose, blood pressure, and weight, due to the insulin resistant action of steroids. You may need a change in your medications—your steroids, blood glucose–lowering medications, or blood pressure medication. Your glucose, blood pressure, and weight will usually return to normal after you stop these medications. Do not stop taking steroids abruptly, as this can cause serious problems. If you feel you must stop these medications, talk with your health care provider about how you should taper them down.

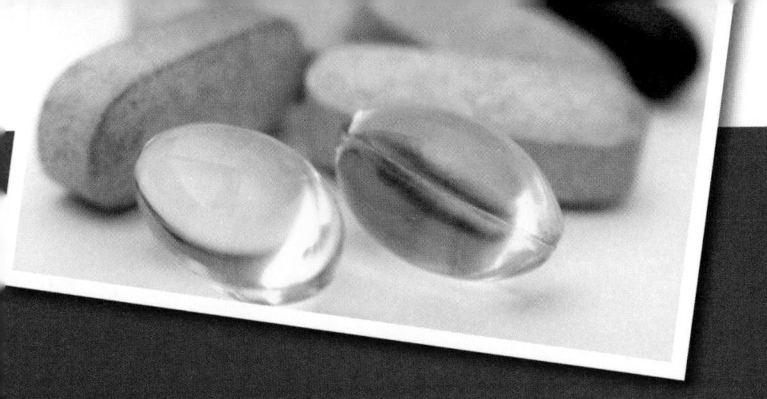

CHAPTER 10

No Prescription Needed

In the world we live in today, medicine and treatment don't always mean a trip to the doctor. Along with all the great medical research that has advanced over the years, there are also new research and findings that verify the positive effects of alternative and complimentary medicines. Other treatments, including dietary supplements and over-the-counter medications, are now considered an important part of health management. Some of these directly affect your diabetes management, some work indirectly, some don't affect it at all, and some may adversely affect it. Learn more about both sides of the story, so you can make the best choices for what you want to take to manage your diabetes.

What You'll Learn:

- People with diabetes use more complementary or alternative medications than people who don't have diabetes
- The difference between complementary and alternative medicine
- The regulations that guide the sales of dietary supplements
- Information about commonly used dietary supplements for diabetes care
- How to take dietary supplements and over-the-counter medications safely

Complementary and Alternative Medicine

The National Center for Complementary and Alternative Medicine (NCCAM) defines complementary and alternative medicine (CAM) as treatments and health care practices not widely taught in medical schools, not generally used in hospitals, and not usually reimbursed by insurance companies. CAM therapies cover a broad range of healing philosophies, approaches, and treatments. CAM health care practitioners use the term "holistic" because they consider the whole person—physically, mentally, emotionally, and spiritually.

Alternative therapies are those used instead of standard medical practice. Complementary therapies are those combined with other alternative or conventional therapies.

NCCAM categorizes CAM into five different domains: biologically based practices, energy medicine, manipulative and body-based practices, mind-body medicine, and whole medical systems. This chapter focuses on the biologically based practices. Biologically based practices include, but are not limited to, botanicals, vitamins, minerals, herbs, and fatty acids. These items are in the category of dietary supplements.

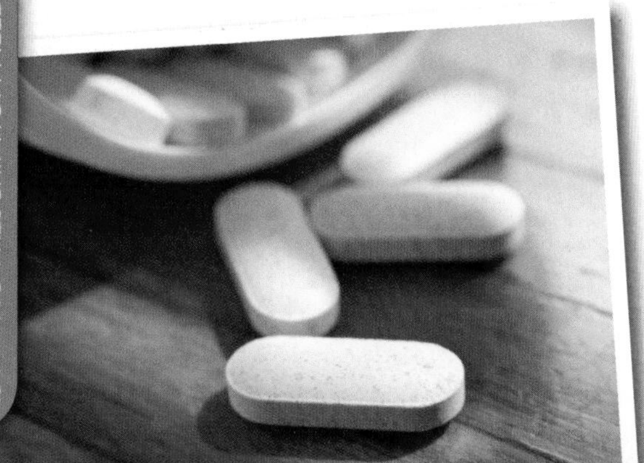

By the Numbers

People with Diabetes and Complementary or Alternative Medication Supplements

People with diabetes are 1.6 times more likely to use a complementary or alternative medication supplement than people who don't have diabetes. Of the people who do use these supplements, less than 40% tell their health care providers. Although many believe these will help their diabetes management, many people don't realize that they might cause harm instead.

Dietary Supplements

The Food and Drug Administration (FDA) traditionally considered dietary supplements to be composed only of essential nutrients, such as vitamins, minerals, and proteins. The Nutrition Labeling and Education Act of 1990 added herbs, or similar nutritional substances, to the term dietary supplement. Through the Dietary Supplement Health and Education Act (DSHEA), Congress expanded the meaning of the term dietary supplements beyond essential nutrients to include such substances as ginseng, garlic, fish oils, psyllium, enzymes, glandulars, and mixtures of these.

The DSHEA established a formal definition of dietary supplement using several criteria. A dietary supplement:

- is a product (other than tobacco) that is intended to supplement the diet that bears or contains one or more of the following dietary ingredients: a vitamin; a mineral; an herb or other botanical; an amino acid; a dietary substance for use by man to supplement the diet by increasing the total daily intake; or a concentrate, metabolite, constituent, extract, or combinations of these ingredients.

- is intended for ingestion in pill, capsule, tablet, or liquid form.
- is not represented for use as a conventional food or as the sole item of a meal or diet.
- is labeled as a "dietary supplement."
- includes products such as an approved new drug, certified antibiotic, or licensed biologic that was marketed as a dietary supplement or food before approval, certification, or license (unless the Secretary of Health and Human Services waives this provision).

Many dietary supplement companies claim their products can improve your diabetes. It is wise for you to get your information from some place other than the company, store, or person who sells supplements.

Common Supplements Used By People With Diabetes

Although people use many dietary supplements to manage diabetes, some of the most commonly used ones are cinnamon, chromium, Alpha-Lipoic Acid (ALA) or Lipoic Acid (LA), magnesium, Omega-3 fatty acids, and Vitamin D. Each supplement works in its own way, and all of these can be found in over-the-counter forms.

Tell your health care providers about all the supplements you take, including prescription

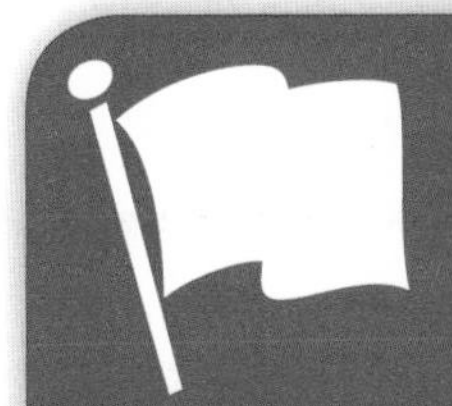

RED FLAG

Supplements and Type 1 Diabetes

If you have type 1 diabetes, and someone tells you their supplement will allow you to stop taking insulin, don't believe it! Unless you have a successful pancreas transplant or hear of a cure through reputable organizations, such as the ADA, you will always need to take insulin.

Psst...

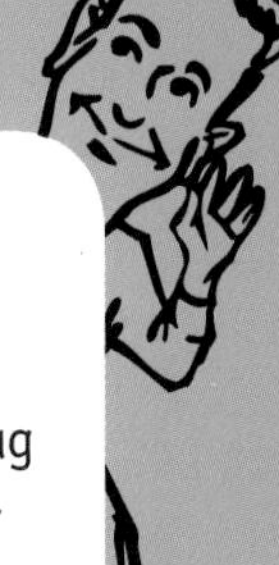

Regulation of Dietary Supplements

In the United States, the Food and Drug Administration (FDA) is responsible for dietary supplements. Supplements are marketed and regulated differently than prescribed medicines. The FDA does not approve dietary supplements before they are allowed on the market, but the FDA can take a dietary supplement off the market if problems occur. The FDA now requires all supplement containers to come with a Supplement Facts label.

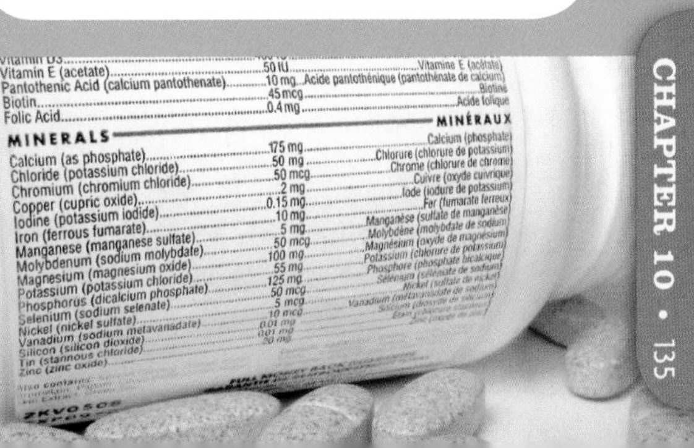

Wonder?

Why do so many people with diabetes use dietary supplements?

The reasons people with diabetes use dietary supplements include:

- The hope of managing diabetes without medications What many people don't realize is that dietary supplements are not always safe and/or effective.
- Perceived or real side effects from prescriptions. People either believe they will experience, or have actually experienced, more side effects from taking prescription medications than from taking dietary supplements.
- A need to have control over their health. People can choose their treatment rather than have someone prescribe a treatment for them.
- Increased cost of prescription medication. Dietary supplements are not always less expensive than prescription medication, especially if you take a lot of them and if they are not effectively managing your diabetes.
- Dissatisfaction with traditional medicine.

and over-the-counter medications and dietary supplements. Buy reputable brands of dietary supplements and over-the-counter medications. Natural does not necessarily mean safe. Many prescription drugs and poisons come from natural sources. Prescription medications go through science and standards to be made safe for human consumption. A good rule of thumb: If it sounds too good to be true, it usually is, so be cautious.

CINNAMON

Cinnamon has sprinkled its way into many venues over thousands of years, from being used in embalming processes, to healing sore throats, and now as a possible treatment for diabetes. Researchers have discovered that in laboratory settings the outcomes for cinnamon helping lower blood glucose have been mixed. Some of the research has been positive, and some has not shown any benefit.

The latest study on cinnamon supplementation for diabetes was reported in the January 2008 issue of *Diabetes*. An analysis of several human studies, which involved 282 subjects, showed no significant benefits of cinnamon supplements on A1C levels, fasting blood glucose (FBG) levels, or lipid parameters. The conclusion at this time? Cinnamon does not appear to improve A1C, FBG, or lipid parameters in people with type 1 or type 2 diabetes.

If you are currently taking cinnamon, and you feel that it helps lower your blood glucose, it's important to know all of the facts.

- There are different kinds of cinnamon. Cassia cinnamon is the kind you usually find in the grocery store and in supplements.

- Cinnamon naturally contains a compound called coumarin, which is a blood thinner. It should not be a problem if you are lightly sprinkling it on your food, or use a cinnamon stick in your coffee or tea daily, but if you are regularly taking more than this, tell your health care provider.
- Be aware of, and report, any unusual bruising, bleeding, black stools, nosebleeds, or faint feelings.
- You SHOULD NOT TAKE more than a sprinkle on your food or a stick in your coffee or tea if you are taking a blood thinner.

CHROMIUM

Chromium is an essential trace mineral the body needs to maintain normal blood glucose levels. Chromium may help lower blood glucose levels and improve blood lipids in people with type 2 diabetes. In 2004, a study was published in *Diabetes Care*, showing that men with diabetes and heart disease had lower toenail chromium levels compared with healthy men. The study revealed that long-term clinical studies are necessary to determine if chromium supplementation is beneficial for people with diabetes. At this time, there are no long-term clinical trials underway, and research results have been mixed; therefore, the ADA cannot recommend chromium.

The form of chromium that has been found to have the most benefit is chromium picolinate. Dietary sources of chromium are found in small amounts in foods like egg yolks, whole grains, green vegetables, bran cereals, and processed meats.

Most studies use chromium at 200 to 600 mcg per day. Doses of up to 1,000 mg per day have been used with no toxic effects. A reasonable supplemental dose is 400 mcg per day. Antacids and calcium carbonate can reduce the absorption of chromium. If you are also taking these, take them at a different time of the day from when you take your chromium.

ALPHA-LIPOIC ACID (ALA) OR LIPOIC ACID (LA)

Alpha-lipoic Acid (ALA), also known as Lipoic Acid (LA), is considered a potent antioxidant and may help prevent the damage that free radicals can do to various tissues in the body. ALA is normally made in the liver, and small amounts circulate in the body.

Some studies show that ALA may help improve your insulin sensitivity and may slow

DEFINITIONS:

antioxidant: a chemical substance that helps protect against cell damage caused by free radicals.

free radicals: a naturally occurring molecule that is essential to many biological processes; its high reactivity may be associated with cancer, heart disease, emphysema, and other conditions.

the progression of kidney damage. Other studies have found ALA to lessen the pain of diabetes nerve disease. It has been used in Germany for years to decrease the pain associated with peripheral neuropathy. Foods contain only small amounts of alpha-lipoic acid. If you take alpha-lipoic acid, the typical dose is 600 mg once or twice a day.

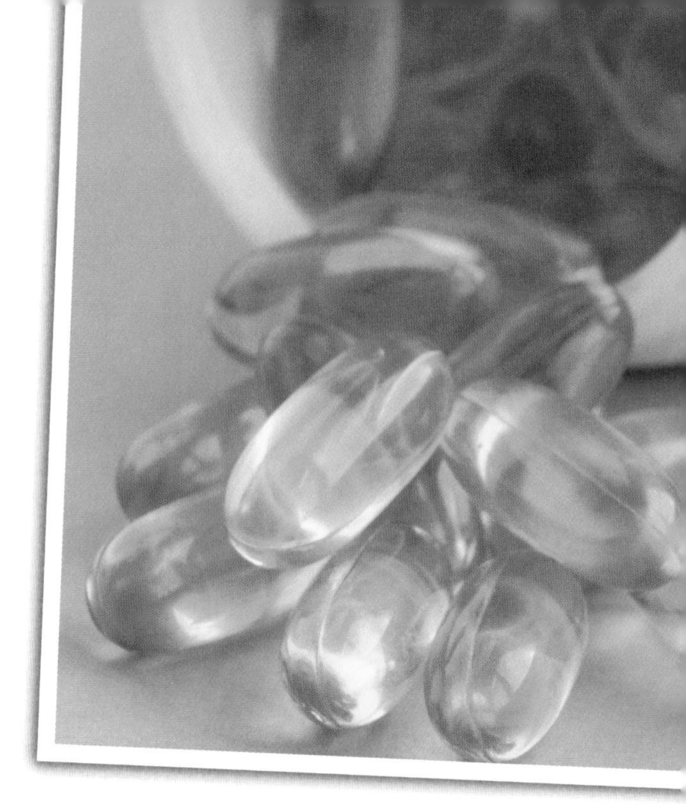

MAGNESIUM

Magnesium (Mg) is an essential trace mineral needed for over 300 biochemical reactions in your body. It is important for muscle contraction (your heart is a muscle), and nerve conduction, and to maintain the appropriate tone of your blood vessels. Many people with diabetes have low magnesium; however, this is difficult to see in your lab work because magnesium resides inside your cells, and blood tests measure the magnesium in your blood, not your cells. Studies have been done on the impact of magnesium on glucose levels with people who have diabetes, but the results are mixed and, when favorable, are minimal. Magnesium supplementation may help protect your heart, kidneys, and nerves, but more science is needed. Dietary sources of magnesium include green leafy vegetables, legumes, grains, seeds, nuts, meats, coffee, and dark chocolate. Do not take magnesium supplements if you have kidney problems.

OMEGA-3 FATTY ACIDS

Omega-3 fatty acids are essential fatty acids, which means they are essential to your health. Your body does not make them, so you must obtain them from food or dietary supplements. At this time, there are no studies to show that omega-3 fatty acids decrease your blood glucose; however, they have been shown to reduce triglycerides and protect your blood vessels, two problems associated with diabetes. Omega-3 fatty acids have also been shown to help depression. People with diabetes have twice the rate of depression of people without diabetes.

The two active ingredients in omega-3 fatty acids are Eicosapentaenoic Acid (EPA) and Docosahexaenoic Acid (DHA). Dietary sources of omega-3 fatty acids include salmon, mackerel, tuna, halibut, and other marine life, such as algae and krill. They can also be found in grass-fed beef, some eggs, certain plants, and nut oils. If you are taking omega-3 fatty acids, the ADA recommends you eat fish (particularly fatty fish) at least two times a week.

People taking more than 3 grams of omega-3 fatty acids from capsules should do so only under a physician's care. High intakes could

TIPS + TACTICS

Working Omega-3 Fatty Acids Into Your Life

- ***People without documented coronary heart disease (CHD):*** *Eat a variety of (preferably fatty) fish at least twice a week. Include oils and foods rich in alpha-linolenic acid (flaxseed, canola, and soybean oils; flaxseed and walnuts).*
- ***People with documented CHD:*** *Consume about 1 gram of EPA+DHA per day, preferably from fatty fish. EPA+DHA in capsule form could be considered in consultation with the physician.*
- ***People who need to lower triglycerides:*** *2 to 4 grams of EPA+DHA per day provided as capsules under a health care provider's care.*

*Source: AHA (*www.Americanheart.org*)*

cause excessive bleeding in some people. Pregnant women and mothers, nursing mothers, young children, and women who might become pregnant should not eat several types of fish, including swordfish, shark, and king mackerel. These individuals should also limit consumption of other fish, including albacore tuna, salmon, and herring.

Wonder?

Should I take a daily multivitamin?

The ADA recommends that healthy people at low risk for nutritional deficiencies meet their nutritional requirements with food, and does not generally support the use of dietary supplements for people with diabetes. The supplements they do recommend are the same as those recommended for the general public. The ADA notes that people who are at increased risk for micronutrient deficiencies, such as those following very low calorie diets, the elderly, strict vegetarians, and other special populations, may benefit from adding multivitamin supplements. Ask your health care provider if this is a good option for you.

VITAMIN D

Vitamin D is a fat-soluble vitamin that is naturally present in very few foods, added to others, and available as a dietary supplement. It is produced in your body when ultraviolet rays from sunlight hit your skin and trigger vitamin D synthesis. Vitamin D obtained from sun exposure, food, and supplements is biologically inactive and must undergo two chemical reactions in your body to activate it. The first occurs in your liver and converts vitamin D to 25-hydroxyvitamin D [25(OH)D], also known as calcidiol. The second occurs primarily in your kidneys and forms the physiologically active 1,25-dihydroxyvitamin D [1,25(OH)2D], also known as calcitriol.

Vitamin D has many health benefits, including its contribution toward the possible prevention of type 1 diabetes. There is evidence of the positive effects of vitamin D

TIPS + TACTICS

Taking over-the-counter medications

- *Don't wait to be sick; do your homework now. Start reading labels of the over-the-counter medications you usually take. If it says it may affect your diabetes, ask your pharmacist or other health care provider what you should take if you need this type of medication.*
- *Look for alternatives. Read labels for cough lozenges and syrups, and choose those that are not sweetened or are sweetened with sugar substitutes.*
- *Understand that aspirin, acetaminophen, and other over-the-counter medications can affect your diabetes management.*
- *Check your blood glucose and blood pressure often when you are taking over-the-counter medications to see how these medications affect your diabetes management. If the supplement claims it affects your blood glucose or your blood pressure, monitor your blood glucose and blood pressure to see how it affects you.*
- *If a product says diabetes on it, the price can be higher than the exact same product that doesn't say diabetes on it. Read labels to see the ingredients. You may save some money.*

on insulin resistance, prevention of cardiometabolic syndrome, and type 2 diabetes [also check out *Chapter 1*, page 5]. Other studies have shown the positive effects of vitamin D on longevity, heart disease, neuromuscular problems, depression, obesity, bone health, and cancer.

Very few foods in nature contain vitamin D. The flesh of fish (such as salmon, tuna, and mackerel) and fish liver oils are among the best sources. Small amounts of vitamin D are found in beef liver, cheese, and egg yolks. Some mushrooms provide vitamin D in variable amounts. Fortified foods provide most of the vitamin D in the American diet. Almost all of the U.S. milk supply is fortified with 100 IU/cup of vitamin D.

By the Numbers

Recommended daily intake of Vitamin D*

Age	Men	Women	Pregnancy/ Lactation
Birth–13 years	5 mcg (200 IU)		
14–18 years	5 mcg (200 IU)	5 mcg (200 IU)	5 mcg (200 IU)
19–50 years	5 mcg (200 IU)	5 mcg (200 IU)	5 mcg (200 IU)
51–70 years	10 mcg (400 IU)	10 mcg (400 IU)	
71+ years	15 mcg (500 IU)	15 mcg (500 IU)	

**The American Academy of Pediatrics (AAP) recommends 10mcg (400 IU) of vitamin D per day in pediatric and adolescent populations.*

CHAPTER 11

The Importance of Catching Your Z's

Life has changed, and so have our sleep patterns. People are working more, doing more, and, in order to fit it all in, sleeping less. In 2008, the National Sleep Foundation (NSF) reported the standard 8-hour business day is no longer the norm for America. NSF's 2008 Sleep in America poll reports that the average American's workday is now 9 hours and 28 minutes. The average time spent in bed is 6 hours and 55 minutes, with 6 hours and 40 minutes spent actually sleeping. Who would have dreamed that lack of sleep or too much sleep could cause you to be overweight, have type 2 diabetes, or have high blood pressure?

Despite what many people think, sleep is not discretionary. It is something you need for good health, and sleep experts are quickly discovering more connections between sufficient sleep and health. You may be having sleep problems and not even know it. Read on to learn more about the importance of getting enough sleep and how this relates to pre- and type 2 diabetes and their related conditions.

What You'll Learn:

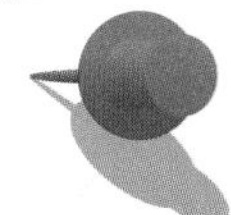

- What sleep has to do with preventing and treating type 2 diabetes
- Number of people with pre-diabetes and type 2 who have sleep apnea—a common sleep disorder
- How much sleep is recommended for people in different age groups
- Why it is important you get the right amount of sleep
- How sleep apnea combined with diabetes can have dangerous health consequences
- How to know if you have a sleeping problem, and how to get help for it

Why Your Body Needs Sleep

Contrary to what many people think, sleep is not optional. Like food and water, it is a necessity. Rats deprived of sleep die within 2-3 weeks, similar to the timeframe of death due to starvation for rats. Many people falsely mistake sleep as "downtime," a time when their brains shut down and their bodies rest. The truth is, during sleep your brain is hard at work.

Lack of sleep keeps your organs from functioning at the highest level and interferes with your body's ability to produce insulin and also to fight off illness. Lack of sleep also increases your risk for heart attacks, strokes, high blood pressure, and depression.

A sleep study conducted at Columbia University Hospital in New York from 1982 to

By the Numbers

Hours of Sleep

The National Center for Health Statistics published a study, Sleep Duration as a Correlate of Smoking, Alcohol Use, Leisure-Time Physical Inactivity, and Obesity among Adults: United States, 2004-2006. The study reported that, despite evidence of the health implications of insufficient sleep, a large number of Americans do not routinely get optimal sleep. It is estimated that 70 million Americans are affected by chronic sleep loss or sleep disorders.

- 6 in 10 U.S. adults (63%) usually slept 7 to 8 hours in a 24-hour period
- 1 in 10 adults (8%) slept less than 6 hours
- 2 in 10 (21%) slept 6 hours
- 1 in 10 (9%) slept 9 or more hours

Factors That Can Prevent a Good Night's Sleep

- High or low glucose levels from diabetes
- Caffeine in coffee, soft drinks, or tea
- Prescription and over-the-counter medications. Certain pain relievers, decongestants, steroids, some heart and blood pressure medications, and other medications or illegal drugs
- Asthma or bronchitis, due to breathing difficulties or the medications
- Arthritis, congestive heart failure, sickle cell anemia
- Schizophrenia, bipolar disorder, anxiety disorders, stress, and depression
- Large meals or exercise before bedtime. Studies show that exercise in the evening delays the extra release of melatonin at night that helps the body fall asleep
- Over-scheduling
- Alcohol, which allows you to fall asleep more easily, but prevents deep sleep and REM sleep
- Problems that cause you to urinate more often
- Snoring

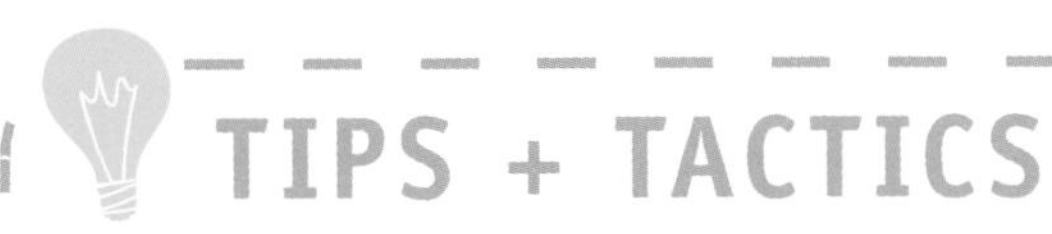

TIPS + TACTICS

Tips to Help You Sleep Better

- *Avoid napping during the day; it can disturb your normal pattern of sleep and wakefulness.*
- *Avoid stimulants such as caffeine, nicotine, and alcohol too close to bedtime. While alcohol is well known to speed the onset of sleep, it disrupts sleep in the second half as you begin to metabolize the alcohol, causing you to wake up.*
- *Engage in vigorous exercise in the morning or late afternoon. Relaxing exercises like yoga can be done before you go to bed to initiate a restful night's sleep.*
- *Eating right before sleep can be disruptive; stay away from large meals close to bedtime.*
- *Ensure adequate exposure to natural light during the day. This is particularly important for older people who may not venture outside as frequently as children and adults. Light exposure helps you maintain a healthy sleep-wake cycle.*
- *Establish a regular relaxing bedtime routine. Try to avoid emotionally upsetting conversations and activities before trying to go to sleep.*
- *Associate your bed with sleep. It's not a good idea to use your bed to watch TV, listen to the radio, or read.*
- *Make sure that your sleep environment is pleasant and relaxing. The bed should be comfortable, and your room should not be too hot or cold or too bright.*

Source: National Sleep Foundation (*www.sleepfoundation.org*)

1992 showed that people who aren't getting enough sleep are at a much higher risk for diabetes. Participants who slept five or fewer hours were significantly more likely to have developed diabetes when they returned for the follow-up study. The study discovered significant relationships between short sleep duration and obesity and hypertension.

Other sleep studies done over the past several decades have shown that sleep is not just a uniform block of time when you are not awake. It is now known that sleep has distinct stages that cycle throughout the night in predictable patterns. How well rested you are, how well you function, and your risk for health problems depend not just on your total sleep time, but also on how much of the various stages of sleep you get each night.

Along with medical problems, a lack of sleep can also impact your ability to focus, pay attention, or respond quickly. It is also related to faulty decision making and more risk taking; impaired learning and memory; and mood problems and depression. Aim to get between seven and nine hours of solid sleep every night.

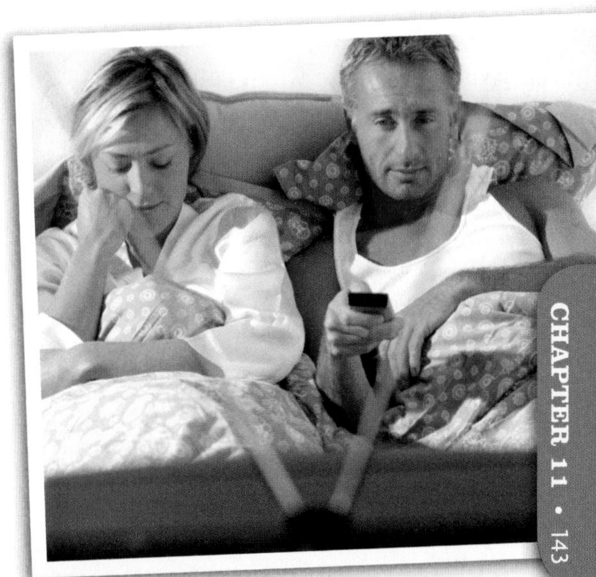

Wonder?

Does diabetes affect how much sleep I get, or does how much sleep I get affect my diabetes?

Unmanaged diabetes can disrupt your sleep and can affect how much sleep you get. If your blood glucose is high, you might get up to urinate more often. You might feel hungry or thirsty, causing you to wake up to get something to eat or drink. If your blood glucose is low, that can also wake you up. If blood glucose highs or lows are a problem for you, discuss changing your bedtime blood glucose goals with your health care provider. If you are not sure what's causing what, check your blood glucose when you wake in the middle of the night or wear a continuous glucose monitor. Once you and your health care provider know what the problem is, you can make the adjustments you need. And once you sleep better, your blood glucose levels will probably be in better control because you will be spending more time in your needed sleep stages.

Stages of Sleep

Non-REM Sleep		Rapid Eye Movement (REM) Sleep
Stage 1	Light sleep; easily awakened; muscle activity; eye movements slow down	Usually occurs about 90 minutes after you fall asleep; cycles along with the non-REM stages throughout the night. Eyes move rapidly, with eyelids closed. Breathing is more rapid, irregular, and shallow. Heart rate and blood pressure increase. Dreaming occurs. Arm and leg muscles are temporarily paralyzed, so you cannot act out the dreams you are having.
Stage 2	Eye movements stop; slower brain waves, with occasional bursts of rapid brain waves	
Stage 3	Considered deep sleep; difficult to awaken; brain waves slow down more, but still have occasional rapid waves	
Stage 4	Considered deep sleep; difficult to awaken; extremely slow brain waves.	

Sleep Needs Change Over Your Lifetime

The evidence continues to mount that health problems such as obesity, insulin resistance, and type 2 diabetes are related to not getting enough sleep and sometimes related to too much sleep. A lack of sleep can cause numerous health problems to people of all ages. As you get older, the amount of time you need for sleep and your sleep patterns will change.

Children spend more time than adults in these deep-sleep stages, which explains why children can sleep through loud noises and why they might not wake up when they are moved from the car to their beds.

By the Numbers

Sleep Needs Over the Life Cycle

Infants/ Babies*	0–2 months	10.5–18.5 hours
	2–12 months	14–15 hours
Toddlers/ Children*	12–18 months	13–15 hours
	18 months–3 years	12–14 hours
	3–5 years	11–13 hours
	5-12 years	9–11 hours
Adolescents	8.5–9.5 hours	
Adults	average 7–9 hours	

**Total time includes naps*

Source: *www.sleepfoundation.org*

During adolescence, a big drop occurs in the amount of time spent in deep sleep, which is replaced by lighter, stage 2 sleep. Between young adulthood and midlife, the percentage of deep sleep falls again—from less than 20% to less than 5%, one study suggests—and is replaced with lighter sleep (stages 1 and 2). From midlife through late life, people's sleep has more interruptions with wakefulness during the night. This disruption causes older adults to lose more and more of stages 1 and 2 non-REM sleep as well as REM sleep.

Older people don't need less sleep, but often they get less sleep or find their sleep is not as refreshing. This is because as people age they spend less time in the deep, restful stages of sleep and are more easily awakened. Older people are more likely to have illnesses and take medications that disrupt their sleep. Sleep disorders become more common with age.

There are more than 70 sleep disorders that affect 40 million Americans today and account for an estimated $16 billion in medical costs, not counting costs due to lost work time and other factors. The four most common sleep disorders are insomnia, sleep apnea, restless leg syndrome, and narcolepsy.

Sleep disorders are particularly common in people with type 2 diabetes. These problems can lead to or escalate existing problems with depression, weight gain, poor blood glucose control, and heart disease. Many people with type 2 diabetes also have sleep disorders, such as sleep apnea.

Psst...

Get a Few More Minutes of Sleep Out of Your Night

Getting more sleep may seem impossible. Life can be so full of activities that sleep is often the first thing to go. While a few more minutes per night may not seem to make a difference, it's a start, and every little bit can help. Start by moving your bedtime up by 10 minutes. In a few weeks, shift the time up by another 10 minutes, and repeat each month until you've reached your goal. Just like exercise, start slowly and build up. You'll be getting more sleep before you know it, and will likely see better control of your blood glucose and blood pressure.

Sleep Apnea and Type 2 Diabetes: A Dangerous Combination

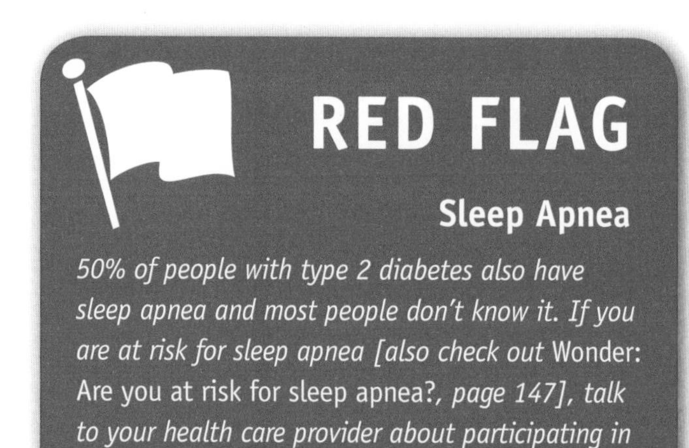

Sleep apnea (Obstructive Sleep Apnea) is a sleeping disorder in which breathing stops briefly or becomes shallow during sleep. Currently, about 50% of people with type 2 diabetes also have sleep apnea. Sleep apnea is very dangerous because it can increase your blood glucose levels and blood pressure and increase your risks for heart disease, strokes, and death. If left untreated, sleep apnea can also cause memory problems, weight gain, erectile dysfunction in men, and headaches. Common symptoms of sleep apnea are daytime sleepiness, snoring (although snoring doesn't always mean sleep apnea, and you don't have to snore to have sleep apnea), morning headaches, dry mouth, sleeping during inappropriate times of the day, depression, high blood pressure, and weight problems. Sleep apnea can occur in anyone, young or old, male or female, including children. Even though sleep apnea is a big problem in the U.S., nearly 80% of people with sleep apnea remain undiagnosed and untreated. Sleep apnea may require the use of a CPAP machine to keep nasal passages open or possibly surgery; however, more moderate cases can often be controlled by losing extra weight and making changes to your sleeping habits.

The only way to actually know if you have sleep apnea is to participate in a sleep study. Talk with your health care provider if you believe you have a sleep disorder. If you are unsure if you have a sleep disorder, find out if you are at risk [also check out *Wonder: Are you at risk for sleep apnea?*, page 147]. If several of the conditions on this list apply to you, don't just ignore them. Talk to you health care provider, and ask to be referred to a sleep clinic for an evaluation. You will then meet with a sleep specialist who will evaluate your sleep history and most likely have you come in for a sleep study (polysomnogram) [also check out *Studies While You Sleep*, page 147]. This non-invasive study will involve you spending one or two nights at a sleep clinic.

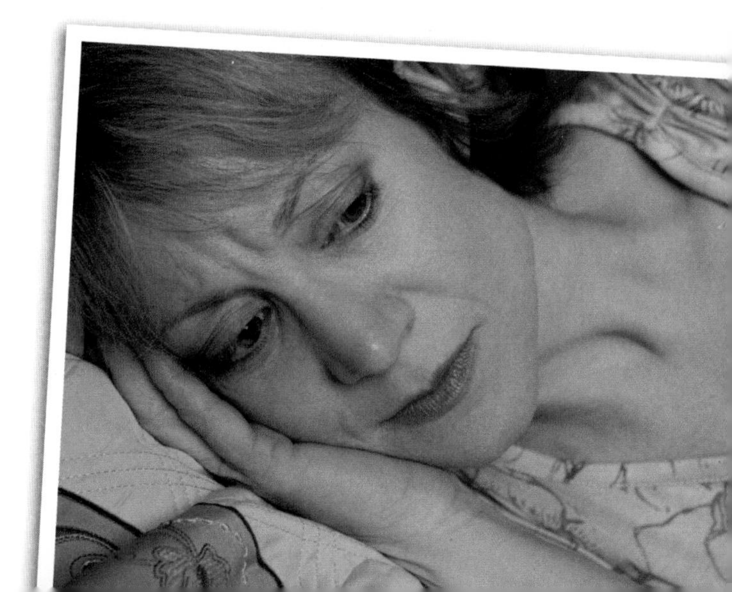

Wonder?

Are you at risk for sleep apnea?

Sleep apnea can occur in anyone, young or old, male or female, including children. These factors put you more at risk:

- **Age.** Sleep apnea occurs two to three times more often in adults over 65 years old.
- **Type 2 diabetes.** Approximately 50% of people with type 2 diabetes have sleep apnea.
- **Ethnicity.** African Americans, Asians, and Latinos have a high incidence of sleep apnea.
- **Family history.** Having a family member with sleep apnea increases your risk.
- **High blood pressure.** Sleep apnea is common in people who have high blood pressure.
- **Narrow airway.** Either a naturally narrow throat, or enlarged tonsils or adenoids can block your airway.
- **Neck size.** A neck circumference of greater than 17 inches in men and 16 inches in women is associated with sleep apnea because a thick neck may obstruct your airway.
- **Overweight.** Fat deposits around your upper airway may obstruct your breathing. You do not need to be overweight to have sleep apnea. Thin people do have sleep apnea.
- **Sex.** Being male increases your risk of sleep apnea. Once a woman reaches menopause, the risks are the same for both men and women.
- **Smoking.** Smoking increases your risk of sleep apnea; however, if you stop smoking, your risk decreases.
- **Alcohol, sedatives, and tranquilizers.** These relax the muscles in your throat.

Research shows that proper treatment—using a continuous positive airway pressure (CPAP) machine for at least four hours a night—can lower blood pressure and improve other diabetes health parameters, such as blood glucose. If you are overweight, have type 2 diabetes and/or high blood pressure, snore, or are tired during wake time, you may have sleep apnea.

Studies While You Sleep

Sleep studies are becoming more and more common and are a fairly easy way for your health care provider to determine if you have a sleep disorder. While you sleep, a sleep technologist records your brain wave activity, breathing, heart rhythm, eye movement, and muscle tone via electrodes and monitors placed on your head, chest, and legs. The results of your study will be evaluated by a sleep specialist who will meet with you and tell you the results and recommendations, or the sleep specialist will send the evaluation and recommendation to the health care provider who referred you for the study to discuss the findings with you.

Before your sleep study, find out if the sleep lab or sleep center is accredited by the American Academy of Sleep Medicine. This denotes the highest standards of care. It's also a good idea to contact your insurance company before the sleep study to find out if they will cover the study, at either the center you are referred to or another facility, as well as any treatment you might need if you are found to have a sleep disorder.

Treatments for Sleep Disorders

The good news is that there are treatments to relieve your sleep problems. Your treatment will depend on your problem and range anywhere from weight loss, addressing and making changes in your sleep habits and environment, and dispelling any misconceptions about sleep you may have, to using medications, dental appliances, continuous positive airway pressure (CPAP) machine, and/or having surgery.

Fewer than 10% of people with sleep disorders take medications for the condition; however, there are several newer drugs on the market that can help you get a more restful night sleep. Lunesta, Rozerem, and Ambien are three of the newer sleep aids that can help you sleep, without remaining in the body for long periods of time like older sleep aids. If you decide to try one of these sleeping medications and are on it for more than a few weeks, carefully monitor any unusual symptoms or side effects, and notify your health care provider about them immediately.

Weight loss is recommended as a treatment for sleep apnea if you are obese and overweight. Other treatments for sleep apnea include oral devices and possibly surgery. Oral devices, such as dental appliances, can help keep the airway open during sleep. These devices can even be specifically designed by dentists with expertise in treating sleep apnea. Surgery is another option for treating sleep apnea, particularly if you have enlarged tonsils or adenoids.

The gold standard for treatment of sleep apnea is CPAP machines. CPAP machines deliver a stream of compressed air to a nasal pillow, nose mask, or face mask, and keep the airway open under pressure so that breathing becomes easier and apnea is reduced. They also often reduce or eliminate the snoring that accompanies sleep apnea. CPAP treatment can be a highly effective treatment option for you and can improve your quality of sleep immediately. CPAP therapy has also been found to improve cardiovascular function, which can lower your blood pressure and reduce your risk of heart disease and stroke. If you have been diagnosed with sleep apnea and have not found a mask that fits you comfortably, ask to see others. There's a wide variety available, and there's sure to be one for you. Some people are concerned that the CPAP machine will keep them or their partner awake; however, these machines are very quiet, and partners say they also sleep better when their mate is wearing his or her CPAP.

The National Sleep Foundation reports, "Sleep disorder specialists help an estimated 85 to 90% of their patients get better sleep." There's one catch to this: You must follow recommendations and continue to follow them. If you follow the recommendations of your sleep specialist, and things don't improve the way you think they should, follow up, ask questions, or ask for different therapy if needed. Just don't give up!

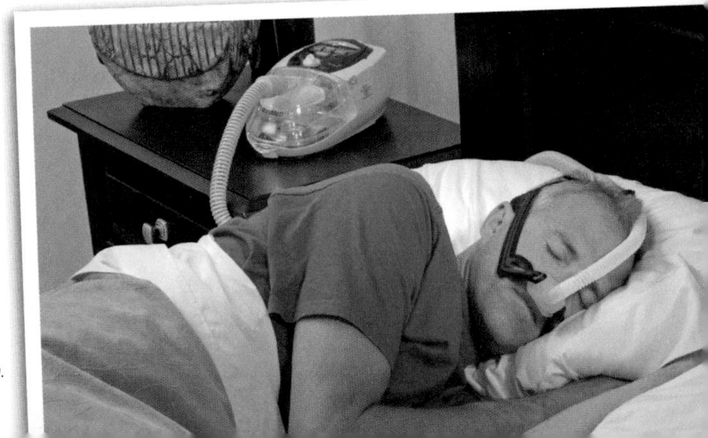

Image printed with permission from ResMed Corporation.

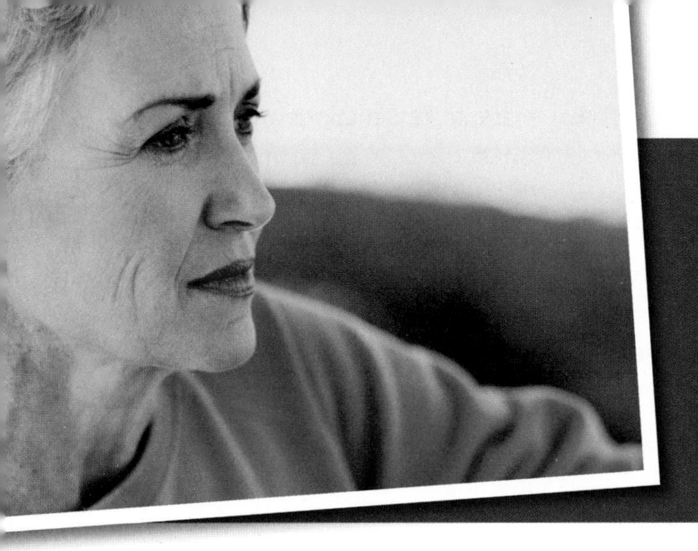

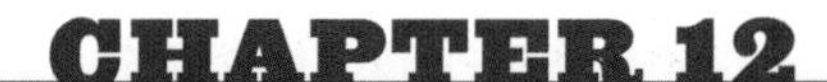

CHAPTER 12

Stress, Depression, and Diabetes

No one would really expect you to be happy about the fact that you have diabetes. It is not unusual for you to feel denial, fear, frustration, sadness, anger, guilt, or overwhelmed and burned out sometime in your life, whether you have diabetes or not. Just because you have felt these things doesn't necessarily mean you were or are depressed. There is a difference between these negative feelings most people feel some time in their life and true depression. Whether you are feeling down, stressed, or you are truly depressed, you will learn that these feelings are all too common with people who have diabetes.

Whether you are stressed, depressed, or anything in between, feeling down can affect the way you take care of your diabetes, and your diabetes can affect the way you think and feel. The good news is that there is help and hope for diabetes and for feeling blue. Read on, understand, and get the help you need.

What You'll Learn:

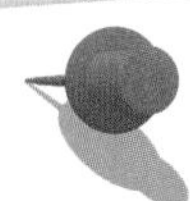

- What stress is and how it affects your blood glucose
- What you can do to identify your stressors
- Some things you can do to decrease stress in your life
- What depression is and how it affects diabetes
- What treatments are available for people who have diabetes and depression
- Why it is important for you to get treatment if you are depressed

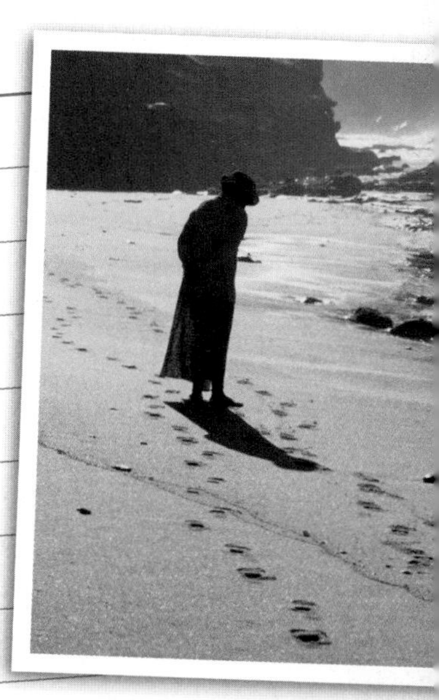

Stress in Your Life?

Everyone experiences stress sometime in their daily life, and contrary to popular belief, stress is not always a response to something negative. You'll see the culprit is not really the stressor, or what it is that's causing the stress, but how your body responds to it. It's about how you cope. You can change how you deal with stress and how stress affects you. Stress can affect your sleep, your blood pressure, your cholesterol, your weight, and more.

Stress results when something causes your body to behave as if it were under attack. Sources of stress can be physical like injury or illness, or they can be mental like problems in your marriage, job, health, or finances. They don't really even have to be considered problems at all. For example, if you have a new job you really like, or you are preparing for a wedding or a new baby, you may not perceive these situations as problems; nevertheless they can still be stressful experiences and affect your diabetes.

When stress occurs, your body prepares to take action. This preparation is called the fight-or-flight response. In the fight-or-flight response, certain hormone levels shoot up, making stored energy—glucose and fat—available to cells. These cells are then primed to help the body get away from danger. In people who have diabetes, the fight-or-flight response does not always work well. Insulin is not always able to let the extra energy into the cells, so glucose can accumulate in your blood, which can result in high blood glucose levels. [also check out *Chapter 15*, page 195].

Many sources of stress are not short-term threats. For example, it can take many months to recover from surgery. Stress hormones that are designed to deal with short-term danger can stay turned on for a long time. These hormones are called counter-regulatory hormones because they fight against insulin. As a result, long-term stress can cause long-term high blood glucose levels.

Many long-term sources of stress are mental. Your mind sometimes reacts to a non-dangerous event as if it were a real threat. Like physical stress, mental stress can be short-term or long-term; however, long-term stress is a lot more hazardous to your health. It's important for your health to do what you can to decrease some of that mental stress from your everyday life.

Stress-Coping Styles

The way you respond to stress is considered your coping style. If you have a problem-solving attitude, you cope by thinking, "What can I do about this problem?" You try to change your situation to get rid of the stress. For example, when you were diagnosed with diabetes, you may have decided to learn all you could about how to manage your diabetes. Or, you may have talked yourself into accepting the problem by saying to yourself, "This problem really isn't so bad after all." In this case, you realized you had to make some lifestyle changes to manage your diabetes, and you took steps to do so. These two methods of coping can be helpful. People who use them tend to have less blood glucose elevation in response to mental stress.

If coping with stress has been a problem for you, your first step is to realize that you can

Myth

Stress always increases your blood glucose

Fact

In research, manipulating stress levels in controlled environments has not consistently caused blood glucose levels to rise. This conflicting information can only mean that stress MAY affect your blood glucose. It may affect it sometimes but not at other times. There are even some people who notice their blood glucose going down during times of stress.

Stress can also contribute to less attention to diabetes self-care. If you're feeling stressed, you might be eating unhealthy foods, drinking more alcohol, taking drugs, skimping on sleep or physical activity, or not taking your medication like you should. Any and all of these things can cause your blood glucose to rise and will affect your health in the long run if not reversed. Remember, it's not the stress itself that affects you, but how your body deals with it. Learn what coping methods work for you and use them regularly to stay healthy and minimize stressful situations.

Wonder?

How do I know how stress affects my blood glucose?

It would be difficult for you to know how all types of stress affect your blood glucose. The best way for you to know is to check your blood glucose often or use a continuous glucose monitoring system. When you do this, you become familiar with what your blood glucose is at different times of the day, so you have a better sense of when something is off. When you record your blood glucose, make a note of how you are feeling. Are you under stress? Have you been feeling under the weather? It's important to record how you feel, so you can have an accurate picture of what has an effect on your blood glucose levels.

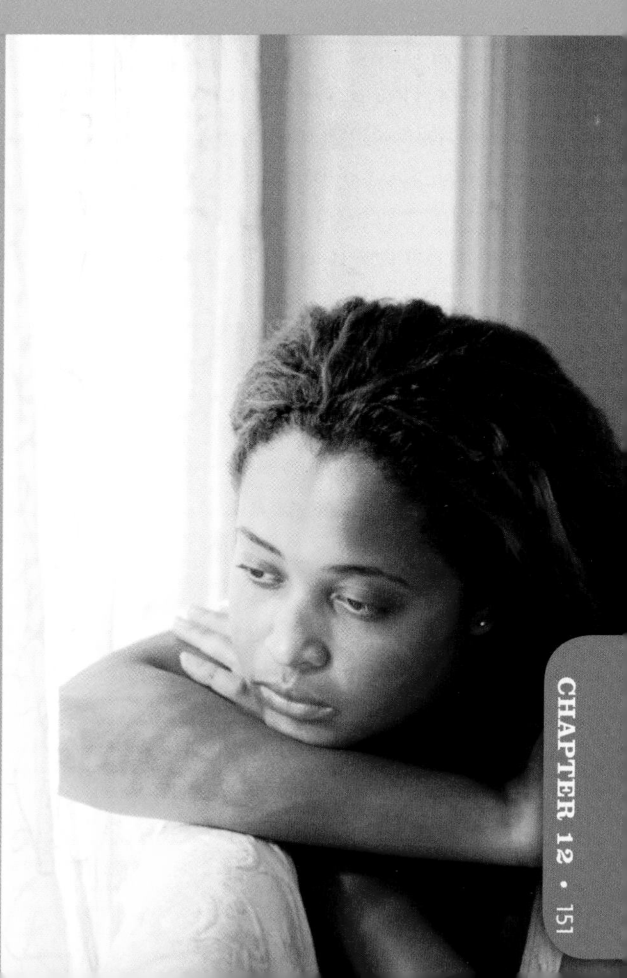

have some control over your reaction to stress. You may not know this now, but you can change how you respond to stress if you want to. You can learn to relax and reverse your body's hormonal response to stress. You can and will most likely need to make some changes in your life to relieve sources of stress.

Preventive action is the best way to change the way you respond to stress in a stressful situation. In other words, the more you learn to relax in life, the better you will cope when stressful situations arise. Learn the simple techniques of some preventive actions to manage stress. If writing or talking about your feelings helps you relax, then keep a journal or talk to someone regularly. If physical activity or breathing exercises work best for you, find a way to work these activities into your daily life. Find out what works for you, and stick with it. Once these become a part of your life, you can use some of these during a time of stress [also see *Tips and Tactics: Preventive Actions to Manage Stress*, right].

Develop Your Diabetes Burnout Plan

Daily diabetes self-care, from monitoring to healthy eating, means you're on the job 24/7. There will be times when things are going great and you'll be able to easily follow your self-care plan, and other times when the daily demands of care or the swings in blood glucose will drain your fortitude. Don't wait for an episode of diabetes burnout. William Polonsky, PhD, a well known and respected diabetes psychologist and President of the Behavioral Diabetes Institute, a nonprofit organization dedicated to helping people with

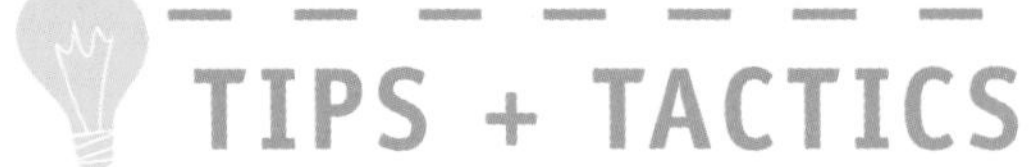

Preventive Actions to Manage Stress

- *Breathing exercises. Take in a deep breath, and push out as much air as you can. Breathe in and out again, this time relaxing your muscles on purpose while breathing out. Do the breathing exercises at least once a day.*
- *Physical Activity. [also check out* Chapter 7, *page 89]*
- *Replace bad thoughts with good ones. Each time you notice a bad thought, purposefully think of something that makes you happy or peaceful.*
- *Journal. Write something every day.*
- *Change your direction or time of day. For example, if traffic upsets you, find a new route to work, or leave home early enough to miss the traffic jams.*
- *Change something at work. If your job drives you crazy, discuss with your boss how to improve things, or possibly apply for a transfer. If things still don't improve, it may be time to look for another job.*
- *Join a group or team you are interested in. Volunteer at a hospital, school, animal shelter, or somewhere that's meaningful to you.*
- *Forgive someone else as well as yourself. If you are at odds with a friend or relative, make the first move to patch things up.*
- *Realize that some sources of stress are never going to go away no matter what you do. Having diabetes is one of those. Still, there are ways to reduce the stresses of living with diabetes. Making friends in a support group can lighten the burden of diabetes-related stresses.*
- *Whatever method you choose to relax, practice it. Just as it takes weeks or months of practice to learn a new sport, it takes practice to learn relaxation.*

diabetes live long, healthy, and happy lives (*www.behaviorialdiabetes.org*), described diabetes burnout in his book for people with diabetes (*Diabetes Burnout*, ADA, 1999). Polonsky discusses the four factors for burnout in the box below, and suggests action plans to help you prevent and manage it.

Deal Directly With Diabetes-Related Stress

When it comes to your diabetes-related stress, deal directly with it. Think about the aspects of your life with diabetes that are the most stressful for you. It might be taking your medication, checking your blood glucose levels regularly, exercising, or eating as you should. If managing your diabetes seems overwhelming, pick out one aspect of your care to work on, and master that before you consider moving on to something else. Remember, small steps make for big changes in your diabetes care plan. Diabetes is something you will be living with for a long time. You don't need to do it all at once, and there's no such thing as a "perfect diabetic" [also check out *Chapter 4*, page 49].

You can get help with any of these issues. Ask a member of your diabetes team for a referral to see a diabetes educator or another specialist who may be able to help you with your particular need [also check out *Chapter 3*, page 35]. If your stress seems so severe that you feel overwhelmed, you may actually be depressed. If so, psychotherapy and/or medications can help you. Whether it's stress or depression, always know there is hope for you to manage it, get over it, and get on with your life in a healthy way.

Diabetes Burnout

Burnout factor:	Example prevention action:
Burnout factor #1: ***It's a hassle and frustration to complete the daily diabetes self-care tasks.***	Whittle down your to-do list. Can you safely check your blood glucose less often? Consider alternating the times you check your blood glucose and cover all the times you need to check in two days rather than one.
Burnout factor #2: ***You don't feel your friends, family, and other pillars of strength supporting you.***	Confide in a supporter: Let someone you are close with know that you are struggling. Let them know what you need—a call or get-together.
Burnout Factor #3: ***You hear yourself thinking and verbalizing negative thoughts.***	Rehearse positive self-talk messages: When you hear yourself reciting negative self-talk, catch yourself. Turn this around with one of your well-rehearsed positive messages.
Burnout factor #4: ***The environments in which you live your life are not supporting your efforts to take care of diabetes.***	Seek supportive settings: Identify environments that assist and support you in taking care of your diabetes. Spend more time in these settings and less time in those that lead you astray.

Source: *Diabetes Burnout* (ADA, 1999).

Depression and Diabetes

People who have diabetes have twice the risk of being depressed than people who don't have diabetes. There are no easy answers about why this is true. "The depression-diabetes interaction is complex and probably bidirectional," said Wayne Katon, MD, professor and vice chair in the department of psychiatry and behavioral sciences at University of Washington Medical School in Seattle. "There is good evidence showing that if you have depression earlier in your life, there's about a 35% increased risk of developing type 2 diabetes. On the other hand, when you compare people with diabetes to age-matched controls without [diabetes], studies have generally shown a two-fold increase in the prevalence of depression among people with diabetes."

Depression is a concern when you have diabetes because if you are depressed you may not care about yourself enough to do what you need to do to take care of your diabetes. This can make your diabetes and your depression worse. If you have negative feelings about having diabetes, this does not necessarily mean you are depressed. But if you have feelings of sadness and hopelessness most of the time for two weeks or more, this is a sign of depression. There are three types of depression: major depressive disorder (MDD), dysthymic disorder, and adjustment disorder with depressed mood.

The underlying reasons why there is such a strong correlation between diabetes and depression are not fully understood. We do know that environmental, genetic, and hormonal factors are involved in both diabetes and depression. Other factors, such as a history of depression, increase your risk for getting diabetes later in life, and there is evidence that both depression and diabetic hypoglycemia may result in brain changes. Research in animal models has shown possible hormonal mechanisms that account for this relationship, including the role of cortisol in both counter-regulatory hormonal mechanisms in diabetes

By the Numbers

Undertreatment of Depression in Diabetes

Depression is undertreated in people with both diabetes and depression. Only 30% of people with diabetes and depression receive adequate antidepressant treatment, and fewer than 20% complete four or more visits for psychotherapy.

DEFINITIONS:

depression: a spectrum of mood disorders characterized by lack of interest in usual activities. It is a treatable illness caused by an imbalance of brain chemicals called neurotransmitters.

cortisol: a hormone produced by the adrenal gland; commercially manufactured as hydrocortisone and used to reduce inflammation.

and depression. No matter the cause, the combination of diabetes and depression adds side effects that make it harder to deal with both diseases. Some of the negatives effects are:

- **Self-Care.** Adults with diabetes and depression don't adhere as well to their diabetes self-care regimen, which includes worsened adherence to medication and lifestyle recommendations.
- **Diabetes Complications.** Depression has a small but significant negative impact on glucose control. Depression is also moderately related to diabetes complications, including retinopathy, neuropathy, and macrovascular and microvascular complications [also check out *Chapter 21*, page 257].
- **Cost.** Both diabetes and depression are associated with increased health care costs. One study has shown that people with diabetes and depression have 4.5 times the health care cost of having diabetes alone.
- **Disability and Mortality.** Having diabetes and depression has been found to be associated with increased functional disability and mortality more than having diabetes without depression.
- **Quality of Life.** Studies have shown lower quality-of-life scores among people who have diabetes and depression than those who have diabetes alone.

Wonder?

I'm feeling kind of down about having diabetes. How do I know if I'm really depressed? And, if so, what do I do?

Identifying depression is your first step. Getting help is the second. If you have been feeling sad, blue, or down in the dumps, check for these symptoms:

- Loss of pleasure. You no longer take interest in doing things you used to enjoy.
- Change in sleep patterns. You have trouble falling asleep, you wake often during the night, or you want to sleep more than usual, including during the day.
- Early to rise. You wake up earlier than usual and cannot to get back to sleep.
- Change in appetite. You eat more or less than you used to, resulting in a quick weight gain or weight loss.
- Trouble concentrating. You can't watch a TV program or read an article because other thoughts or feelings get in the way.
- Loss of energy. You feel tired all the time.
- Nervousness. You always feel so anxious you can't sit still.
- Guilt. You feel you never do anything right and worry that you are a burden to others.
- Morning sadness. You feel worse in the morning than you do the rest of the day.
- Suicidal thoughts. You feel you want to die or are thinking about ways to hurt yourself.

If you have three or more of these symptoms, or if you have just one or two but have been feeling bad for two weeks or more, it's time for you to get help.

Getting Help Is Your Next Step

The good news is that there is help for your depression. If you are feeling symptoms of depression, don't keep them to yourself. First, talk them over with your health care provider, and rule out a physical cause of your depression.

Diabetes that is in poor control can cause symptoms that look like depression. During the day, high or low blood glucose may make you feel tired or anxious. Low blood glucose levels can also lead to hunger and eating too much. If you have low blood glucose at night, it could disturb your sleep. If you have high blood glucose at night, you may get up often to urinate and then feel tired during the day [also check out *Chapter 15*, page 195].

Other physical causes of depression include:

- **Alcohol or drug abuse.** [also check out *Chapter 18*, 229].
- **Thyroid problems.** An under or overactive thyroid can cause you to feel sluggish or anxious and can affect your sleep, appetite, weight, and mood [also check out *Chapter 9*, page 121, and *Chapter 16*, page 207].

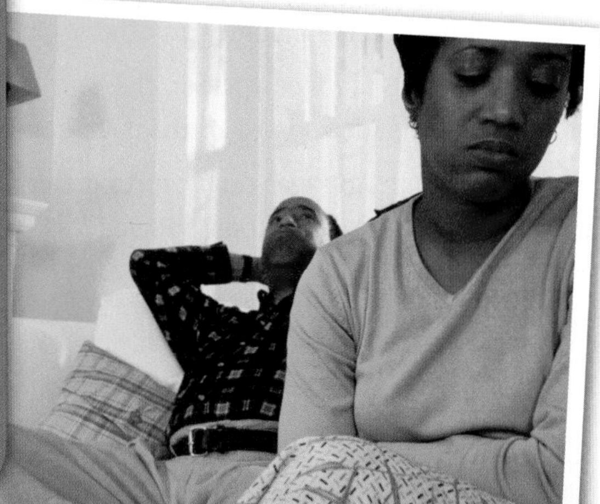

- **Side effects from some medications.** If you think your symptoms are related to side effects from a medication you are taking, do not stop taking it. Stopping some medications abruptly can be dangerous. Work with your health care provider to identify what medications could be causing the problem, and work together to make the necessary changes.

There are two main treatment options for treating depression: psychotherapy and pharmacotherapy. As if taking care of diabetes is not expensive enough, having both diabetes and depression is even more expensive. Many, but not all, mental health therapists are covered by insurance, so check with your health care provider before seeking service.

Psychotherapy

Psychotherapy, also known as talk therapy, is an important treatment option for you if you are depressed. Talk therapy is not just a time for you to talk about your problems, it is also a time when you work with a qualified, licensed, mental health care provider to help find solutions. Your therapist may be a psychiatrist (MD or DO), psychologist (PhD, PsyD, EdD, MS), social worker (DSW, MSW, LCSW, LICSW, CCSW), counselor (MA, MS, LMFT, LCPC), or psychiatric nurse (APRN, PMHN).

Cognitive Behavior Therapy (CBT) is a type of psychotherapy that has been effective in helping people who have diabetes and depression. CBT emphasizes the adoption of coping skills through an understanding of your thoughts, feelings, and behaviors that

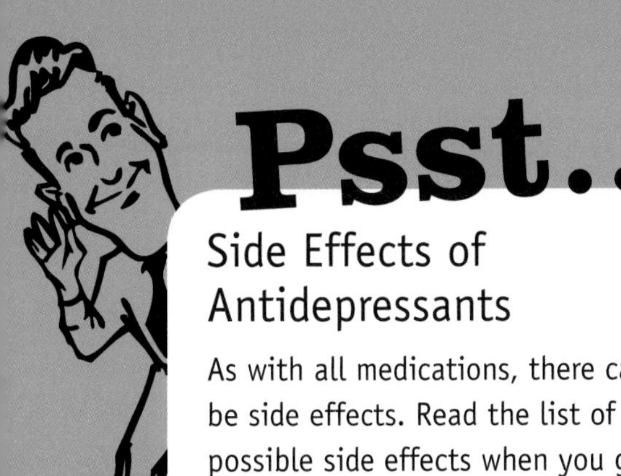

Side Effects of Antidepressants

As with all medications, there can be side effects. Read the list of possible side effects when you get your medication from the pharmacy, and report any side effects to your health care provider. Sometimes, antidepressants may be associated with worsening symptoms of depression or suicidal thoughts or behavior, particularly early in treatment or when you change your dosage. Be sure to talk to your health care provider about any changes in your symptoms. You may need more careful monitoring at the beginning of treatment or upon a change in treatment, or you may need to stop the medication if your symptoms worsen.

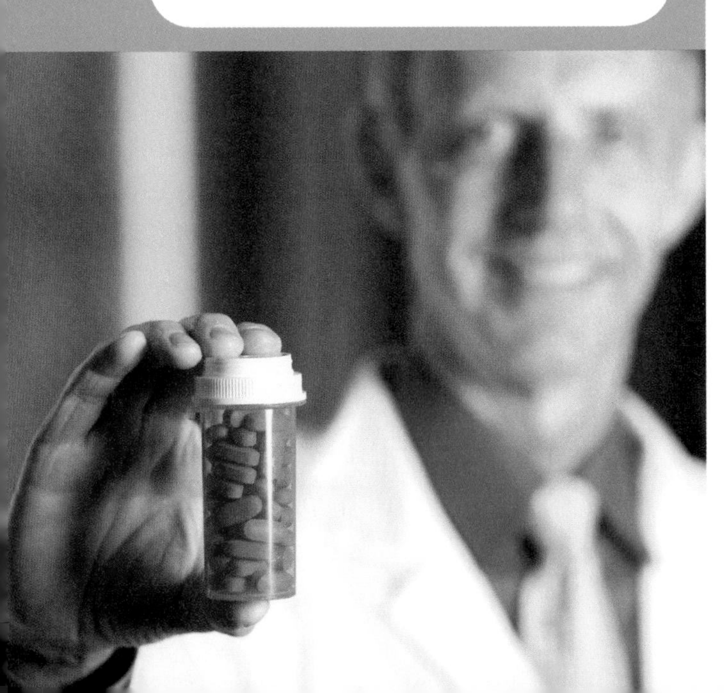

promote or prevent depressed moods. For example, if you have recently retired, you may experience symptoms of depression. Through working with your therapist, you may be able to identify when your depressive symptoms started (right after retirement), and that you are feeling depressed because you no longer feel you are doing something worthwhile. Having identified these possible causes, the two of you can come up with solutions. One solution may be for you to volunteer at a school or hospital to help you feel like you are giving something back.

Pharmacotherapy

Pharmacotherapy is the treatment of diseases with the use of drugs. Antidepressants are a class of drugs used in medicine and pharmacology to treat depression. They may be prescribed to correct imbalances in the levels of chemicals in your brain. These medications are not sedatives, uppers, or tranquilizers and are not habit-forming. Generally, antidepressant medications have no stimulating effect if you are not experiencing depression.

Antidepressants have developed a bad reputation over the years, mainly because people believe they will become addicted to the pills or will not act like their former selves. The truth is that antidepressants are not addictive and will not make you feel any specific way. Their main function is to help make you feel like your former self, before depression became a part of your life. When combined with psychotherapy, there is evidence that antidepressants can help people confront the real problems in their lives that need to be resolved.

Antidepressants may produce some improvement within the first week or two of treatment, but you may not realize the full benefits for two to three months. If your feel little or no improvement after several weeks, talk with your health care provider about making changes in your antidepressant regime. Do not make changes on your own.

For the most part, treating depression with newer antidepressive medications is safe and effective, but some of the older drugs do present challenges if you have diabetes and if you take medications to lower your blood glucose. There are five types of antidepressants used at this time: selective serotonin reuptake inhibitors (SSRIs), serotonin and norepinephrine reuptake inhibitors (SNRIs), sorepinephrine and dopamine reuptake inhibitors (NDRIs), combined reuptake inhibitors and receptor blockers, and tetracyclic antidepressants.

SELECTIVE SEROTONIN REUPTAKE INHIBITORS (SSRIs)

These are usually the first choice of antidepressants recommended because they generally work well with the fewest side effects. It's not exactly clear how SSRIs affect depression. Serotonin is a brain chemical (neurotransmitter) associated with depression. SSRIs seem to relieve symptoms of depression by blocking the reabsorption of serotonin by certain nerve cells in your brain. This leaves more serotonin available in your brain, which results in enhanced neurotransmission—the sending of nerve impulses—and improves your mood. SSRIs are called selective because they seem to affect only serotonin, not other neurotransmitters. Some SSRIs out on the market are:

- Citalopram (Celexa)
- Escitalopram (Lexapro)
- Fluoxetine (Prozac, Sarafem)
- Paroxetine (Paxil, Paxil CR)
- Sertraline (Zoloft)

SEROTONIN AND NOREPINEPHRINE REUPTAKE INHIBITORS (SNRIs)

SNRIs are a type of antidepressant medication that increases the levels of both serotonin and norepinephrine by inhibiting their reuptake into the cells in your brain. It is thought that these increased levels enhance neurotransmission and elevate your mood. Medications in this group of antidepressants are sometimes known as dual reuptake inhibitors. Examples of SNRIs are:

- Duloxetine (Cymbalta)—also indicated for relief from peripheral neuropathy
- Venlafaxine (Effexor, Effexor XR)

DEFINITIONS:

norepinephrine: a neurotransmitter released by the brain that has such effects as constricting blood vessels, raising blood pressure, and dilating bronchi.

dopamine: a neurotransmitter acting within the brain to help regulate movement and emotion. Its depletion may cause Parkinson's disease.

CONFIDENTIAL

Research Brief

The verdict is still out as to whether being depressed increases your risk for developing diabetes or if pharmacologic treatment with antidepressants causes diabetes. Two recent studies point to antidepressants being the culprit. A study published in *Diabetes Research & Clinical Practice* (May 16, 2008) reported University of Alberta's Dr. Lauren Brown's findings. Dr. Brown was analyzing data from Saskatchewan health databases and found that people with a history of depression had a 30% increased risk of developing type 2 diabetes. She then studied the medical history of 2,400 people who were taking antidepressants to determine whether there was a clear correlation between depression and type 2 diabetes. Brown found that the risk of diabetes almost doubled for the patients who were using two types of therapies at the same time, tricyclic antidepressants (TCAs) and selective serotonin reuptake inhibitors (SSRIs). Brown believes these results demonstrate an increased risk of type 2 diabetes in people with depression, and emphasize the need for regular screening for type 2 diabetes in people with depression, particularly those taking more than one antidepressant. Brown also encourages diabetes and depression organizations to educate their members about this link.

In a recent issue of *Diabetes Care* (2008;31:420–6), there was analysis to assess the association between elevated depression symptoms or antidepressant medicine use on entry to the Diabetes Prevention Program (DPP) and the risk of developing diabetes during the study [also check out *Chapter 2*, page 23]. They had all 3,187 participants complete a report about their use of antidepressant medication. Baseline antidepressant use was associated with diabetes risk in both the placebo and intensive lifestyle arms. Continuous antidepressant use during the study (compared with no use) was also associated with diabetes risk in the same arms. Among metformin arm participants, antidepressant use was not associated with developing diabetes.

NOREPINEPHRINE AND DOPAMINE REUPTAKE INHIBITORS (NDRIs)

NDRIs increase the levels of neurotransmitters norepinephrine and dopamine by inhibiting their reuptake into cells. It is thought that these increased levels help enhance neurotransmission and thereby improve and elevate your mood. An example of an NDRI is Bupropion (Wellbutrin, Wellbutrin SR, Wellbutrin XL).

COMBINED REUPTAKE INHIBITORS AND RECEPTOR BLOCKERS

Combined reuptake inhibitors and receptor blockers are dual-action antidepressants. They act on your brain cells in two ways—they inhibit the reuptake of neurotransmitters into your nerve cells, and they block your nerve cell receptors. This leaves more of these neurotransmitters available in the brain, which elevates your mood. These are some combined reuptake inhibitors that are only available in generic form:

- Trazodone
- Nefazodone
- Maprotiline

TETRACYCLIC ANTIDEPRESSANTS

Tetracyclic antidepressants prevent neurotransmitters from binding with nerve cell receptors called alpha-2 receptors. This indirectly increases the levels of norepinephrine and serotonin in the brain, and that may improve and elevate mood. Mirtazapine (Remeron, Remeron SolTab) is an example of a tetracyclic antidepressant.

OLDER TYPES OF ANTIDEPRESSANTS

There are two other kinds of antidepressants that are older but are still used regularly to treat depression. They are tricyclic antidepressants (TCAs) and monoamine oxidase inhibitors (MAOIs). TCAs inhibit the reuptake of serotonin and norepinephrine. They also inhibit reabsorption of dopamine, as well as block certain cell receptors, which accounts for many of their side effects. TCAs were among the earliest antidepressants in the 1960s, and they remained the first line of treatment for depression through the 1980s, before newer antidepressants arrived. They continue to be effective today, although with more side effects than the newer antidepressants. A few TCAs on the market are:

- Amitriptyline
- Amoxapine
- Desipramine (Norpramin)
- Doxepin (Sinequan)
- Imipramine (Tofranil)
- Nortriptyline (Pamelor)
- Protriptyline (Vivactil)
- Trimipramine (Surmontil)

If I Only Knew . . .

There was help for me . . .

I had been living with diabetes for some time when I became depressed. My blood glucose was going up because I wasn't eating right. I wasn't doing the things I knew to do because I didn't care. When you're depressed, you don't care about yourself, nor do you care about or trust people. My diabetes educator listened to me and didn't judge me. She was more concerned about my depression than my diabetes, because if I didn't feel better, I wouldn't take care of my diabetes. She told me there was hope. She recommended a psychiatrist who helped some of her other patients. Before long, I started feeling like myself again. I started to eat healthy and became more active. As my mood improved, so did my blood glucose control. Had I known there was help for me, I would have sought psychiatric help sooner.

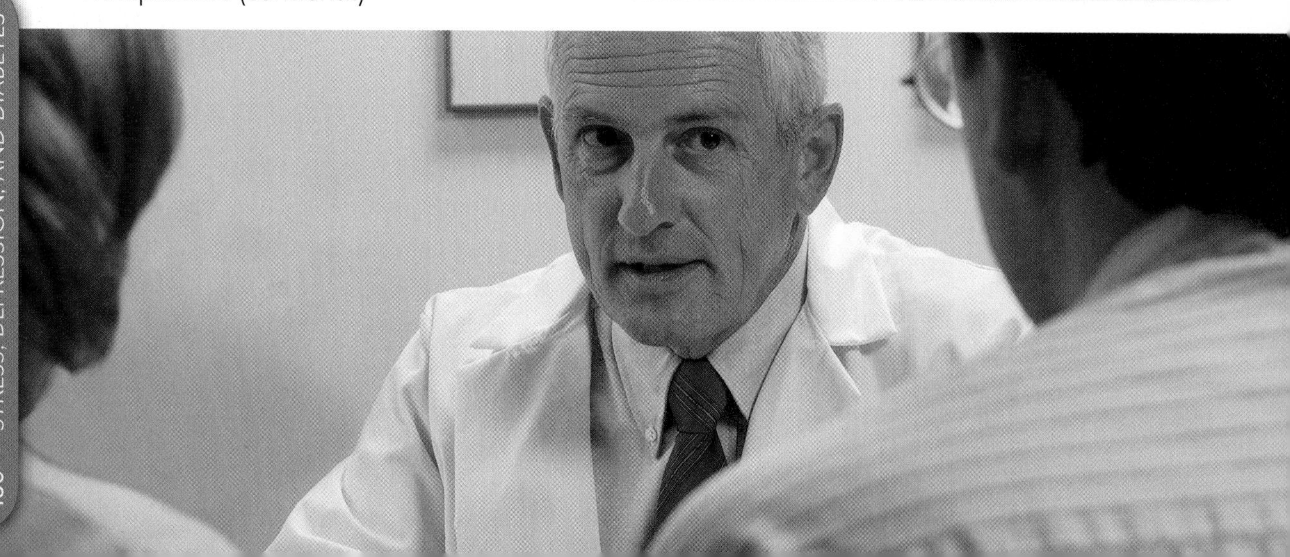

It is thought that MAOIs relieve depression by preventing the enzyme monoamine oxidase from metabolizing the neurotransmitters norepinephrine, serotonin, and dopamine in your brain. As a result, these levels remain high in the brain, boosting mood. The problem with these is that if you eat certain foods with MAOIs, you can experience severe side effects; therefore, today MAOIs are reserved for people whose depression hasn't been relieved by other antidepressants. Some MAOIs are:

- Phenelzine (Nardil)
- Tranylcypromine (Parnate)
- Isocarboxazid (Marplan)
- Selegiline (Emsam)

Non-Medical Treatment Options for Depression

In many cases, non-medical treatment is usually discussed before medical treatment. If you are truly depressed, it is important that you get professional help. There are additional steps you can take to help you fight your depression and get back to feeling like yourself again. Some non-medical treatment options for depression are:

- Blood glucose management. High blood glucose levels, low blood glucose levels, and rapidly fluctuating blood glucose levels can affect how you feel and think. Managing your blood glucose levels to your target ranges can help you feel more alert, energetic, and more positive [also check out *Chapter 15*, page 195].
- Physical activity. It doesn't have to be much, and it doesn't have to be long. Any kind of physical activity should help you feel better, especially if you are a couch potato. Whether you enjoy it at the time or not, regular physical activity may generate biological changes in you to help relieve your depression [also check out *Chapter 7*, page 89].
- Find a confidante. Isolation often goes hand in hand with depression. Even when you are surrounded by a loving family, it is easy to feel that no one understands what you are going through. Find someone you can confide in, and make the most of their support [also check out chapter 3, page 35].
- Do not self-medicate. This means with prescribed or over-the-counter medicine, illicit drugs, alcohol, or any other type of mood-altering substance. You may think some of these things will help you, but in reality they can only make things worse. For example, you may think alcohol makes you feel better, when in reality it is a considered a depressant, not an antidepressant [also check out *Chapter 18*, page 229].

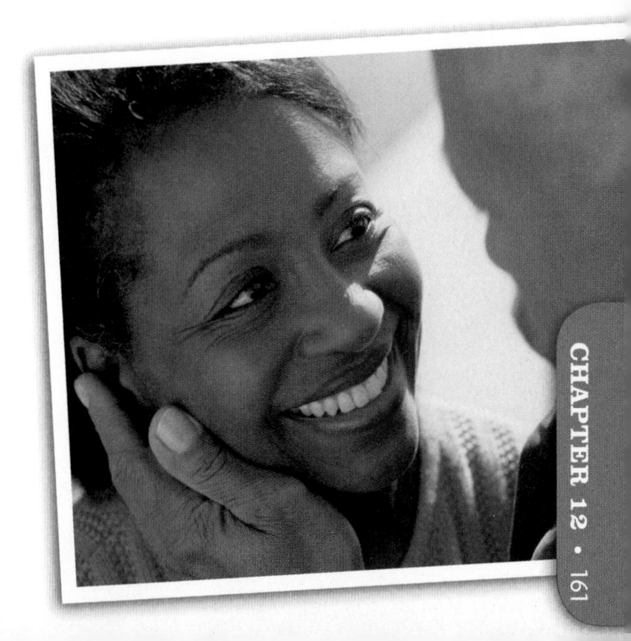

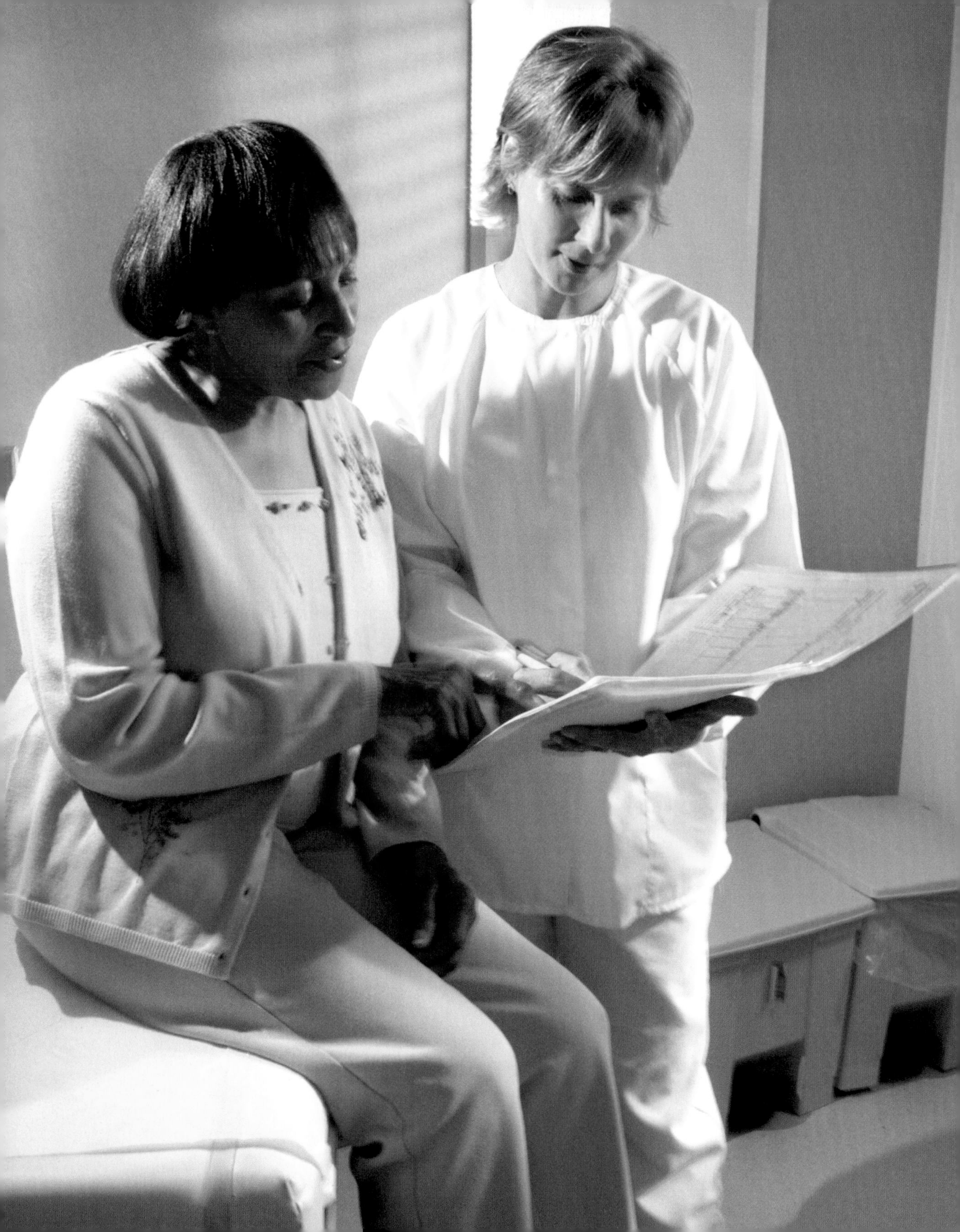

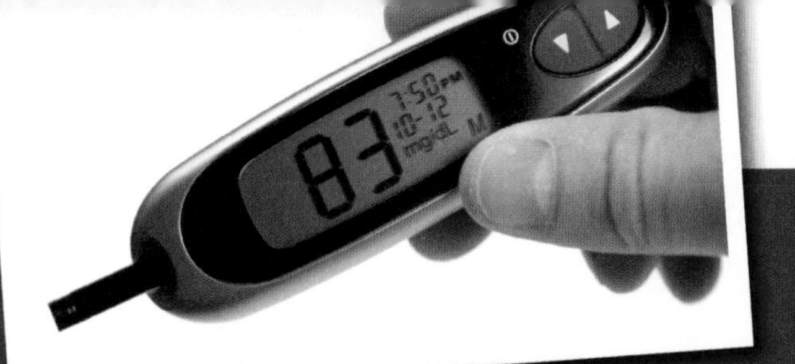

CHAPTER 13

Monitoring Glucose and Blood Pressure Matters

Over the last 20 years or so, it's become clear that getting and keeping your glucose and blood pressure into target ranges can help you prevent or delay the onset of diabetes complications. What's also happened over these years is that it's become possible for you to regularly monitor your blood glucose and blood pressure on your own, if need be. As technology continues to advance, the age of continuous glucose monitoring is coming into its own. Learn about the available technology to monitor your blood glucose and blood pressure as well as how often and what times of day to check these important health parameters. Monitoring matters in your quest for better blood glucose management and better health.

What You'll Learn:

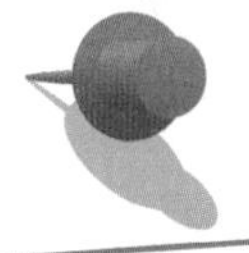

- Why it's important to monitor your glucose levels on your own
- The supplies you'll need to monitor your glucose levels
- How often and when to check your glucose levels
- Tips to make the most of your monitoring results
- The difference between blood glucose monitoring and continuous glucose monitoring
- The importance of home blood pressure monitoring and whether or not you need to do it

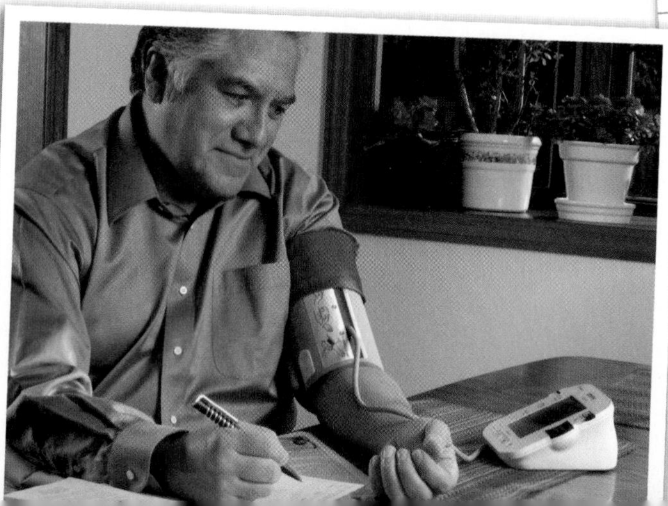

Wonder?

Why do I need to monitor my blood glucose levels?

Monitoring your glucose levels gives you immediate feedback and data to help you in two ways:

1. It helps you make immediate decisions about your diabetes care. For example, do you need to treat a low blood glucose level or manage a series of high blood glucose levels.
2. A review of your blood glucose records over the past fews weeks or months helps you and your health care provider determine whether your diabetes care plan is working or needs some adjustments to help you hit your blood glucose targets more often. This information can help you:
   - Achieve and maintain your target glucose goals
   - Prevent and detect low glucose (hypoglycemia) levels (if you are at risk)
   - Prevent and detect high glucose (hyperglycemia) levels
   - Prevent rapid and large fluctuations of glucose levels
   - Evaluate your personal glycemic response to types and amounts of foods, physical activity, medications, and more

Blood Glucose Monitoring Comes of Age

It's important to take a step back in history and realize that prior to the late 1970s, the ability to check your blood glucose at any time of day or night was something people only dreamed of. At that time, people with diabetes and their health care providers were relegated to checking their urine glucose, which simply told them if their blood glucose was high, very high, or sky high. Over the last 30 years, blood glucose meters have gotten smaller, faster, and easier to use and require a tinier-than-ever amount of blood. Today, you can get a result in a mere five seconds and many meters fit in a small carrying case, which makes them very portable—thus hardly something to use only at home.

For starters, it's important to understand what blood glucose meters are and what they monitor. With the information you obtain from monitoring, you can best manage your diabetes, prevent or delay complications, and live a long, healthy life [also check out *Chapter 21*, page 257].

By the Numbers

Blood glucose ranges for adults with diabetes as recommended by the ADA:

Glycemic Control: A1C < 7%

Preprandial plasma glucose (before a meal): 70–130 mg/dl

Postprandial plasma glucose (1 to 2 hours after a meal): <180 mg/dl

Check with your health care provider if you need a more personalized target blood glucose range.

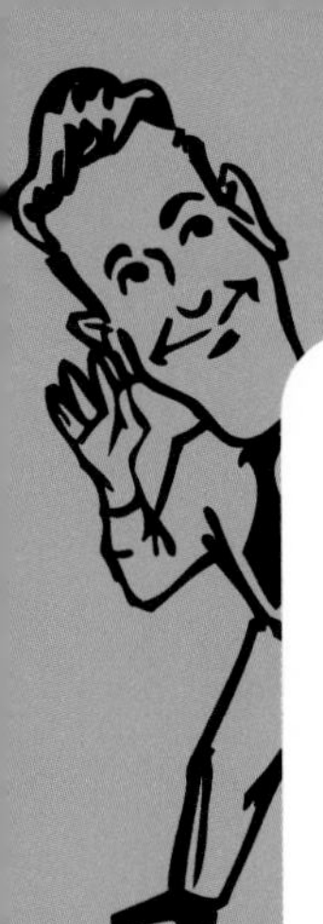

Psst...

To start using your meter, you will need these items, which usually come in all blood glucose monitoring kits:

- Meter
- Blood glucose strips
- Lancet: a small device with a very small needle that goes in a lancing device to prick your skin.
- Lancing device: a spring-loaded device that your lancet goes into. This helps make obtaining a sample of your blood easier and less painful.

User guide: Although the procedure for checking your blood glucose is mainly the same for all monitors, there are differences. Follow the steps in your meter's user guide.

What Is a Meter and How To Use It

A blood glucose monitor (meter) is an FDA-approved, small, portable device that you use to check your blood glucose levels. After pricking your skin (usually the side of a finger, but there are other approved sites, such as the forearm, palm of your hand. and others) with a lancet, you place a tiny drop of blood on a test strip that partially goes in the meter. The meter quickly (usually within 5 seconds) displays the blood glucose level as a number on the meter's digital display. In general, you want your blood glucose to fall into the recommended target ranges of 70–130 mg/dl before meals or <180 mg/dl one to two hours after meals. These are the target goals set by ADA, but talk to your health care provider to find out what numbers are right for you, and how often you should test your blood glucose.

Most blood glucose meters today test whole blood but report the number as a plasma reading. Older meters were whole blood–calibrated and reported the number as whole blood. When you get your blood tested at the laboratory, it tests your plasma—the part of your blood that contains glucose. New meters are plasma-calibrated to provide you with a number more closely related to your reading at the laboratory.

Most of the large manufacturers of blood glucose meters provide easy-to-use instructions for using your meter. Companies also provide 24/7 service, so you can talk to someone if you have problems or questions at any time. This toll-free phone number is usually on the back of your meter itself. Most companies that make meters also have a website with instructions for use. This, too, can be a good resource to learn from [also check out *Psst: Online Resources for Blood Glucose Meters*, page 166].

Although detailed instructions come with your meter, you should be taught to use your meter by your health care provider or by someone from where you purchased your meter. If you bought it at a pharmacy, ask your pharmacist to teach you how to use it. If there is no one where you purchased your supplies, ask whether there is a diabetes

Psst...

Online Resources for Blood Glucose Meters

Software and websites are available that contain one or more of the following: carbohydrate counts of foods and ability to track intake, a way to track blood glucose results by downloading the meter, integration and analyze of data, or ability to communicate about the data online with a health care provider.

- ***www.mycareteam.com*:** MyCareTeam is a website that allows you to upload your blood glucose readings and transmit them over the Internet for health care providers and family members to have access to.
- ***www.dia-log.com*:** This site provides tracking logs and an ability to download results from blood glucose meters. For food and carbohydrate tracking it links with *www.myfooddiary.com*.
- ***www.diabetespilot.com***
- ***www.healthengage.com***
- ***www.numedics.com/diabetespartner***

Every meter company has a website, so check yours out.

educator or a diabetes education program available in your community. A diabetes educator can teach you how to monitor your blood glucose properly as well as share tips from experience to make it easier for you. In fact, it's a good idea to have a diabetes educator check your blood glucose–monitoring technique once a year. You can always refer back to your meter's instructions for more help, and if you have a question or a problem you can't get resolved, call the toll-free number to speak with someone in customer support. These people are trained to answer most any question you may have.

TIPS + TACTICS

Make Sure Your Meter is Working Properly

- *Check your results against the lab results of your health care provider to make sure it's accurate.*
- *Know whether your meter reads plasma or whole blood.*
- *If your meter needs to be coded, make sure it is coded correctly.*
- *Use control solution as per your meter's user guide.*
- *If you feel your monitor is malfunctioning, call the toll-free number on the back of your meter to speak with customer service. They will help you troubleshoot. If they can't resolve your problem, they will most likely send you a new meter.*

Choose the Best Monitoring System For You

When it comes to buying the right meter for you, there are several options you need to consider first. There are a wide variety of blood glucose meters to choose from, so determine what features are important to you. Some meters are made for people who have poor eyesight. Most meters come with memory so you can store your results in the meter itself. The ADA does not endorse any products or recommend one meter over another. If you plan to buy a meter, here are some things to consider.

COST. Factor in the cost of test strips when evaluating your meter purchase. The cost of the strips are quite similar; however, some insurance companies will only pay for a certain brand of meter and strips, or they may pay more for one brand over another. This matters because this will determine your out-of-pocket cost. Call your health plan before you purchase a meter, and ask if they prefer a certain brand of meter and strips, and how you should purchase them to get the best price. You might save money using your health plan's mail-order pharmacy. If your health plan does not pay for blood glucose–checking supplies, rebates are often available toward the purchase of your meter. Many health care providers will even give you a blood glucose monitor, but you still have to consider the cost of the matching strips and lancets, so shop around. Costs vary depending on the brand and where you purchase your strips.

SIZE AND USER-FRIENDLINESS. Is it convenient and easy to use? If you prefer an unobtrusive meter that can be used discreetly, you'll want to consider something small and easy to use. If you have vision problems, look at the screen to see whether you can actually read it clearly.

TREND DATA AND COMPUTER COMPATIBILITY. Does the meter interface with a computer and allow you to download results directly to your home and/or your health care provider's computer?

BATTERY LIFE AND AVAILABILITY. How long is the battery life? Does the meter use a common type of battery that is easy to find?

BLOOD SAMPLE SIZE. How much blood does the meter require?

ALTERNATIVE SITE TESTING. Will the meter allow you to test blood from a site other than your fingertips? Some meters allow you to take blood from your forearm or other sites. Understand that the most accurate reading is from your fingertips, particularly if it is at certain times such as when your blood glucose may be falling or rising rapidly. When done correctly, most people find that checking from their fingertips is not really a problem

BELLS AND WHISTLES. Glow-in-the-dark cases, talking meters that "tell" you your blood glucose, backlighting, internal strips, and swappable faceplates are just a few of the other features today's blood glucose meters offer.

Your certified diabetes educator or pharmacist is a good source of information on which blood glucose monitoring system may be right for you.

Wonder?

How can I tell whether my meter is reading accurately?

After you understand how to use a blood glucose meter, make sure the one you are using is accurate. Compare your meter reading to a lab test. A blood glucose monitor's test result is considered clinically accurate if the levels are within +/– 20% of an accepted reference result, which is usually a lab test. The only real way to be certain your meter is accurate is to compare the reading taken at the same time you take your lab test. If your blood glucose at the lab is 100mg/dl, your meter is considered accurate if the result of that reading is 80–120mg/dl.

Lancing Devices and Lancets

A lancet is a pointed piece of surgical steel contained in plastic that you use to prick your skin to obtain a drop of blood. Lancets come in different widths called gauges. A higher gauge and a finer needle equals a smaller perforation into your skin and less pain. Some people are not able to get an adequate sample with a small-gauge lancet, and therefore they need to use a slightly wider one.

There are as many lancing devices and lancets as there are meters, and some are easier to use than others. Some lancing devices can be used with several different brands of lancets, and some only use the brand that matches. Try the lancets and lancing device that come with your meter first. Most of the lancing devices have a way to adjust how deep the lancet will prick your skin. If the skin on the testing area is soft, you should be fine pricking your skin at a lower level; however, if your skin is dry and somewhat thickened—like the fingers of a construction worker or guitar player—you will probably need to set it on a higher number to get an adequate drop of blood. Also, if you prick a certain area over and over again, that area will become hardened and tougher to obtain a sample from. You may need to try another type of lancing device and possibly another size of lancet.

When to Check Your Blood Glucose

The ADA suggests that people taking multiple insulin injections or using insulin pump

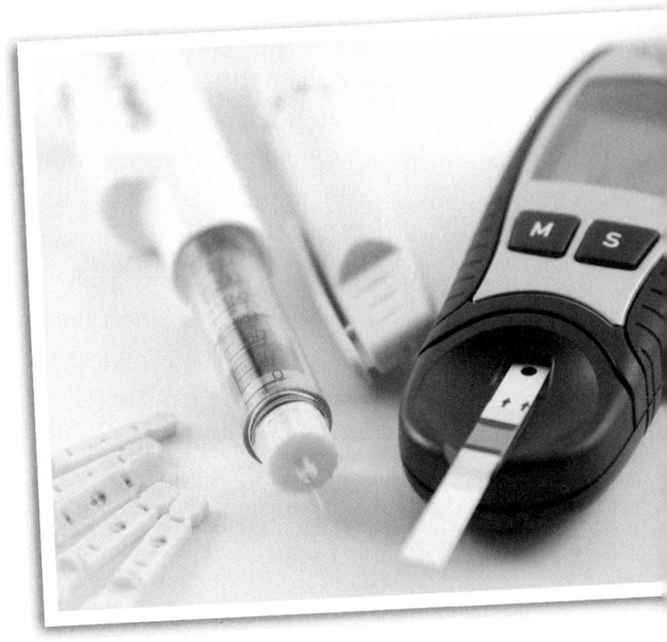

Wonder?

I can't seem to get enough blood on my strip to check my glucose. I waste a lot of strips. It's getting expensive. What should I do?

To obtain an adequate blood sample size, make sure your hands are warm. When your hands are cold, your blood vessels are more constricted, and it is difficult to get a good sample. Warm your hands by washing them in warm soap and water, rinse in warm water, and dry well. If your hands are still not warm enough, hold them in a warm towel a few moments before you check. It also helps to let your hand hang down at your side or to shake your hands like you would a thermometer prior to pricking your fingertips. After you puncture your skin, gently "milk" it from your knuckle to your fingertip to help you get a blood sample. You may need to change your lancing device and size of lancet. If these simple actions don't work, call the toll-free number on the back of your meter. The customer-support team can usually help you and might even send you some free strips to replace the ones you were not able to use. Always feel free to discuss this problem with your health care provider. One way or another, there is help for you.

therapy, such as those with type 1 diabetes, some pregnant women with diabetes, and people with type 2 diabetes who take multiple injections of insulin daily, should test three or more times each day.

There is no official recommendation for testing frequency for people with type 2 diabetes who use blood glucose–lowering medications other than insulin or who control their diabetes with a healthy eating plan and exercise only. The ADA states that blood glucose monitoring may be appropriate in order to achieve blood glucose targets.

Ask your health care provider how often you should check your blood glucose. Your health care provider may recommend checking your blood glucose before or after every meal, before bedtime, early in the morning, before physical activity, or to do a combination of these. Developing a routine for checking your levels will allow you to learn the patterns (ups and downs) of your blood glucose. With this information, and in consultation with your health care provider, you can work to get your numbers where they should be at specific times each day.

Be strategic about when and how often you check your blood glucose. If you have type 2 and do not take insulin, there is no set amount of times you should test your blood glucose per day; however, if you are taking a blood glucose–lowering medication that can cause hypoglycemia [also check out *Chapter 15, page 195*], it's a good idea to check more often. Complications occur from wide swings of blood glucose levels and long-term high blood glucose levels, so you also want to check for these as well, so you can be proactive rather than reactive, which is nearly impossible to do if you do not know your blood glucose levels.

Observe the Big Picture

Pattern management is a term used to describe the process that allows you and your health care provider to evaluate "the big picture" of your blood glucose readings. When you practice pattern management, you consider the actions and activities that affect your blood glucose. Getting a handle on the ups and downs of your blood glucose helps you learn to be proactive rather than reactive—in other words, it helps you make adjustments before your blood glucose gets out of control rather than managing after the fact, which defeats the purpose. Taking action proactively can help you minimize wide blood glucose fluctuations.

Information you need for pattern management:

- Your blood glucose targets. For example, 70–130mg/dl before you eat.
- Your blood glucose readings. At least 3 to 10 days of your glucose readings, including the date and time of day. These readings should be the same time of the day. For example, fasting blood glucose and two hours after eating breakfast, lunch, and dinner. That would be four readings a day.
- Your food record. A written record of the food you have eaten, including the type, amount, and time you ate.
- Your physical activity record. A written record of any physical activity you did, including the date, time of day, type, and intensity.
- Your medication(s) record. A written record of any medication you took that

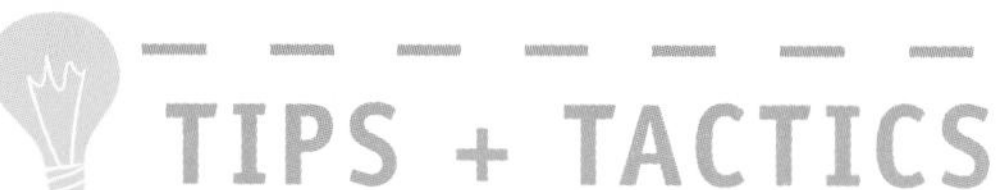

Less painful blood glucose monitoring

Some people won't check their blood glucose because of pain. Try these tips to decrease the pain of blood glucose monitoring:

- *Prick the side of your finger in the fleshy part by your nail bed. Your fingertips have a lot of nerves, which makes the tips a more painful site to use. Hold the area tight, putting pressure on the area before you prick.*
- *Use a lancing device rather than a lancet alone. If the lancing device you use doesn't make a difference, try another brand. There are a lot to choose from. Your health care provider can help you find one that is less painful.*
- *Don't use alcohol. Using alcohol is not only drying to your skin, but also any trace of alcohol can cause pain and stinging when you pierce the skin. It may also affect your reading if not rinsed and dried well. To avoid infections, try to make sure your hands are clean before you prick your skin for a check.*
- *Use a new lancet every time, or change it at least once a day. The duller the lancet, the more painful.*
- *Change fingers or use the same site on the same finger over and over again. Some people find it less painful to change where they test, yet some people find that checking at the same site forms a callous and makes it less painful.*
- *Use an alternate site. Some meters have been FDA-approved for alternative site testing (AST). If you choose to try this, follow the instructions that come with your meter. AST is not always as accurate as finger testing. This is especially true when your glucose is rapidly changing, such as after you eat, after taking insulin, or during and after vigorous exercise.*

lowers or affects your blood glucose. Include the name, dosage, date, and time(s) of day.

- Your events record. A written record of any event that may have affected your blood glucose (e.g., stress, illness, travel) [also check out *Chapter 14*, page 181].

Some people use a log book to fill in this information, some health care providers have forms they like people to use, some people make their own forms, and some people use the printouts from their meter, or use programs available online [also check out *Psst; Online Resources for Blood Glucose Meters*, page 166]. It is difficult to assess patterns, make necessary adjustments, and assess your response without recording your blood glucose results in some manner. It is not helpful to you or your health care provider to just scroll through the memory of your meter. Yes, you get a sense of the results, but not the what, when, and where information. It is this information that puts context around your results and helps make adjustments in your diabetes care plan.

If you're looking for an example of tracking pattern management, use the chart on page 172 as your guide. With the information gathered for pattern management, it becomes easy for you to identify the out-of-range numbers as well as the causes. One way to mark blood glucose results that are too high or too low is to use two different colored highlighters. Use this information to work with your health care provider to make the necessary changes you need to make to best manage your diabetes.

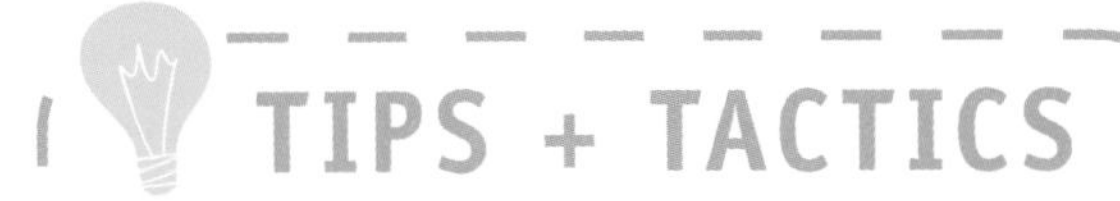

When you need to check your blood glucose more often

There are times when you may need to check your blood glucose more often than you normally do. These times are:

- *When your A1C or eAG is above target. Checking your blood glucose more often allows you to get timely information about your blood glucose patterns. With your records in hand, you and your health care provider will have the information to make informed changes.*
- *When there is a change in your diabetes medication(s), eating, or physical activity habits. More frequent checking will alert you to the effect of these changes on your blood glucose, and you and your health care provider can use these to further adjust your diabetes care plan.*
- *When you are physically or emotionally stressed. You will be able to see how this affects your blood glucose so you can adjust an aspect of your diabetes care plan.*
- *When you have other health conditions or are started on medications to treat another condition with a medication that may affect your blood glucose.*
- *When you have several high or low blood glucose levels in a row or at the same time of the day. Although you don't want your blood glucose to be too high or too low, you want to be aware of, treat, and prevent these highs or lows as soon as possible.*

Pattern Management

Below is an example of a person's blood glucose record for a week. The best way to analyze your patterns is to write down your observations and discuss them with your health care provider. If your numbers are within your target range, keep doing what you're doing. If they are too high or too low, determine whether your food, physical activity level, medications, or other actions or activities might be causing the imbalance.

An example of pattern management with sample readings

Target BG-Before Meals 70–130mg/dl, 1–2hours after meals < 180mg/dl

Day	Fasting	After Breakfast	After Lunch	After Dinner
Sunday	150	228	140	280
Monday	128	240	100	170
Tuesday	112	270	60	198
Wednesday	94	202	126	202
Thursday	102	226	146	157
Friday	123	278	125	206
Saturday	99	204	182	197
Pattern?	**OK**	**HIGH**	**OK**	**HIGH**

Let's say this is your record. Your fasting blood glucose is within range other than one day, Sunday morning. So, these look okay. All after-breakfast glucose levels are elevated. You would make sure the before-meal level was not elevated. If not, then look at the carbohydrate content of breakfast. It that is high, make adjustments to lower it and check again. If that's not the problem, it may be due to being sedentary, or not enough blood glucose–lowering medication. The after-lunch levels are acceptable, except the 182. You would ask yourself the same questions: have you eaten too much food, gotten too little activity, or taken too little medication? Since it is okay more than 80% of the time, it's okay. The after-dinner readings are elevated over 80% of the time, so once again you'll want to figure out what you think the problem is and adjust. Some adjustments you will be able to make on your own, and some you will want to work on with your health care provider. As you become more comfortable with your blood glucose management, you will gain the confidence to make more adjustments on your own; however, this depends mostly on the blood glucose–lowering medications you take.

Take these records with you when you visit your health care provider so you can review them together and make the necessary corrections. When despite all your efforts, your patterns don't improve, don't wait for your next appointment that may be weeks or months away. Speak up, don't put it off. Call your health care provider. Let him or her know your levels are out of your target. Ask whether you should discuss this over the phone, email, or fax your information over, or just set up an earlier appointment to make changes in a timely manner.

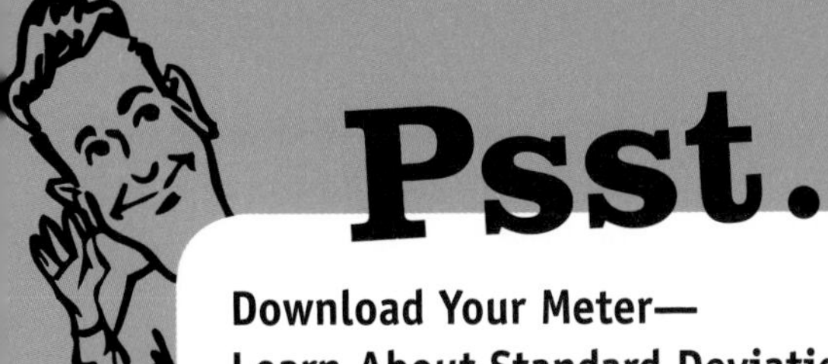

Psst...

Download Your Meter—Learn About Standard Deviation

Most meters come with software, which allows you to download your results and do some analysis. You can get all kinds of records, graphs, and pie charts to help you see the bigger picture. One important reading you will get on most meter downloads is your standard deviation. Standard deviation is a statistical measure of the spread or difference between your lowest to highest blood glucose result—the glucose variability.

The more your glucose varies up and down, the more glucose variability you have, and the larger your standard deviation. One theory about the development of diabetes complications points to glucose variability [also check out *Chapter 21*, page 257]. Your goal should be to keep your standard deviation as small as possible by keeping your glucose level in a fairly level range rather than the wide swings. Several experts recommend that your standard deviation multiplied by 2 should be less than your average glucose number. For example, if your average after-lunch glucose is 150mg/dl, and your standard deviation is 50, 50 times 2 equals 100, which is less than 150, so this is acceptable. On the other hand, if your standard deviation is 100, it's too high because 100 times 2 equals 200, which is higher than the average of 150, and is considered too high.

Wonder?

Will my health care plan pay for the supplies I need to monitor my blood glucose?

Most health care plans provide some coverage for diabetes supplies, but the only way to know is to check with your health care plan. Most plans, including Medicare, cover your meter, strips, lancets, and lancing devices. Coverage has continued to improve over the past decade. If you don't have coverage for your blood glucose–monitoring supplies, shop around for the best prices on meters and strips [also check out *Chapter 19*, page 237].

Continuous Glucose Monitoring (CGM)

Just as technology rang in the era of blood glucose–monitoring devices a little more than 30 years ago, a new era of monitoring technology called continuous glucose monitoring (CGM) is dawning in diabetes care. Today, CGM is in its infancy. The first generation of continuous glucose monitoring systems (CGMS) are here, and there are three FDA-approved systems on the market. They are not approved to replace blood glucose monitors, but to be used in conjunction with them.

A CGMS is made up of three parts: a sensor, a transmitter, and a receiver that reads and records your glucose numbers on a minute-to-minute basis. The sensor needs to be

Research Brief

CONFIDENTIAL

Early Blood Glucose Management Pays Off! DCCT and UKPDS—Ten Years Later...

Two landmark studies, the Diabetes Control and Complication Trial (DCCT) and the United Kingdom Prospective Diabetes Study (UKPDS) both proved that intensive glucose management matters to prevent complications of diabetes.

The Epidemiology of Diabetes Interventions of Complications (EDIC) Study followed the people who participated in the DCCT [also check out *Chapter 2*, page 23]. Researchers also continued to follow the participants of the UKPDS. Both the EDIC and the UKPDS 10-year follow-up showed that early blood glucose control matters. Although the differences between the intensive groups and the conventional groups were small, as time went on, early blood glucose management decreased complications in the long run. Some experts have called this "metabolic memory" or "the legacy effect" because it seems that your body remembers the early "good" blood glucose control to protect you from eye, kidney, and nerve damage as well as a heart attack or stroke.

Since the UKPDS also followed blood pressure, the 10-year follow-up of the blood pressure segments of the study showed no "metabolic memory or legacy effect" when it comes to blood pressure. In order to prevent complications related to high blood pressure, although early management matters, you need continuous control of blood pressure to prevent the complications of elevated blood pressure. These results do not mean that you should only be concerned about early management of your blood glucose, but they do mean that managing both your blood glucose and your blood pressure does matter in the long-term.

changed every three to seven days, depending on the brand. The CGM measures glucose in your interstitial fluid—the fluid among your cells—rather than your blood. This difference presents some issues that you need to be aware of, such as the lag time between the two.

With the information you receive from CGM, you can track trends, which means you can see whether your glucose is rising or falling. You can also set points at which you will receive alarms to alert you if your glucose is rising or falling too quickly, as well as if you are above or below your targets. This is very helpful when you are not sure whether you need to take immediate action to correct your blood glucose or not, and if you have hypoglycemia unawareness.

Today, CGMs are mainly being used by people with type 1 or 2 diabetes who take insulin. CGM is beginning to be covered by more, but certainly not all, health care plans. You may find your health care plan is assessing on a case-by-case basis and you may need to provide blood glucose records, a letter of necessity from your health care provider, and more. As time goes on, and there are more devices, more people who want them, and more research and more experience about their cost-savings benefits, health care plan coverage will likely improve.

If you are interested in a CGM, technology is moving fast, and devices continue to get smaller. More accurate and easy-to-use devices will likely be available in the next few years. Stay tuned to diabetes magazines and websites to track happenings with this exciting technology.

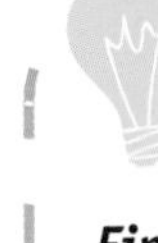

TIPS + TACTICS

Find the right blood pressure monitor for you

- *Buy an accurate monitor. There are many blood pressure monitors to choose from, but not all of them are accurate. Accurate blood pressure monitors will say, "Independently Validated for Proven Accuracy" on the box.*
- *Know the price range. Accurate blood pressure monitors range from $20.00 to $150.00. The average price is about $70.00.*
- *Choose the type of blood pressure monitor that is best for you. The automatic ones are easier to use and more accurate, but they cost more.*
- *Take your blood pressure based on the instructions that come with your blood pressure monitor.*
- *Take your home blood pressure monitor with you to your next appointment with your health care provider. Check to make sure your blood pressure monitor and your health care provider's monitor have similar readings.*

Monitoring Your Blood Pressure at Home

Because heart disease is the number-one complication of diabetes that leads to increased health problems and death, it is important to know if you have high blood pressure and how to manage it. The ADA recommends that you have your blood pressure checked at every routine diabetes visit. Along with blood pressure checks at the office, anyone with a history of high blood pressure or who is taking blood pressure medications should consider buying a home blood pressure monitor.

Monitoring at home is very important for people with high blood pressure because early-morning high blood pressure can be a serious problem if left untreated. In fact, the American Heart Association (AHA), the American Society for Hypertension (ASH), and the Preventive Cardiovascular Nurses Association (PCNA) recently published a "Call to Action" recommending home blood pressure monitoring. They recommend home blood pressure monitoring to diagnose high blood pressure, and for people who have high blood pressure or have a condition related to high blood pressure. They also recommend you use a monitor that uses an electronic sensor. Learn more at *http://www.americanheart.org/presenter.jhtml?identifier=3058553.*

RED FLAG

Health Care Plans Don't Pay for Blood Pressure Monitors

Most health care plans do not pay for blood pressure monitors. With the average cost being about $70.00 for a blood pressure monitor that lasts many years, it is good insurance for you to buy one. This device can help you and your health care provider manage your blood pressure and prevent complications of diabetes and high blood pressure. Just think, spending $70.00 can prevent you from having a stroke or other complications of diabetes. What a deal!

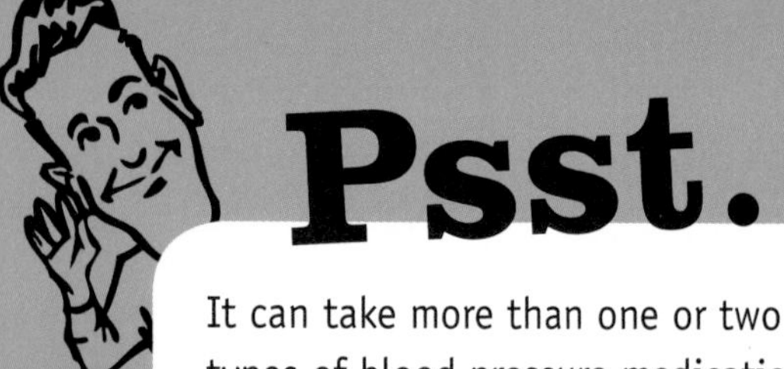

Psst...

It can take more than one or two types of blood pressure medication to manage your blood pressure. If one doesn't work, don't stop taking it, and don't give up. Remember, managing your blood pressure is as important as managing your blood glucose when it comes to the prevention of diabetes complications [also check out *Chapter 9*, page 121, and *Chapter 21*, page 257]. Work with you health care provider to increase medication to get your blood pressure under control.

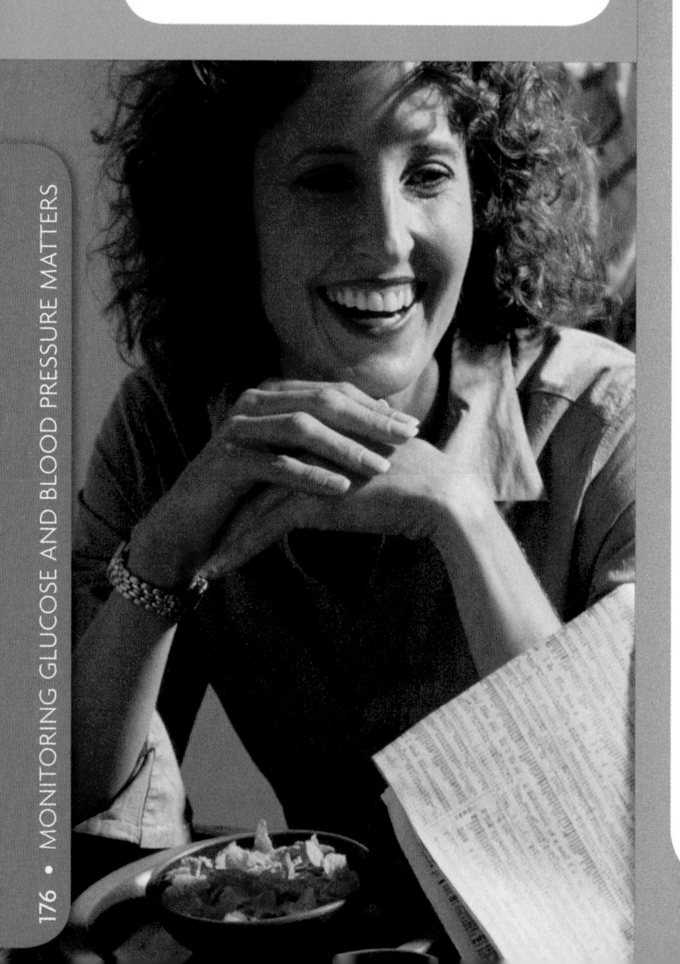

Wonder?

Are there other self-care actions I should take daily to take care of my diabetes?

Yes! Managing diabetes to stay healthy day to day and year to year puts a lot of responsibility on you to implement daily self-care actions. Remember, take it one day at a time. Set realistic goals, and do what you can do.

- Try to be active a total of 30 minutes most days. Ask your health care provider about the activities that are best for you [also check out *Chapter 7*, page 89].
- Take your medicines as prescribed [also check out *Chapter 8*, page 101, and *Chapter 9*, page 121].
- Check your blood glucose according to the schedule you and your health care provider agree on. Maintain your blood glucose records, and analyze these regularly [also check out *Chapter 15*, page 195].
- Look at your feet regularly for cuts, blisters, sores, swelling, redness, or sore toenails. Report any changes to your health care provider right away.
- Brush and floss your teeth every day.
- Get and keep your weight, blood pressure, and lipids under control.
- Don't smoke [also check out *Chapter 18*, page 229].

Section 3

When Life Happens

In a perfect world, you would have healthy foods prepared for you, and they would be on the table ready for you to dig in. Restaurant menus would be filled with healthier offerings. There would be plenty of spare time to get those 30 minutes of walking in each day. You'd have no stresses about the cost of health care or taking time off to spend unlimited time with your numerous diabetes health care providers. These providers would take unlimited time with you, mulling over your recent lab tests, glucose records, and behavioral-change goals and accomplishments, and you would be able to connect with them as need be via fax, e-mail, and the Internet. Lastly, your school, work, and/or family life would be stress-free.

But the world is not perfect. Money doesn't grow on trees, and daily life contains its stresses and strains and ups and downs. Managing diabetes adds to the complexities of daily life in many ways. Rather than shying away from recognizing these realities, *Real-Life Guide to Diabetes* faces them head-on here in Section 3—When Life Happens. Managing diabetes today is a balancing act between doing what needs to be done to care for your diabetes to stay healthy and doing and accomplishing your day-to-day tasks and life-long goals, whatever they may be.

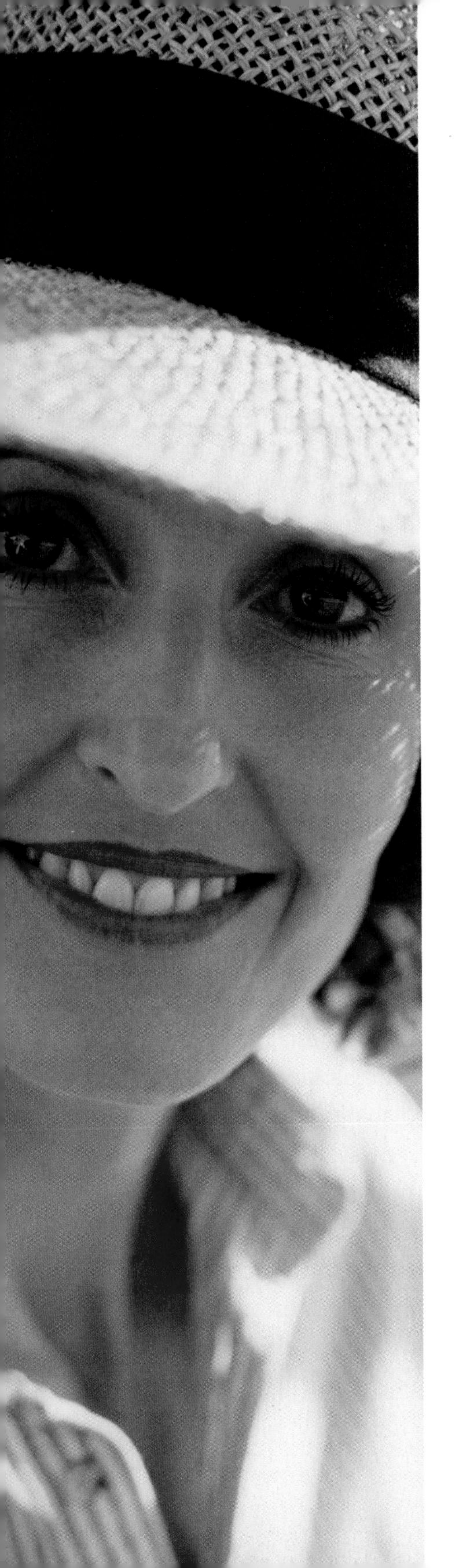

A brief look at the chapters in Section 3—
When Life Happens:

Chapter 14

When Life Veers Off Schedule: Life doesn't necessarily go as planned everyday. There are positive changes to your schedule, such as going on vacation or out to a relaxing and delicious restaurant meal, but there are also the negatives, sick days (you or a loved one) and emergency situations. Learn how to plan and be ready for these times when life simply veers off schedule.

Chapter 15

Glucose Highs and Lows: No matter how well you fine-tune your diabetes care plan, you will likely experience times when your blood glucose is too high or too low. Learn the signs and symptoms of these situations, and be prepared to prevent or manage them.

Chapter 16

Lose Weight, Keep It Off: Losing weight and keeping those pounds off is an important aspect of diabetes care, especially with pre- or type 2 diabetes. You'll learn the countless benefits of weight loss for your health and diabetes control. You'll get a sense of how much weight you need to lose and will become aware that, once you are diagnosed with type 2 diabetes, you'll likely need to take blood glucose–lowering medication in addition to working on trimming those pounds and pumping those legs. Learn about weight-loss medications and surgery and gain insights from the latest research on long-term weight control.

Chapter 17

Your Sexual Health: A complex topic, both emotionally and physically. Learn about different types of intimacy and how diabetes can affect your sex life day to day. Learn how to have a satisfying sex life while you manage your diabetes.

Chapter 18

Tobacco and Alcohol: How They Mix with Diabetes: It's essential to deal with these two commonly used vices because many people, though not ideal for health, use one or both of them. You'll learn both the positive and negative effects of alcohol, along with the negative effects of smoking on your diabetes and your health and how to reduce or remove the use of alcohol and cigarettes in your life.

Chapter 19

Health Care Plans and Money Matters: Diabetes is a costly disease to manage—from visits to your health care providers, to medications, monitoring equipment, special tests, and more. Learn about what to look for when you shop for a health care plan. Learn which diabetes supplies and services are typically covered and how to make sure you get the coverage you deserve.

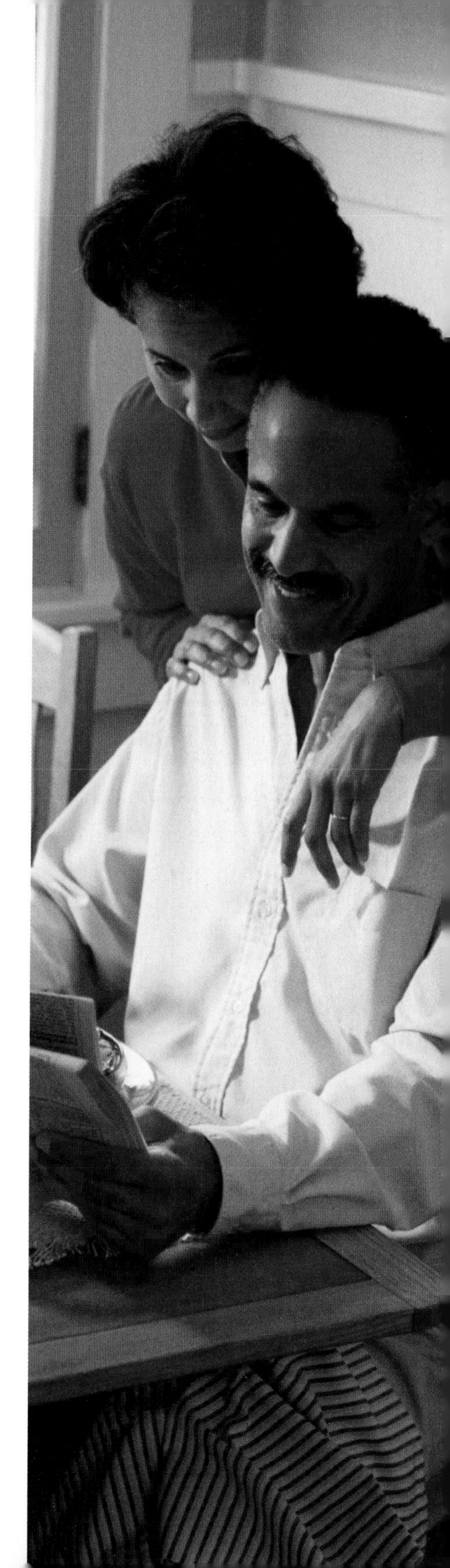

Chapter 20

Know Your Rights, Don't Be Wronged: Having diabetes means you may encounter discrimination in your life travels, from school or job discrimination, to being told you can't carry your diabetes supplies into a public venue. You'll learn about your rights, how to protect them, and about how the ADA is applying its four-step process to help keep you from being wronged: educate, negotiate, litigate, and legislate.

Chapter 21

Prevent and Delay Long-Term Diabetes Problems: Unfortunately, health problems associated with having diabetes exist. Fortunately, you and your health care providers can take actions to prevent and delay these problems. Learn about the various types of diabetes complications and what to do on your own, at health care visits, and in everyday life to keep those complications at bay.

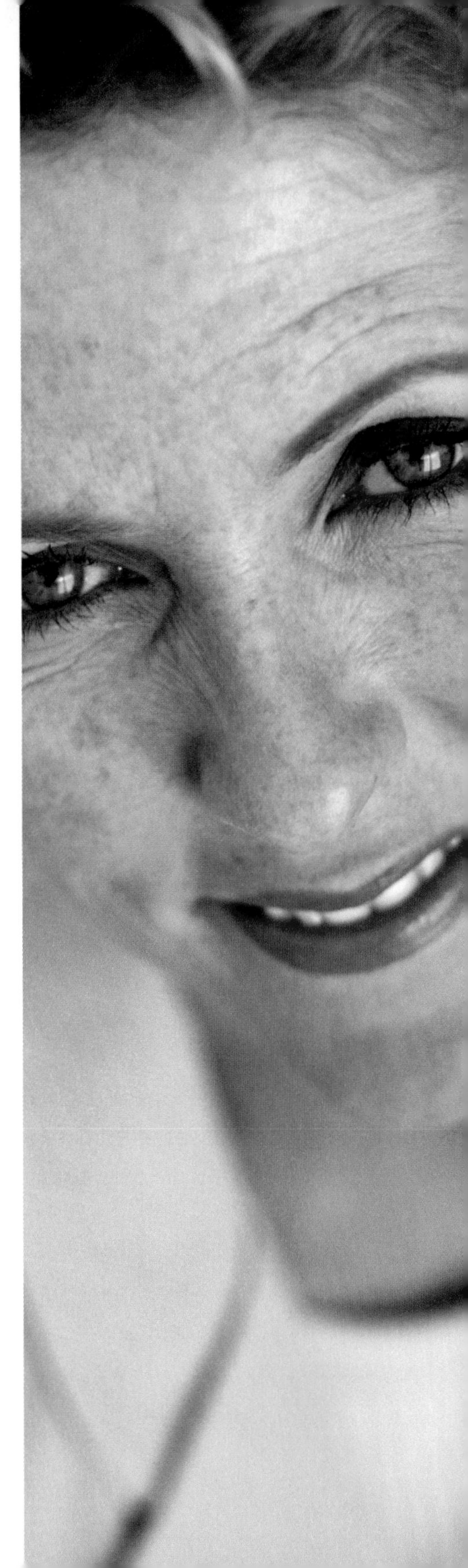

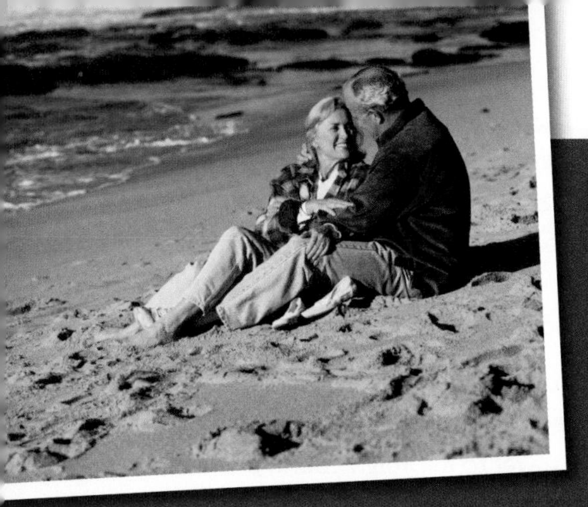

CHAPTER 14

When Life Veers Off Schedule

No two days are quite the same when it comes to real life, yet diabetes care tends to demand a structured schedule. Very few people want, or are able to, live a rigid life, which demands that meals be eaten, medications be taken, and exercise be done at the same time each day, all in the name of keeping your blood glucose and other parameters in control.

Things happen in life that can get you off your schedule for a few hours, such as getting stuck in traffic, experiencing hypoglycemia during a work meeting, or a missed or delayed meal. Life can be different for a few days or longer because of a trip you have been looking forward to, an unplanned trip to take care of an ill loved one, an illness, or a milestone celebration. Some of these events you can anticipate and deal with, and others you can't. When you have diabetes, and particularly if you take blood glucose–lowering medication that can cause your blood glucose to be out of your target range, it's important to be prepared for any and all of these situations.

What You'll Learn:

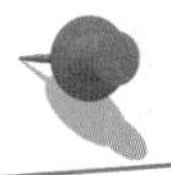

- Tips for traveling with diabetes
- Tips for taking care of yourself and your diabetes when you are sick
- How to prepare for and act in emergencies situations and disasters
- How to adapt to sudden changes in your schedule
- Tips to manage your food, physical activity, and medications when you are "off schedule" for whatever reason

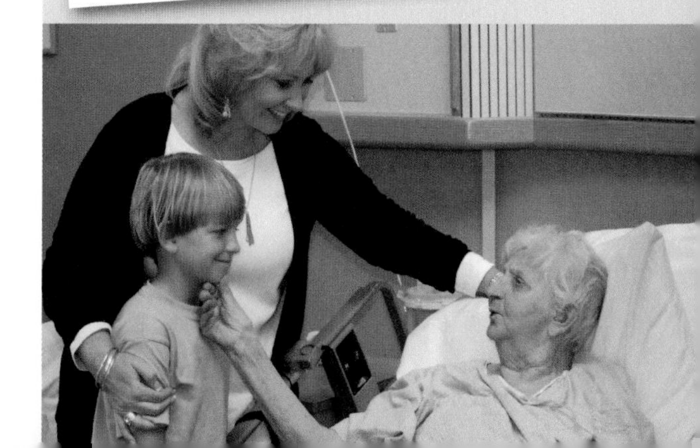

Before You Travel

Although your reasons for travel can be different, most kinds of travel can cause you to be "off schedule" in some way, causing stress to your body and your mind. The best approach to travel is to always be prepared by planning for as much of the trip as you can. Ask questions of health care providers, friends with diabetes who travel, travel agents, and people who have been to the location you're going to visit. Be ready for the unexpected, including delayed or cancelled flights, lost luggage, and illnesses. Do not assume that you will be able to buy your diabetes supplies at your destination. Take what you need and pack extra. As a person with diabetes, you should always pack at least twice as much medication and glucose-checking supplies as you think you need. Make sure to pack at least half of your supplies in your carry-on bag so that your medications and supplies are always with you.

TIPS + TACTICS

Snacks to Carry

No matter what kind of trip you're going on, it's a good idea to carry at least one or more of these portable snacks.

- *Nuts are healthy for you and the portion-controlled packages help you not overeat. Buy the prepackaged one-ounce size of nuts.*
- *String cheese works well because it is typically individually packaged and is low in fat.*
- *A small apple, orange, peach, or pear is easy to carry.*
- *Pretzels or popcorn*
- *Individual packages of trail mix*
- *Nutrition bars*

Make sure to get a letter and any prescriptions you will need from your health care provider before you travel to a foreign country. The letter should explain what you need to do for your diabetes, such as if you take oral medications and or injections to lower your blood glucose. It should list your medications, the supplies you need, and any other medications or devices you use. It should also include any allergies you have or any foods or medications to which you are sensitive, and it should have your health care provider's signature.

Your prescriptions should be for your medications and supplies. Take more than enough medicine and supplies to last you through your trip. Prescriptions are good to have in case of emergency. In the U.S., prescription rules vary from state to state. The prescription laws may also be very different in other countries. If you're going out of the country, visit the International Diabetes Federation's website at *www.idf.org* for more information on international prescription laws.

No matter where you go, wear a medical ID bracelet or necklace that shows you have diabetes [also check out *Chapter 15*, page 195]. Carrying an identification card in your wallet is also a good idea; however, wearing a medical ID is preferable, since there are times you can be separated from your wallet, and emergency personnel will look for ID on your

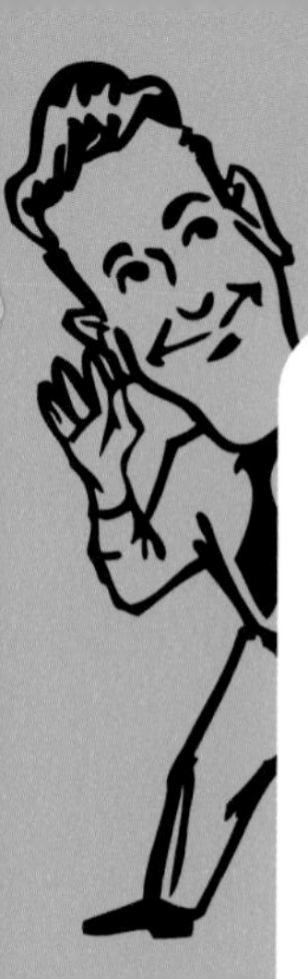

Psst...

Don't Forget Your Feet

When you have diabetes, it doesn't matter where you are going, or for how long, when it comes to your feet. It's always important to take very good care of your feet. Wear comfortable, well-made shoes that protect your feet—running or walking shoes of a breathable material are the best choice. On a trip, be sure to take several pairs of shoes, so you can change them throughout the day and keep blisters from forming. Also, if you are flying, try to get up and move every half hour or so. When you are sitting more than an hour, move your feet as if you are drawing circles with them. It's good to keep circulation flowing to your feet when you can't walk around.

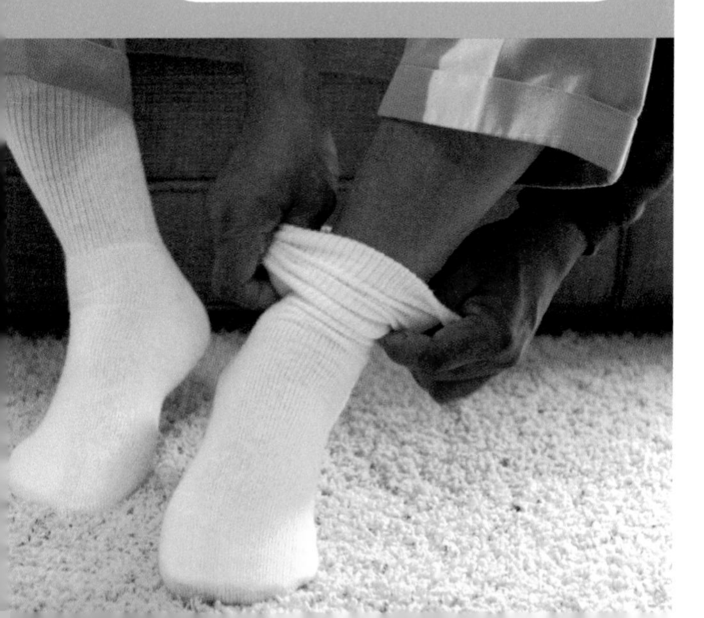

Your Diabetes Carry-On Bag

- Blood glucose monitor and urine testing supplies. Be sure to include extra batteries and strips for your blood glucose monitor.
- All of your medications, both to lower glucose and other medications as well as the supplies you'll need to take them (include extra just in case).
- Other medications, such as glucagon, anti-diarrhea medication, antibiotic ointment, and anti-nausea meds.
- Well-wrapped, airtight snack pack of cheese or peanut butter crackers, fruit, a juice box, nuts, cheese sticks, and some form of carbohydrate to treat low blood glucose.
- If you wear a pump or a continuous glucose monitor, take extra supplies for these, including batteries.
- A diabetes identification card. Wear identification but also carry the card in your bag.

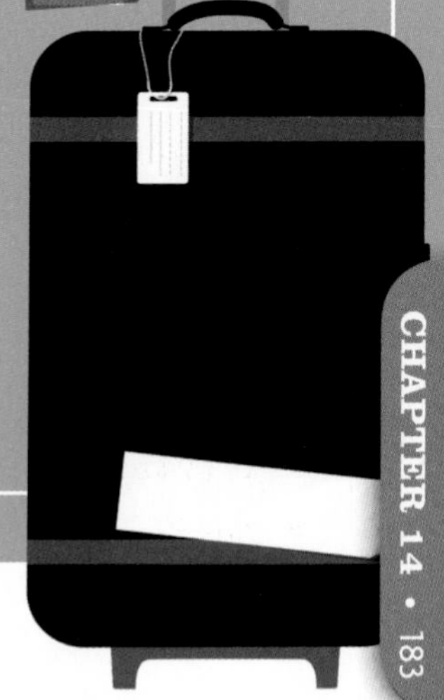

body rather than in your wallet or purse. If you will be in a foreign country where English is not commonly spoken, learn how to say, "I have diabetes" and "sugar or fruit juice, please" in the language or languages of the countries you'll visit in case you have a low.

Getting Your Diabetes Supplies through Airport Security

One of the most stressful parts of traveling is finding out what you can take with you on an airplane and how to notify airport personal about your diabetes needs. Even worse, the rules at airports constantly change, so it can be difficult to keep up with the current restrictions.

Currently, small quantities (up to 3 oz) of liquid toiletries will be allowed through airport security checkpoints along with large volumes of liquid and gel to treat hypoglycemia. These need to be in a quart-sized

If I Only Knew . . .

Anything can happen . . .

Things happen. I've broken insulin bottles, left them in hotel rooms, had my blood glucose monitor stolen, and panicked when I tried to explain in another language that I have diabetes. And let's not forget when I was stuck on an airport runway for hours with no food! Now I never travel without extra supplies, medications, and snacks (four prepackaged peanut butter cracker sandwiches that are cheap and lightweight, and fit into any size bag). I also bring along my prescriptions and health care providers' phone numbers. When I travel out of the country, I've learned to bring measurements in that country's equivalents, so it's easy to read labels. I also make up my own emergency card in the country's language. It says, "I have diabetes," with all my emergency contact information listed. I keep it on my person, especially if I'm touring by myself.

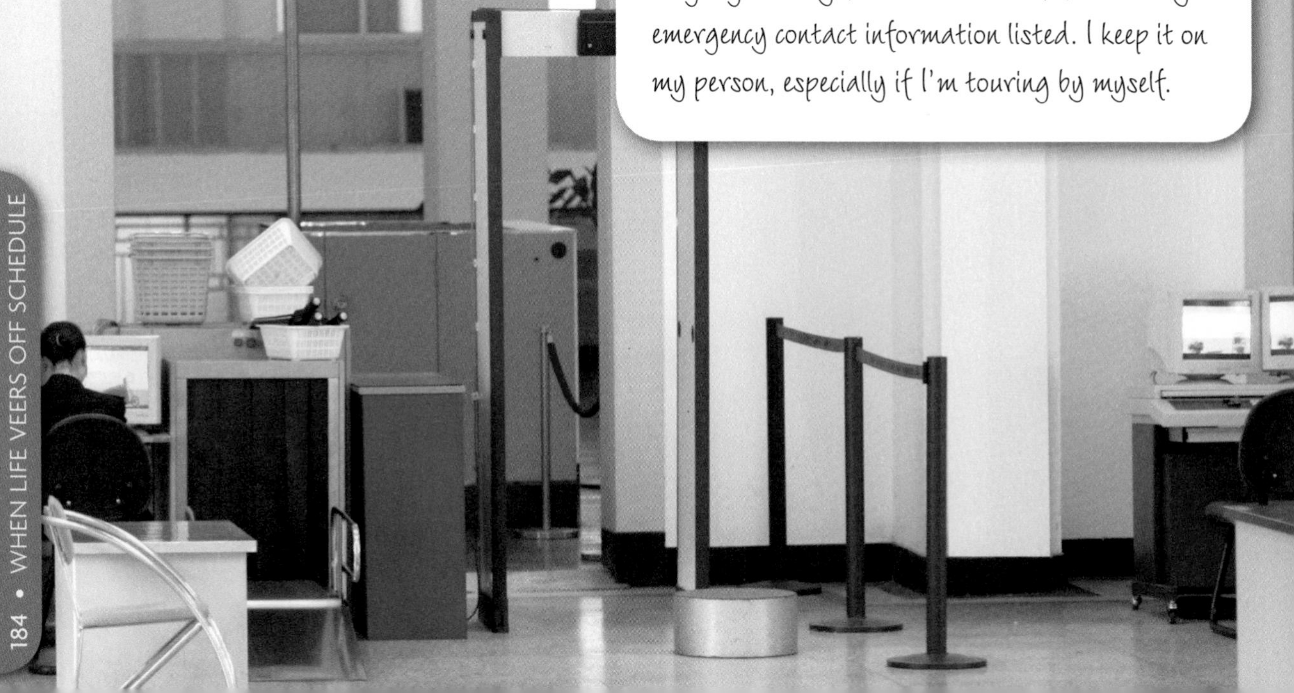

TIPS + TACTICS

TSA Recommendations

TSA recommends that travelers with disabilities and medical conditions may want to consider the following:

- *Arrive at the airport 2–3 hours prior to your flight so you have more than enough time to get through security.*
- *Review TSA's website for travel updates (*www.tsa.gov*).*
- *Take required prescription labels for medication.*
- *Take prescriptions for medical devices when possible.*
- *Pack medications in a separate, clear bag and place in your carry-on luggage.*
- *Be patient with lines, delays, and new screening procedures.*

Contact TSA

If you have an immediate need while being screened, you should ask for a screener supervisor. You may also contact the TSA Contact Center to report unfair treatment or to obtain additional information by calling toll-free 866-289-9673 during the following hours of operation (all times are Eastern Standard Time):

- Monday thru Friday 8 a.m.–10 p.m.
- Saturday, Sunday, and Holidays 10 a.m.–6 p.m

For more information, go to TSA's website (*www.tsa.gov*).

plastic bag that zips closed. Please note that the Transportation Security Administration (TSA) specifically states that passengers with insulin and other liquid diabetes medications are permitted to board airplanes with their medications, supplies, and equipment.

TSA recommends that if you travel with prescription liquid medications such as insulin, pramlintide, exenatide, or a glucagon emergency kit, you should make sure your medications are clearly identified with a prescription label matching your name. Although TSA doesn't require that you have a prescription label, it is a good idea to have one and it can expedite the security process. TSA does allow you to carry multiple containers of glucose gel to treat low blood glucose; however, it would make more sense for you to bring nonliquid forms of carbohydrates to treat hypoglycemia, such as glucose tablets, Life Savers, gumdrops, or raisins.

Under normal conditions, your medications can safely pass through x-ray machines at airport terminals. If your insulin remains in the path of the x-ray longer than normal, or if it is repeatedly exposed to x-rays, be careful. Prolonged exposure to an x-ray can affect the stability of your insulin. If you have concerns about x-rays, you can request hand-inspection. Insulin should never be placed in checked baggage. Passenger baggage stored in cargo holds is subject to powerful x-rays. It also could be affected by severe changes in pressure and temperature. Inspect your insulin before injecting each dose. If you notice anything unusual about the appearance of your insulin or that your insulin needs are changing, call your doctor.

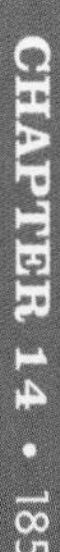

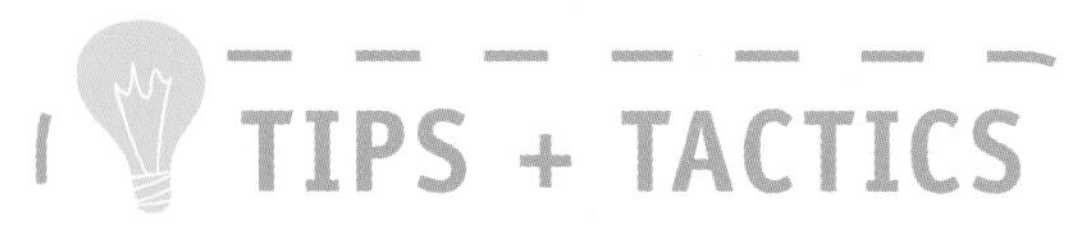

Choice of Visual Inspection Over X-ray

Few people are aware that you have the option of requesting a visual inspection rather than an x-ray inspection of your medications and diabetes-associated supplies. If you request a visual inspection, keep these things in mind:

- *Request a visual inspection before the screening process begins; otherwise, your medications and supplies will undergo x-ray inspection.*
- *Separate your medication and associated supplies from your other property in a pouch or bag.*
- *Label your medications so they are identifiable.*
- *You will be asked at the security checkpoint to display, handle, and repack your own medication and associated supplies during the visual inspection process in order to prevent any contamination or damage.*
- *Understand that any medication and/or associated supplies that cannot be cleared visually must be submitted for x-ray screening. If you refuse, you will not be permitted to carry your medications and related supplies into the sterile area.*

Keeping Your Life Running When Your Schedule Must Shift

The key to managing your blood glucose is to take time to pre-plan and set yourself up as well as possible for as many situations as you think you may face, no matter how big or small. Your life doesn't stop for diabetes, but it's still good to know how to deal with these small snafus when they occur.

Hypoglycemia that occurs when you are driving can dramatically increase your risk for a car accident (and/or hurting someone else). As always, it's best to be prepared. This is a good example of why it's always good to have your glucose monitor and some portable source of carbohydrate with you. If you find yourself in this situation, here's what to do:

- If you have your meter, check your blood glucose (it should be 70–130 mg/dl). If it's lower than this, treat with 15 grams of carbs.
- If you don't have your meter, but you do have food, eat something. It's better to be safe than sorry.
- If you don't have your meter or anything to eat, and you have another person in the car who is able to drive, switch drivers.
- If you don't have anyone else in the car, pull over at the closest store or gas station you see. Find a food that contains carbohydrate to raise your blood glucose for the remainder of your trip.
- Don't continue driving until the hypoglycemia has passed.

People spend a great majority of their time

TIPS + TACTICS

Remember to Take Your Medications

- *Get yourself a medi-planner. A medi-planner is a box that helps you organize your medications for particular days and times of the day. Keep this with you so you can check and see if you have taken your medications for that day.*
- *Link taking your medications with something else you do; like brushing your teeth or eating.*
- *Ask a loved one to call you at a certain time every day to remind you to take your medications.*
- *Use a calendar or chart to mark down your medications when you take them.*
- *Talk with your health care provider. If you are taking one type of medication several times a day, ask whether there is a long-acting medication you can take once a day so it is easier to remember.*

at work, so it's reasonable to believe you will experience hypoglycemia at some time or another on the job. You may want to keep your diabetes private from your coworkers, which can be difficult if you experience a low.

Say you're in a meeting and begin to feel like you need to eat, or else your blood glucose will drop. How can you deal with that situation without calling attention to yourself? The easiest thing to do would be to excuse yourself, go to the bathroom, check your blood glucose, and eat 15 grams of carbohydrates if you have them with you. But what if you're not prepared? Most work sites have some sort of cafeteria or, at the very least, vending machines. If all else fails, you may just need to speak up and find out whether a person near you has any mints or anything else to tide you over until you have access to food. Once again, being prepared with food and your blood glucose meter is your best bet [also check out *Chapter 15*, page 195].

Forgetting to Take Your Medicine

Forgetting to take your medication is a concern and can happen more often than you think, especially when you are traveling or are off your usual schedule. If you have type 1 diabetes and you forget your insulin, it can quickly become dangerous. You can go into diabetic ketoacidosis in a few hours [also check out *Chapter 15*, page 195]. If you have type 2 diabetes, your blood glucose will likely rise higher than it should be; however, you are unlikely to develop a serious medical problem that will require immediate assistance. Don't take it too lightly though, because if forgetting your medications becomes a habit, you will put yourself at greater risk for long-term diabetes complications.

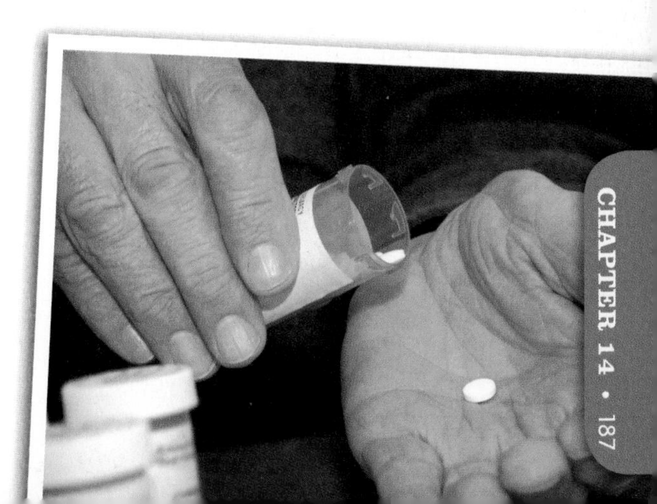

When You're Under the Weather

Being sick can make your blood glucose levels higher and lower than normal because it can throw your entire system out of whack. The best way to prevent a minor illness from becoming a major problem is to work out a plan of action for sick days ahead of time. Then, when you become sick, you will already know what to do and will have the supplies on hand to do it. When you're sick, your body is under stress. In order to deal with this stress, your body also releases hormones that help it fight disease; however, these hormones can raise blood glucose levels and can interfere with the blood glucose–lowering effects of your medications [also check out *Chapter 15*, page 195]. As a result, when you are sick, it is harder to keep your blood glucose in your target range.

Taking Medicines and Eating When You Are Sick

You may need to make some adjustments in your food, physical activity, and medications when you are sick. You may need more or fewer medications, or you may need a different kind while you are sick. If you are vomiting and are on insulin, don't stop taking your insulin, especially your long-acting insulin (Lantus or Levemir). You may need it because your body makes extra glucose when you are sick. If you take other medications, including those that lower your blood glucose, and you are able to take them, do. In either case, check your blood glucose more often than you usually would and call your health care provider if your levels are outside your

TIPS + TACTICS

When to Call Your Health Care Provider

You do not need to call your team every time you have a sniffle or blood glucose level that's a bit elevated, but you will want to call if certain things happen. For example:

- *You've been sick or have had a fever for a couple of days and aren't getting better.*
- *You've been vomiting or having diarrhea for more than 6 hours.*
- *You have moderate to large amounts of ketones in your urine.*
- *Your glucose levels are higher than 240 even though you've taken the extra insulin your sick day plan calls for* *[also check out* Chapter 15, *page 195]*.
- *You take pills for your diabetes, and your blood glucose level climbs to more than 240 before meals and stays there for more than 24 hours* *[also check out* Chapter 8, *page 101]*.
- *You have symptoms that might signal ketoacidosis or dehydration or some other serious condition (for example, your chest hurts, you are having trouble breathing, your breath smells fruity, or your lips or tongue are dry and cracked).*
- *You aren't certain what to do to take care of yourself. When in doubt, always check it out.*

Be ready to tell someone what medicines you've taken and how much, how long you've been sick, whether you can eat and keep food down, whether you've lost weight, and what your temperature, blood glucose level, and urine ketone level are. To be prepared, keep written records of all these things as soon as you become sick and keep your notebook handy.

normal target ranges. If you don't normally take insulin, you may need to take it while you are sick and under greater stress. You may be able to resume your normal medications as you get better [also check out *Chapter 8*, page 101, and *Chapter 15*, page 195].

Eating and drinking can also be a big problem when you're sick, but it's important to stick to your normal eating plan if you can. Drink lots of non-caloric liquids, such as water or diet sodas, to keep from getting dehydrated. It's easy to run low on fluids when you are vomiting or have a fever or diarrhea. Now is the time to discuss a sick-day plan with your health care provider rather than when you are sick and don't know what to do. It's always better to be proactive than reactive.

If you are able to eat and drink, try to take in your normal number of calories with foods that are easy on your stomach, like regular gelatin, crackers, soups, and applesauce. If these mild foods are too hard to eat, you may have to stick to drinking liquids that contain carbohydrate. Try to drink 8 ounces at least every three to four hours. Other high carbohydrate liquids and almost-liquids include juice, frozen juice bars, sherbet, pudding, creamed soups, fruit-flavored yogurt, and broth. To prepare for sick days, have on hand at home a small stock of non-diet soft drinks, broth, applesauce, regular gelatin, and other handy sick-day snacks.

Medicines to Watch Out for When You Are Sick

You may want to take over the counter medicines when you are sick. If you have a cold, you may want to take a cough medicine. Small doses of medicines with sugar are usually okay, but, to be on the safe side, ask your pharmacist or health care provider about sugar-free medicines and medications that won't raise your blood glucose or your blood pressure.

Many medicines you take for short-term illnesses can affect your blood glucose levels, even if they don't contain sugar. For example, aspirin in large doses can lower your blood glucose levels. Some antibiotics lower glucose levels in people with type 2 diabetes who take diabetes pills. Decongestants and some products for treating colds raise your blood glucose levels as well as your blood pressure.

Handy Sick-Day Snacks

Keep the following food and drinks on hand for sick days. Each contains 10 to 15 grams of carbohydrates.

- 1 double-stick popsicle
- 1 cup Gatorade
- 1 cup soup
- 1/2 cup fruit juice
- 1/2 cup regular soft drink (not diet)
- 6 saltines
- 3 graham crackers
- 1 slice dry toast (not light bread)
- 1/3 cup frozen yogurt
- 1/2 cup regular ice cream
- 1/2 cup sugar-free pudding
- 1/2 cup mashed potatoes

Source: Diabetes Care When You're Sick, *by Rachel Gifford, RN, MSN, CDE, and Belinda P. Childs, ARNP, MN, BC-ADM, CDE,* Diabetes Forecast, *February 2005.*

A Trip to the Hospital

No matter how hard you try to stay away, you will most likely be hospitalized a few times in your life. Be proactive, so you'll be ready when and if the time comes. Whether it's a planned hospitalization or an emergency, prepare and keep your recent medical information together in a document, and let your loved one(s) know where it is, so they can take it to the hospital. This document should include your type of diabetes and your current list of medications, including the dosage, route, and time of day you take your medications. Although most hospitals don't allow you to take your own medications from home, take at least a 2-day supply of your meds just in case what you take is not available. This will give the hospital time to get what you need.

Take your blood glucose meter with the understanding that the staff will most likely check your blood glucose with their meter. If you feel low or high or want to check it at any time, you can. They may have to double-check it with the hospital's meter, but at least you are being proactive. If you are on blood glucose–lowering medications, keep a piece of fruit or glucose tablets at your bedside in case you need it before the staff can get it to you. If you take these, tell the staff so they can record it.

When your medications are brought to you, ask the nurse the name of the medications you are receiving. If something sounds unfamiliar, or if you think you are missing something, speak up. Medication errors do happen. When you are ready to go home, make sure you have a medication list that tells you what you are taking and how often to take it.

Wonder?

I am scheduled for surgery and was told not to eat or drink anything after midnight the night before. Can I still take my medicines? If so, can I drink water or eat if I need to take food with my medications?

If you are told to fast, ask for how long, and whether or not that means you should take water with your medications. Make sure all your health care providers know you have diabetes and the entire list of medications (blood glucose–lowering and others) you take. If you are to take your medications, talk with your health care provider to find out whether you need to adjust them during this time. Once again, be proactive. No one else will ask these questions for you, so get the answers you need for any questions you have.

The reason you are in the hospital will dictate whether you will or will not be eating during your stay. Either way, remind your health care providers and hospital staff that you have diabetes. If you are not eating, you will most likely be receiving intravenous (IV) fluids. If you are eating and don't feel you are getting the correct foods, ask to speak with a registered dietitian.

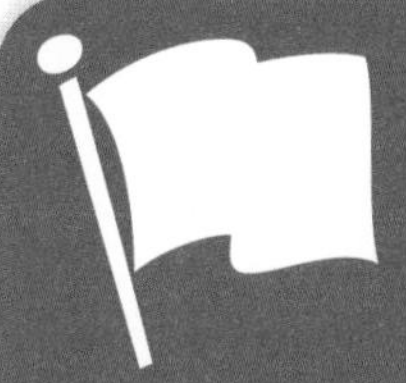

RED FLAG

Disaster Emergency Kit

Don't wait for a disaster to hit, prepare a disaster kit now so you will be ready if a natural disaster ever strikes. Because your prescriptions and medications can change, make sure to inspect your kit at least twice a year so it is up to date. Pick dates when you'll remember to do it (birthdays, anniversaries, etc). Your kit should include at least a week's worth of:

- *oral medicine(s)*
- *injectable medications*
- *injectable medication–delivery supplies*
- *lancets*
- *extra batteries (for your meter, pump, or continuous glucose monitor)*
- *list of emergency contacts*
- *quick-acting source of glucose*
- *moist towlettes, hand cream, and lip balm*
- *a notebook and pen*

Disasters and Emergencies

An emergency or disaster can happen at any time. Whether it's the weather or a terrorist attack, take a few minutes today to gather supplies and discuss your diabetes with your family, friends, and coworkers to help you stay healthy under these stressful circumstances [also check out *Chapter 3*, page 35]. The best resource in these situations is to prepare a disaster kit with everything you need in case of an emergency.

Store at least one week's worth of diabetes supplies in an easy-to-identify container in a location that is convenient to get to in an emergency. If you are a parent of a child with diabetes, keep copies of physician's orders that may be on file with the child's school or day-care provider. When you are away from home, consider discussing your diabetes with those around you, and tell them where your emergency supply kit is stored.

Consider wearing medical identification that will enable colleagues, school staff members, or emergency medical personnel to identify

Wonder?

Can people with diabetes fast for religious or health reasons?

People often fast for religious or health purposes. If you have diabetes, talk to your health care provider about fasting before you begin. Discuss how long you plan to fast. If you are taking blood glucose–lowering medications, your health care provider can advise you on how to adjust your medications while fasting.

and address your medical needs. Emergency medical personnel look for a bracelet or a necklace. If you are a parent of a school-age child with diabetes, ask your child's school to identify staff members who will assist your child in an emergency evacuation.

Do what you can to prevent dehydration. You may not feel thirsty, but ask for water or other no-calorie fluids. You should always have some type of carbohydrate source with you. You don't want your blood glucose high, but it may be a bit higher than your usual targets during times like these [also check out *Chapter 8*, page 101, and *Chapter 15*, page 195].

During emergencies, infectious diseases can be a concern, which can ultimately affect your feet. If you can, avoid walking through contaminated water or injuring your feet. Your feet should be inspected visually on a regular basis (at least daily) for any cuts, sores, blisters, or other problems so you can get proper care. If you have any signs of infection (swelling, redness, and/or drainage from a wound), tell relief workers so you can get immediate medical help.

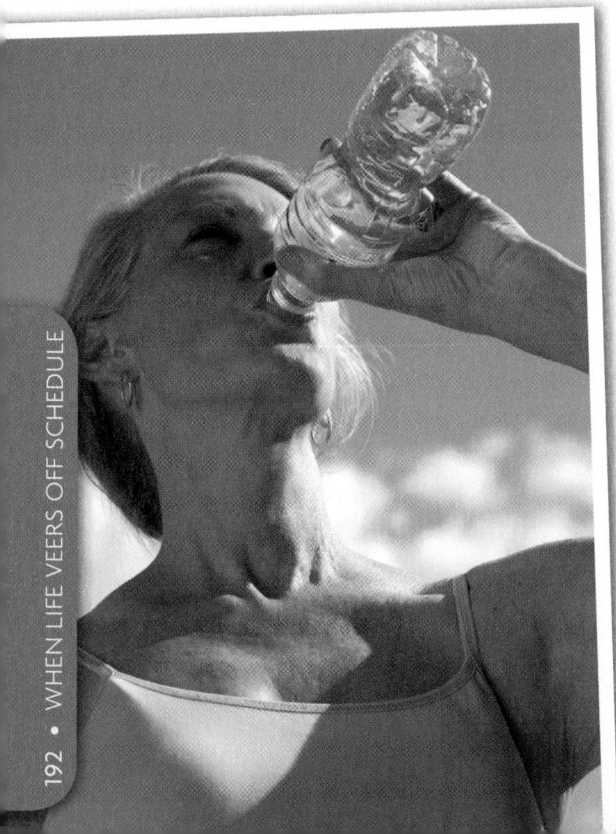

Understanding the medications you are on is one of the most important things you can do to prepare for an emergency [also check out *Chapter 8*, page 101, and *Chapter 9*, page 121]. General advice can only be given here, since some people take no medications, some take oral medications, and some take injectables. If you take insulin, and it's not available, your carbohydrate intake should be reduced. If you have no access to insulin, the most important priority is to maintain an adequate intake of fluids to avoid dehydration. As soon as insulin becomes available, you need to return to your usual insulin regimen, but keep in mind that your insulin requirements may be different due to the stress. Work with the medical staff to see whether you need to make adjustments.

In the affected areas, pharmacies may allow you to get your medications without a prescription if you have your pill bottles. You may take medications for high blood pressure and cholesterol. If you have been without them, these should be restarted. If you have been taking a diuretic, ask the health care personnel helping on the disaster whether you should continue this. If adequate fluids are not available, this can increase your risk of dehydration [also check out *Chapter 9*, page 121]. For more information, visit the CDC Help for People with Diabetes Affected by Natural Disasters at *www.cdc.gov/diabetes/news/hurricanes.htm.*

TIPS + TACTICS

Manage Food at Festive Occasions

Try one or more of these tips to help you manage food when unhealthy foods and beverages abound:

- *Don't arrive famished. It's a set up to overeat.*
- *Peruse the foods being served. Think through your game plan, and set it in motion.*
- *Use a smaller plate, if available, at a cocktail party or buffet.*
- *Fill up on any healthier foods you can find, and enjoy bits and bites of less healthy foods you want to sample.*
- *Implement portion-control tips that work for you at home and in restaurants.*
- *If the function is a potluck affair, bring something healthy that you enjoy.*
- *At a buffet-type function, position yourself far away from the food to limit overeating.*
- *Limit alcohol intake to limit calories and potential problems with high and low blood glucose (depending on the medication you take).*
- *Keep a non-caloric beverage in hand to limit alcohol and food intake, such as club soda or mineral water, water, diet soda, or ice tea.*

When Your Eating Plan Is Derailed

There are days when your schedule goes according to plan, and you eat your meals at ideal times. Then there are other days...they may be weekend days when your reservation for a restaurant meal is earlier or later than your usual meal time, you observe a religious celebration, or partake in a special occasion, such as a family reunion, birthday, or neighborhood barbecue. As you well know, the list of when your eating plan may be off schedule can be endless. That's just the reality of life!

Think about doing the best you can in these situations. Don't beat yourself up for what you couldn't do or how you got off track. Pat yourself on the back for the positive actions you were able to take, and learn from the negative actions. Think about what you could have done differently, to be more successful next time. Could you have adjusted the amount or timing of your medication, not have arrived so hungry, or consumed less alcohol?

The biggest concern in delaying meals is low blood glucose. If you take a blood glucose–lowering medication that can cause your blood glucose to get too low, you'll need to make adjustments, such as eating a snack or taking your medications a little later.

If you take a rapid-acting insulin, take these medications a few minutes before you start to eat rather than at your usual meal time. If you take the oral pills repaglinide or nateglinide, which lower blood glucose after you eat, then you should take these medications a few minutes before you start to eat rather than at your usual meal time. If you take a pre-mixed combination of insulin, it becomes more important for you to eat on time to prevent low blood glucose. (Note: A disadvantage of these insulin regimens is that they do not allow much flexibility in meal times.) If you regularly need more flexibility in your schedule, talk to your health care providers about this need.

Learn from your experiences. Because of the large variation in responses to blood glucose from food and insulin among individuals, you can learn how to fine-tune your control by recording your experiences for future reference. Keep notes of your responses to various foods and activities in a notebook, computer file, or logbook. Although perfect control is impossible, your personal experiences can help you adjust to many different situations you encounter in everyday life [also check out *Chapter 13*, page 163].

When Your Physical Activity Is Off Schedule

Physical activity causes you to use your insulin more efficiently, whether it is the insulin your body makes or the insulin you take. Therefore, when you are off schedule, this means that if you are more active, you are at a higher risk for a low blood glucose level. If you are less active than usual, your blood glucose will most likely be higher. Keep these principles in mind during times of more or less physical activity. Monitor more often to see how your blood glucose is reacting so you will know how to manage your diabetes during these times [also check out *Chapter 7*, page 89].

DEFINITION:

counter-regulatory hormones: hormones made by various organs in your body that raise your blood glucose level in response to stress or other reactions.

When Your Body Is Off Schedule

Besides your schedule being off, there are times your body is off schedule. If you are a woman, you will find that pre-menstrual and menstrual cycles will affect your blood glucose as well as peri-menopause and menopause. Man or woman, you may just be sick, in pain, on a new medication, or stressed. Your counter-regulatory hormones may kick in at these times and cause havoc with your diabetes management [also check out *Chapter 15*, page 195]. You will need to be aware of these times, monitor more often, and use the principles you have learned when you work with your health care provider and adjust for your bodily changes [also check out *Chapter 17*, page 219, and *Chapter 19*, page 237].

Psst...

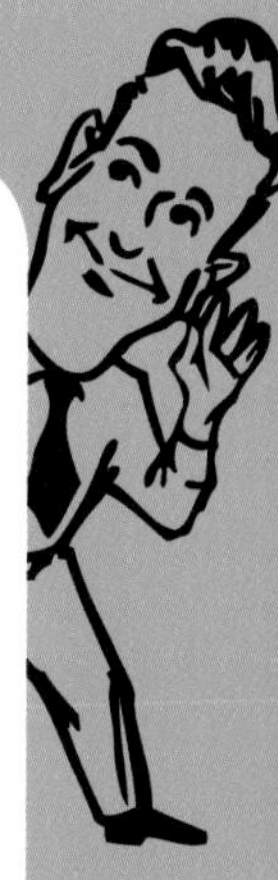

Need a Change in Your Blood Glucose–Lowering Meds?

A positive change in the management of diabetes is that there are new oral and injectable blood glucose–lowering medications, including new types of insulin that better mesh with the realities of life today. Several of these medications help your health care providers and you work out a medication schedule that best controls your blood glucose while allowing you the flexibility you need to live your life in the manner that best suits your needs. If you are off schedule regularly in your life, discuss this with your health care providers. They need to know your habits and lifestyle to help you find a medication plan that suits you [also check out *Chapter 8*, page 101].

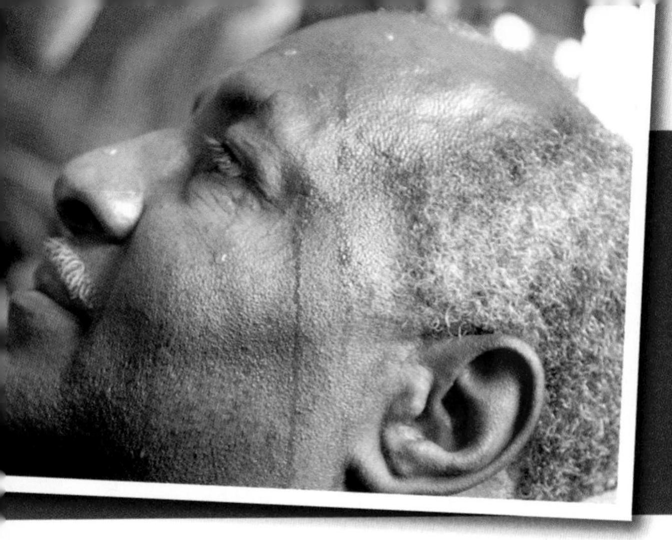

CHAPTER 15

Glucose Highs and Lows

Managing the ups and downs of your blood glucose level is an everyday challenge. How high and low your blood glucose goes depends on whether you have type 1 or 2 diabetes, how well your blood glucose is controlled, and the blood glucose–lowering medications you take. All factors considered, people with type 2 typically have less dramatic swings in their blood glucose levels than people with type 1. The challenge people with type 2 often face is high blood glucose levels that are sustained over prolonged periods of time, without even knowing or experiencing symptoms. Any prolonged exposure to high blood glucose levels can cause damage to the body's tissues and organs, and eventually may cause one or more diabetes complications.

The key to controlling your blood glucose is to check your blood glucose levels regularly. You have a life to lead and shouldn't have to spend it being worried about blood glucose lows or highs. The tips in this chapter will help you understand, recognize, and treat the symptoms of high and low blood glucose to minimize their interference with your life.

What You'll Learn:

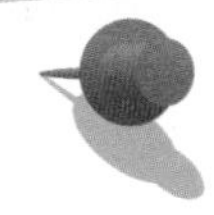

- Common signs and symptoms of mild, moderate, and severe hypoglycemia (low blood glucose)
- How to prevent hypoglycemia before it happens
- Your individual risk for hypoglycemia
- Tips and tactics for treating hypoglycemia
- How to detect and manage hyperglycemia (high blood glucose)
- How to act as your own advocate to keep your blood glucose levels under control over the years

Your Risks For Hypoglycemia

Your individual risk for hypoglycemia depends on the type of diabetes you have and the blood glucose–lowering medications you take. Not everyone with diabetes is at risk for hypoglycemia. You are at risk only if you take insulin or take one or more of the other blood glucose–lowering medications that can cause your glucose to get too low. If you have type 2 diabetes and take no blood glucose–lowering medications or only take ones that aren't known to cause lows, you have no risk of hypoglycemia.

According to research, if you have type 2 diabetes and are taking one or more blood glucose medications that can cause low blood glucose, you may experience mild to moderate hypoglycemia with symptoms almost 16 times per year. Severe low blood glucose will still be infrequent—about once every five years. The longer you have diabetes, the more likely you are to require blood glucose–lowering medications, which causes your chances of hypoglycemia to be higher.

If you have type 1 diabetes and take insulin, you are the most at risk for hypoglycemia and may experience mild to moderate hypoglycemia, on average, about 43 times a year. You may have a severe low blood glucose reaction around twice a year.

As you can see, your frequency of hypoglycemia depends on your type of diabetes and which medications you are on. On page 197 is a graphic of the blood glucose–lowering medications that will or won't cause hypoglycemia.

Myth

Everyone with diabetes has frequent low blood glucose reactions

Fact

No! The frequency of low blood glucose reactions usually depends on the type of diabetes you have and the blood glucose–lowering medicines you take.

How Hypoglycemia Works

Hypoglycemia is the technical name for low blood glucose when your blood glucose level is less than 70 mg/dl. Keep in mind that it isn't always necessary for your blood glucose to dip below 70 mg/dl for you to experience symptoms of hypoglycemia. You may have signs and symptoms if you have just begun to get your blood glucose under control or if you take a blood glucose–lowering medication that can cause low blood glucose.

Repeated hypoglycemia is not a cause of long-term diabetes complications; however, the lack of glucose available for your brain and the rest of your body can be dangerous and put you at risk of other complications. You might not respond as quickly when you are driving or using mechanical devices. This can be dangerous if your thought processes and reflexes aren't as sharp as they usually are. You are at risk for having an accident or saying something you may later regret.

Blood Glucose–Lowering Medicines

Does cause Hypoglycemia		Doesn't usually cause Hypoglycemia	
Category	**Examples**	**Category**	**Examples**
PILLS YOU TAKE BY MOUTH			
Sulfonylureas glimepiride, glipizide, glyburide	Amaryl, Glucotrol, Diabeta, Micronase	Biquanides	Metformin, Glucophage
Meglitinides	Prandin	Glitazones	Actos, Avandia
D-phenylalanine	Starlix	Alpha-glucosidase inhibitor	Precose, Glyset
Dipeptidyl peptidease-IV inhibitors (DPP-4)	Januvia		
MEDICINES YOU INJECT			
Insulin	All types	Exenatide	Byetta
		Pramlintide	Symlin

Note: It is common for people to take more than one medication or a pill that contains two types of medicine. Combining these medicines may cause hypoglycemia.

Stages of hypoglycemia

Stage:	Signs and Symptoms:
Mild	shakiness; trembling; sweating; blurred vision; dizziness (feeling lightheaded); not thinking; clearly; feeling nervous or anxious; being weak; numbness or tingling around mouth and lips; fatigue; headache; sudden hunger; nausea; heart beating fast
Moderate	irritablity; agitation; confusion; lack of coordination; personality change; difficulty speaking
Severe	confusion; becoming unconscious; having seizures or convulsions; unable to treat the low blood glucose by yourself; need help from another person

Hypoglycemia typically occurs for one of four reasons:

- Taking too much insulin or other blood glucose–lowering medication
- Not eating enough food, or delaying or skipping a meal; especially if you are on a glucose–lowering medication
- Being more physically active than usual without taking less medicine or eating more
- Drinking alcohol can cause low blood glucose hours after you drink if you don't eat enough food

At the beginning of a hypoglycemic reaction, you may start to feel dizzy, nauseous, weak, sweaty, or faint. If left untreated, you could experience seizures or even lose consciousness. Different people can experience

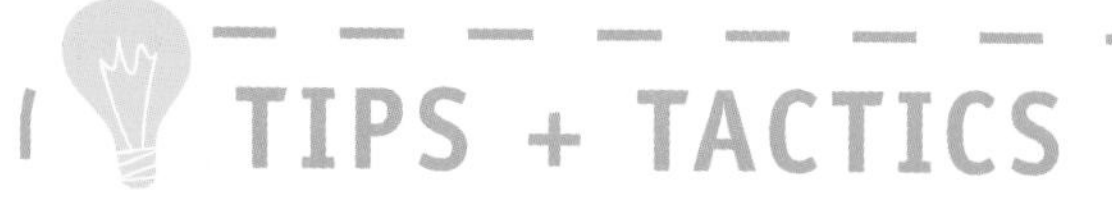

TIPS + TACTICS

Tips to be prepared for blood glucose lows

- *Wear medical identification that identifies you as someone with diabetes—a bracelet or necklace is best [also check out* Psst: Medical IDs to Fit Your Life, *below].*
- *Carry your blood glucose meter and supplies at all times. If you have signs and symptoms, you'll be able to check for hypoglycemia.*
- *Keep treatments for lows in places where you spend a lot of time: desk drawers, your nightstand, purse, backpack, and glove compartment of your car.*
- *Check your blood glucose before you drive a vehicle. Make sure your levels are in a safe range.*
- *If your blood glucose is low before bed, consume 15 grams of carbohydrate to prevent nighttime hypoglycemia.*

Psst...

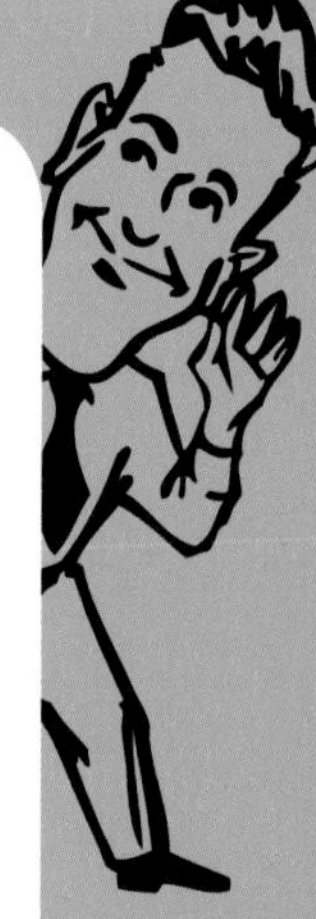

Medical IDs to Fit Your Life

Gone are the days where wearing a medical identification tag meant a thick, unattractive, heavy bracelet. Today's IDs are smaller and more attractive, and can fit almost anywhere. Medical IDs today include temporary tattoos, wristbands, cell phone tags, or beaded bracelets. They can be worn around your wrist, ankle, or neck, or even attached to the front of your shoes. While fashion is great, don't forget the function of the medical ID: It needs to be seen in case of an emergency, so make sure it's located somewhere that emergency personal will notice right away. Along with wearing it somewhere visible, make sure you choose an ID that you will be able to wear all the time. Ask yourself these questions: Is it comfortable to wear? Is it durable enough to survive everyday life?

No matter what shape or size ID you choose, make sure it's large enough to contain all of your vital information. It needs to include your name, medical condition, and at least one phone number for a dependable emergency contact. Order your identification bracelet or necklace today at *www.diabeteswellness.net, www.laurenshope.com, www.coolmedid.com, www.medicassist.com, www.medicids.com,* or *www.medicalert.com.*

different symptoms, so it's important to understand what signals your body is sending you during a low blood glucose reaction.

While most instances of hypoglycemia start with similar symptoms, there are three very different stages of hypoglycemia: mild, moderate, and severe. Your symptoms may start off as mild, but if left untreated, they can progress and even lead to unconsciousness or seizures, which can be dangerous.

How to Treat Mild and Moderate Hypoglycemia

According to the ADA, the best treatment for a mild or moderate low blood glucose reaction is to consume 15 to 20 grams of pure glucose (such as glucose tablets or gel). A source of pure glucose is better than carbohydrate from a food or beverage, such as chocolate or peanut butter because it will raise blood glucose faster; however, if you find yourself without a source of pure glucose (tablets or gel), 15 grams of any source of carbohydrate should help raise your blood glucose level back to normal.

When you have mild to moderate hypoglycemia, you should still be aware enough to treat yourself. When your blood glucose is low, it's easy to over-treat or over-eat because you may be panicked and very hungry. Try to resist because over-treating or over-eating will just raise your blood glucose too high.

Diabetes experts, including the ADA, encourage you to use the following 15/15 guideline for treating hypoglycemia. (This guideline is not intended to replace any instructions you have received from your health care provider.)

Step 1: If you have checked your blood glucose and it is below 70 mg/dl, or you have signs and symptoms of low blood glucose, consume 15 grams of carbohydrate [also check out *Red Flag: Portable Sources of 15 Grams of Carbohydrate*, this page].

Step 2: Wait 15 minutes, then check your blood glucose again. If your blood glucose is still low, consume another 15 grams of carbohydrate.

Step 3: Recheck your blood glucose 15 minutes later.

Continue this cycle until you see your blood glucose rise. (If you don't have a meter with you, continue this cycle until you start feeling better.) Once your blood glucose is back up into your target range, get back to the activity you were engaged in. If it will be several hours before you eat a meal or snack, and you feel your blood glucose may go too low again, eat a small snack.

RED FLAG

Portable Sources of 15 Grams of Carbohydrate

- *3–4 glucose tablets*
- *1 tube of glucose gel or liquid*
- *Small box (4 ounces) of 100% fruit juice*
- *Hard candy (peppermints, Life Savers, or TicTacs)*
- *Sugar cubes or packets (1 teaspoon – 4 g carbs)*
- *Small box of raisins (2 tablespoons) or other dried fruit*
- *Low or fat-free milk (8 ounces/1 cup)*
- *Regular soft drink (not diet) – ½ cup*
- *1 small piece of fruit*

Myth

Chocolate candy or other high-fat sweets are good treatments for low blood glucose

Fact

The fat in chocolate and other high-fat sweets may actually slow the rise of blood glucose and prolong the low blood glucose reaction.

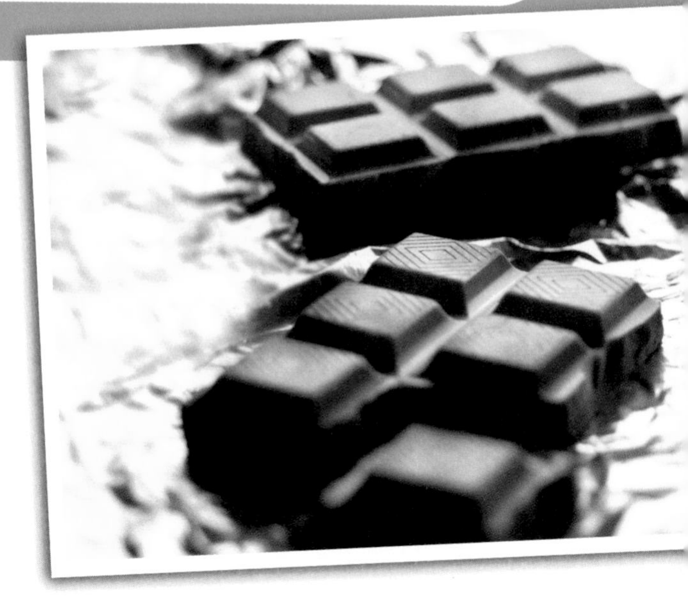

How to Treat Severe Hypoglycemia

Experts define a severe reaction as needing help from another person because of confusion or even unconsciousness. If you are at risk for severe hypoglycemia, make sure your family and friends are aware and know how to help you if this occurs.

The treatment for severe hypoglycemia with unconsciousness is glucagon. Glucagon is a hormone that is normally made in the pancreas and raises blood glucose. The ADA suggests that glucagon be prescribed for anyone who is at risk of severe low blood glucose. Don't wait for severe hypoglycemia to hit; ask your health care provider for a prescription if you are at risk. If you take insulin, you should have glucagon available.

Glucagon needs to be injected. It comes in a kit that you can take with you. Glucagon kits have an expiration date, so make sure to check at least twice a year to make sure that your glucagon hasn't expired. If your family members or friends aren't comfortable giving you glucagon, make sure they know to call 911 immediately if you become unconscious.

Even though you think you can recognize when your blood glucose is low, it's still best to check your blood glucose to verify. Some of the symptoms of hyperglycemia and hypoglycemia are the same. If you are not sure if your blood glucose is high or low, and you don't have a meter with you, treat it as a low. It is not dangerous for you to take 15 grams of carbohydrate if you are high, as it is if you take insulin if you are low.

Preventing Hypoglycemia

The best way to avoid problems associated with hypoglycemia is to understand what causes hypoglycemia and do your best to prevent it. As mentioned earlier in this chapter, the four main causes of hypoglycemia are:

- taking too much insulin or other blood glucose–lowering medication
- not eating enough or skipping meals
- being more physically active than normal
- drinking alcohol without eating

By being aware of your blood glucose and taking action to avoid or manage these situations, you can prevent a majority of hypoglycemia events.

Try not to skip or delay meals. If it seems that you'll have to miss or delay a meal, bring a snack with you or purchase some food. Keep a few portable and perishable snacks close at hand. Crackers, string cheese, pretzels, nuts, and fruit juice are always good to have around.

When it comes to medication, try to take your blood glucose–lowering medication at about the same time every day. If you need a more flexible schedule or you want to learn how to adjust your medicine for those occasions when your mealtimes or activity times will change, ask your health care provider how to best plan around changing schedules.

If you are going to drink alcohol, make sure to eat some form of carbohydrate when you drink, to prevent a low. Check your blood glucose before you go to sleep if you have been drinking. If you blood glucose is low, eat some carbohydrate and protein to prevent nighttime hypoglycemia [also check out *Chapter 18*, page 229].

Wonder?

What is hypoglycemia unawareness?

Hypoglycemia unawareness is a state in which you do not feel or recognize the symptoms of hypoglycemia. If you have frequent episodes of hypoglycemia, you may no longer experience the warning signs. If you have nerve damage, epinephrine is not released on time, and there are no warning symptoms [also check out *Chapter 21*, page 257]. Over time, your body gradually adapts itself to hypoglycemia, so it takes lower blood glucose levels to cause a release of epinephrine and warning symptoms; however, your brain does not adapt to these lower numbers, so your first signal of a low can be confusion or passing out. At that point, you are experiencing a severe low and need help.

The ADA suggests that people who have hypoglycemia unawareness be advised by their health care provider to raise their blood glucose goals for a time period. This action helps prevent severe lows and help your body get resensitized to feel the symptoms of low blood glucose.

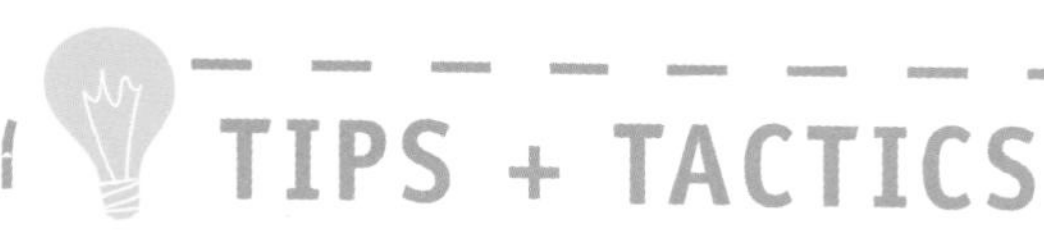

Steps to Take to Prevent Low Blood Glucose if You Delay a Meal

If you take insulin or another blood glucose–lowering medication that can cause low blood glucose, and you delay eating, this can cause your blood glucose to get too low. Take precautions to prevent this by following these steps:

- *Check your blood glucose at the usual time of your meal.*
- *If your blood glucose is high (> 150 mg/dl), you can wait a short time before you eat without concern. But check again if you feel your blood glucose is getting too low before your meal.*
- *If your blood glucose level is around your pre-meal goal (70–130 mg/dl) and you feel it will fall too low before you get to eat, eat some carbohydrate (start with 15 grams) to make sure your blood glucose doesn't go too low before your meal.*
- *If you delay your meal more than one hour, and your blood glucose is around your pre-meal goal, you may need to eat more than 15 grams of carbohydrate to keep it from going too low before your meal.*

Lows During the Night

Hypoglycemia can be dangerous at any time, but there is an extra concern about hypoglycemia during the night when you are asleep. This is called nocturnal hypoglycemia. Studies show that 50% of severe blood glucose reactions happen between midnight and 8:00 a.m. This can happen because sleep stops the output of hormones the body normally puts out to counteract hypoglycemia—these are called counter-regulatory hormones. Most of the time, low blood glucose levels during the night will wake you up; however, this is not always the case, and it can be deadly if your blood glucose gets very low and you don't get treatment. Once again, prevention is your best insurance.

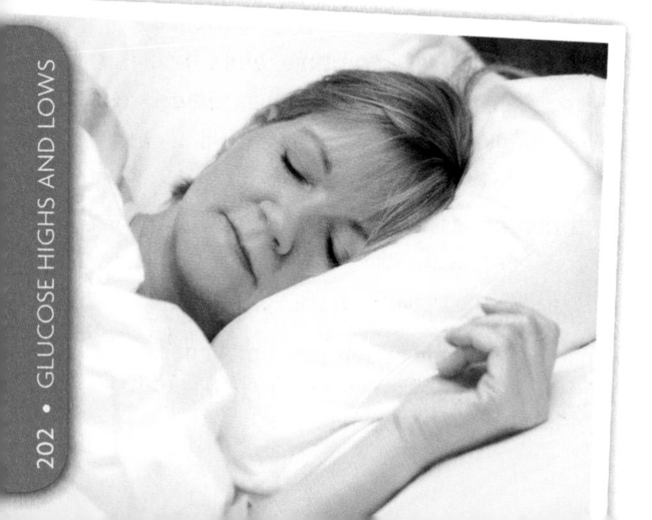

Know your targets. Talk with your health care provider about your personal targets, including bedtime targets, and know your risk for nocturnal hypoglycemia and the best ways to prevent it. Check your blood glucose before you go to bed. Although this is not a guarantee that you won't become hypoglycemic during the night, it does provide you with an opportunity to treat a blood glucose level that is too low to go to bed with [also check out *Chapter 5*, page 59].

Another important note is to report this problem to your health care provider. It is likely that you need to make some changes in your diabetes care plan to minimize or eliminate noctural hypoglycemia.

Hyperglycemia: Glucose on the High Side

Hyperglycemia (or high blood glucose) for extended periods is a major cause of many of the long-term complications that occur in people who have diabetes. For this reason, it's important to know what hyperglycemia is, what its symptoms are, and how to treat it.

Hyperglycemia is the technical term for blood glucose levels that are over 130 mg/dl before meals and over 180 mg/dl 1–2 hours after you eat. If your blood glucose levels are higher than these numbers but not above 250 mg/dl, you might not experience symptoms of hyperglycemia. The most common symptoms of hyperglycemia are frequent urination, intense thirst, fatigue, and hunger; the same symptoms you may have had when you first learned you had diabetes.

A number of things can cause hyperglycemia. If you have type 1 diabetes, you might not have given yourself enough insulin. If you have type 2 diabetes, your body may still make some insulin, but it is not as effective as it should be to keep your blood glucose at normal levels. The stress of an illness or infection, such as a cold or flu, could be the cause, along with other stresses like family conflicts or school or dating problems [also check out *Chapter 14*, page 181, and *Chapter 19*, page 237].

Every hour or day that your blood glucose is higher than your target range, damage can be done to your tissues and organs. It's important to work with your health care provider to develop a plan to get and keep your blood glucose levels under control. Don't assume that because you don't have symptoms of hyperglycemia that you are fine. Be your own advocate and take action, work with your health care provider to progress your therapy, and get your blood glucose under better control [also check out *Chapter 8*, page 101].

Wonder?

Should I only contact my health care provider when my blood glucose is high and I'm not feeling well, or anytime my blood glucose is higher than normal?

That depends on you, your blood glucose targets, and what you and your health care provider decide upon. Ask your health care provider so you will know. Discuss a plan of when you should make contact, along with what to do when your numbers are high. When in doubt, check it out. It never hurts to make the contact.

Risks of Hyperglycemia

With diabetes, the occasional raised blood glucose over 180 mg/dl can be expected from time to time, particularly if you have been stressed or ill, or have not been receiving the correct amount of insulin or blood glucose–lowering medications. The key is to monitor and learn how to keep these episodes at a minimum so you don't experience either short- or long-term complications [also check out *Chapter 21*, page 257].

A brief spell of hyperglycemia may cause you some discomfort but won't have an impact on your long-term health; however, if your blood glucose levels are consistently high, you are at risk for both short-term (acute) and long-term (chronic) complications [also check out *Chapter 21*, page 257].

The most common short-term complications of hyperglycemia are diabetic ketoacidosis (DKA) and hyperosmolar hyperglycemic nonketotic syndrome (HHS). DKA most often occurs in people with type 1 diabetes. HHS is fairly uncommon except in older people with type 2 diabetes.

DKA AND HHS

DKA begins when there is a lack of insulin in your body, which means that you are unable to get glucose into your cells for energy. When this occurs, your body begins to break down fat as an alternative energy source. The by-product of fat breakdown is ketones. Ketones make your body acidic and can cause nausea, vomiting, or abdominal pain. If left untreated, DKA can cause a coma or be potentially fatal, so it's important to seek medical treatment immediately. DKA is fairly easy to treat in the hospital; treatment consists of an intravenous infusion of insulin, along with an infusion of fluids and potassium. While people with type 2 diabetes rarely get DKA, it's typically only necessary to check for ketones if your blood glucose is over 300 mg/dl or if you feel ill.

HHS occurs almost exclusively in people with type 2 diabetes and typically only affects older people. HHS occurs primarily in people who have restricted mobility, such as the elderly or people who cannot take adequate care of themselves. HHS occurs as blood glucose levels get higher and higher, urine output goes up, and dehydration occurs. Extreme dehydration eventually leads to confusion and can eventually lead to seizures, coma, and death. HHS is treated with insulin and large amount of fluids, usually given intravenously to restore fluid balance and blood flow to your brain, heart, kidneys, liver, and limbs, to help prevent a heart attack, stroke, kidney failure, or other problems.

Psst...

Drink, Drink, Drink

When your blood glucose is high, you are at risk for dehydration. When you are dehydrated, you are at risk for high blood glucose. So, pick up that glass of water and drink! If you can't drink water, choose any drink that has no calories and no carbohydrate. When you get older, you may lose your sense of thirst, but drink anyway. If you are unable to walk very well, or are in a nursing home, don't stop drinking for fear you will have to get up and urinate. Make sure there is always water nearby, and drink, drink, drink.

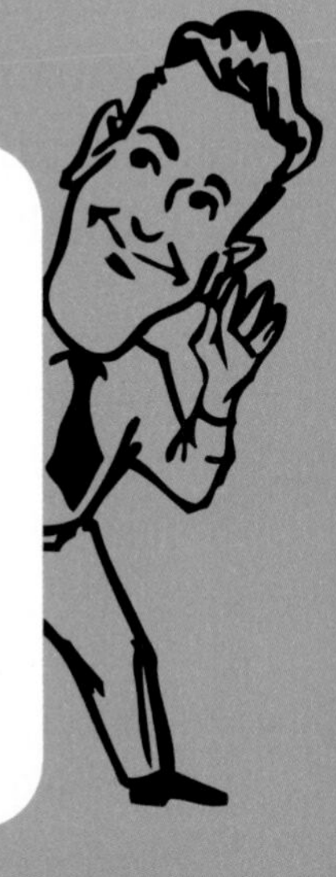

Wonder?

How do I check for ketones?

There are two ways to check for ketones: urine testing and blood testing. Although you can detect ketones in your blood before you will be able to detect them in your urine, at this time, most people check for ketones in their urine. There is only one meter on the market that checks for ketones in your blood.

Test strips for urine ketone testing come in either individually wrapped foil or a bottle (the individually wrapped strips tend to stay good for longer). Collect a sample of urine in a cup or some other clean container, dip the test stick in your urine, remove the stick, wait for the number of seconds suggested by the manufacturer's instructions, and compare it to the color on the instructions. (For more specific instructions, read the manufacturer's instructions.)

Reasons Behind and Treatments for Hyperglycemia

To be able to accurately treat your hyperglycemia, you must first understand what is causing it and be able to take action to keep it from happening. Checking your blood glucose often is the first step to prevention and treatment. Ask your health care provider how often you should check and what your blood glucose levels should be. Checking your blood glucose to prevent and treat high blood glucose early will help you limit complications of hyperglycemia.

The most common causes of hyperglycemia have to do with either a decrease in your physical activity or an increased amount of food consumption. Regulating both of these aspects can help minimize your bouts of hyperglycemia. If you are going to overeat, learn how to adjust your blood glucose–lowering medications (if you can) or your activity level to counteract the additional food.

Stress and hormonal changes in your body can also lead to hyperglycemia. They can work against the insulin in your body to raise blood glucose levels. Women may find that their blood glucose levels are higher at certain stages of their menstrual cycle or during menopause. Monitor your blood glucose levels closely around these changing hormonal times and take action to keep them from affecting you in the long run.

Illness can also cause increased blood glucose levels because glycogen is released into your bloodstream, while increased amounts of cortisol and epinephrine (stress hormones) are released as well. These hormones prevent your insulin from working correctly, which can cause elevated blood glucose levels. If you're sick, be sure to check your blood glucose levels more often than you normally would. This allows you to react quickly and make adjustments to your medications.

If you are doing everything you can, and your blood glucose remains elevated, talk with your health care provider. You may just need an adjustment in your medications or another medication. Just because you were started on one medication, or a particular dose of a medication, remember, type 2 diabetes is a progressive disease. You may need more. It's not that you have done anything wrong, and it's not your fault. Your goal is to get and keep your blood glucose in your target range.

Once you know the reasons behind high blood glucose levels, it will be easier to know how to treat it. The reason behind your hyperglycemia typically determines the treatment for it. If you have been overeating, talk with your heath care provider about ways to get your eating habits under control. The solution may be to decrease your food intake, increase your physical activity, or add medications.

If you can't establish the cause of your hyperglycemia, talk to your health care provider about finding the cause and treating it. Don't keep quiet. You are the one who needs to get your blood glucose under control to prevent the short- and long-term complications.

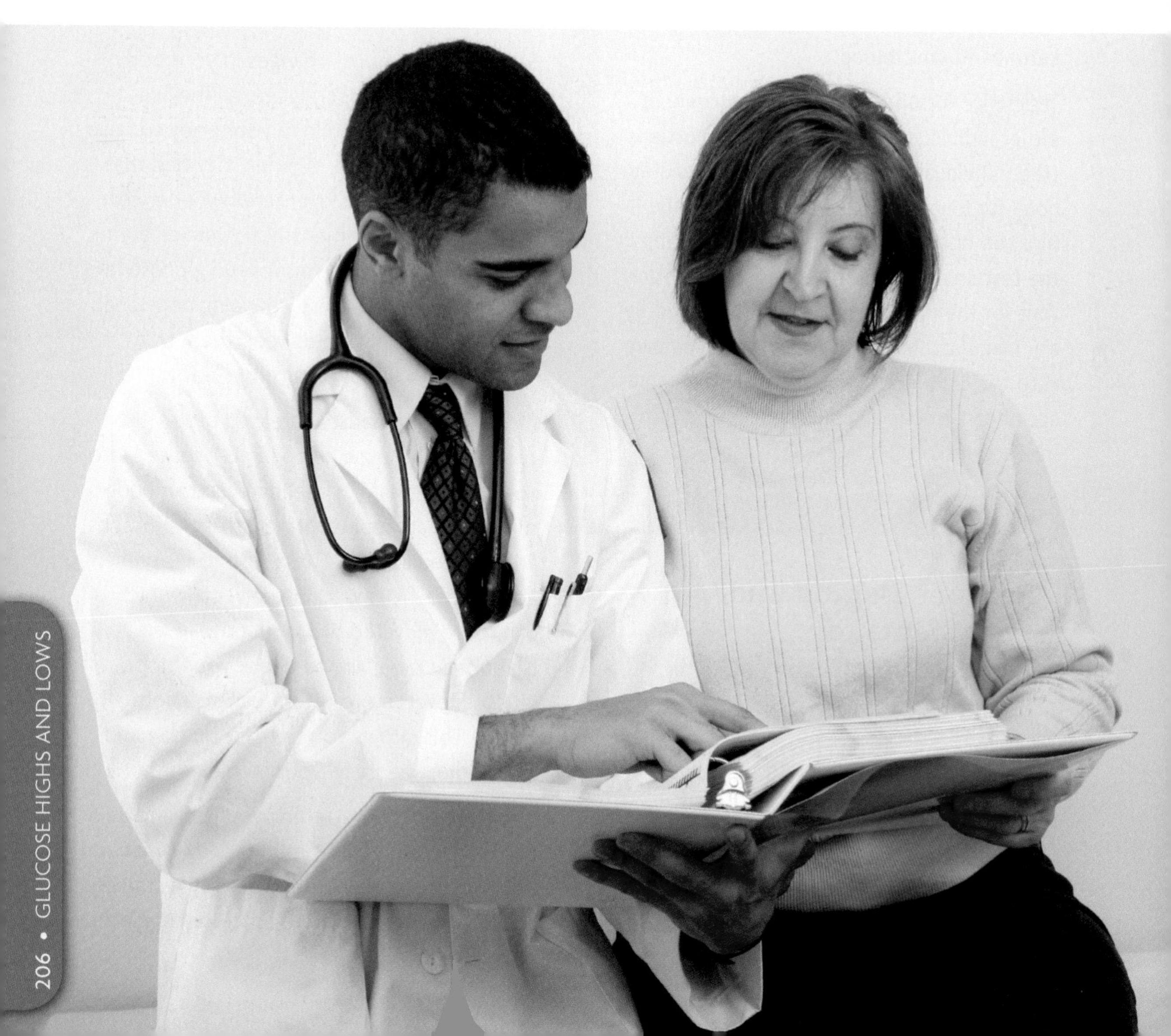

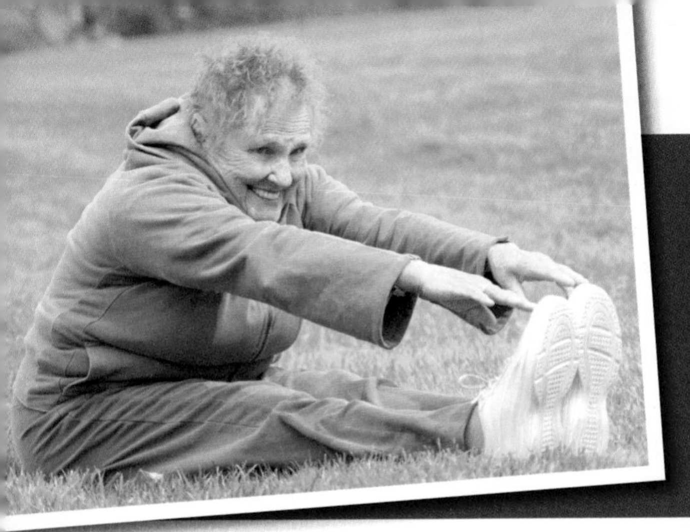

CHAPTER 16

Lose Weight, Keep It Off

It takes a lot more than knowing what to eat, how much to eat, and the amount of exercise you need to lose weight and keep it off. It requires a lot of DOING! Once you've put on pounds during adulthood, it's tougher to shed those pounds and even tougher to keep them off over. There's no magic formula [also check out *Chapter 4*, page 49], but there is good news in store! Research shows that a small amount of weight loss, even 10 to 20 pounds, can prevent and/or delay pre-diabetes and slow the progression of type 2. Weight loss can also provide BIG payback when it comes to your health, longevity, and quality of life. It's better to lose a few pounds and keep it off, than to lose a lot of weight only to regain it quickly.

The benefits of weight loss are abundant. Some benefits affect your health, while others affect social and employment-related aspects of your life, as well as your ability to be active and engaged in life. You can experience one, two, or more of these health benefits by losing just a few pounds (5 to 7% of your starting weight).

It's important to first understand what a healthy weight is for you. If you are overweight or obese, set a realistic weight-loss goal and determine the best way for you to lose that weight and keep it off. Will you be able to lose weight with healthy eating and physical activity alone, or are there weight-loss medications or surgery options you should speak to your health care provider about?

What You'll Learn:

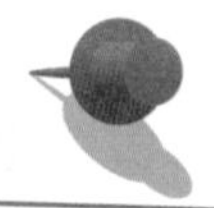

- The many benefits of weight loss
- How weight loss can help you manage your diabetes
- How to know if you're at a healthy weight, overweight, or obese
- How much is enough weight to lose
- The best way to lose weight
- Whether you should take weight-loss medications or are a candidate for weight-loss surgery
- What researchers and people who have succeeded say it takes to keep weight off over time

Body Mass Index (BMI)

Body Mass Index (BMI) has become the primary way that health care providers determine whether you are at a healthy weight, overweight, or obese. Unfortunately, the number of people who have gone from a healthy weight to overweight or obese has been steadily escalating. Being overweight refers to carrying an excess of body weight in the form of excess fat; however, a person can be overweight without having excess fat, such as a large football player.

According to the BMI categories [also check out *Chapter 1*, page 5], you fall into the overweight category if you are 1 to 30 pounds above your healthy weight, and anything more than 30 pounds over your ideal weight is considered obese. Some research suggests that the risk of heart disease and stroke increases progressively with a BMI greater than 20. Research also shows that the location on the body of the excess fat plays a role in health risks. The fat in the abdomen is associated with insulin resistance, so if you're carrying a

Psst...

Health Benefits of Losing Weight and Keeping It Off

- Reduce insulin resistance and increase insulin sensitivity.
- Reduce glucose and need for medication.
- Improve blood lipids and need for medication.
- Reduce blood pressure and need for medication.
- Reduce chance of heart attack and/or stroke.
- Reduce chance of gallbladder disease.
- Reduce problems with bones and joints (orthopedic and arthritis).
- Reduce problems with getting quality sleep (sleep apnea, other breathing problems).
- Reduce some cancers (breast, colon, kidney).
- Reduce stress incontinence (urine leakage).
- Reduce depression.
- Decrease risk with surgery when/if needed.
- Decrease risk during pregnancies.

By the Numbers

The number of American adults and children who are overweight has grown dramatically over the last few decades.

Adults over 20 years of age who are overweight (includes overweight and obese defined by BMI): Total = 134 million (66%)

- Women = 64 million (62%)
- Men = 68 million (71%)

Adults over 20 years of age of are who are obese: Total = 64 million (31%)

- Women = 35 million (33%)
- Men = 29 million (30%)

Children

- About 17% ages 2–19 are overweight
- About 5 million are obese

Source: National Center for Health Statistics (www.cdc.gov/nchs/).

majority of your fat in your abdomen, you are at a greater risk of several diseases [also check out *Chapter 1: How the Shape of Your Body Can Determine Your Health*, page 20].

For most people, it's neither realistic nor necessary to get to an ideal body weight (your weight when you were a young adult or your ideal weight according to those height/weight charts) once you have become overweight or obese. You can derive many health and other benefits by losing a small amount of weight and then working to maintain that small amount of lost weight.

For most people, losing weight is the easy part, and maintaining it is the hard work [also check out *Tips and Tactics: Keep the Weight Off*, page 215]. In fact, it's better to lose a small amount of weight (10 to 20 pounds) and try to maintain this healthier weight over a few months. If you want to lose more weight, try it in a few months. One problem with losing a large amount of weight is that it is difficult to maintain the weight loss and not get into yet another yo-yo cycle. Remember: Any weight you lose is a move in the right direction. In fact, preventing any further weight gain is an accomplishment worth praising [also check out *By the Numbers: Annual Weight Gain*, this page].

By the Numbers

Annual Weight Gain

On average, U.S. adults gain 1 to 2 pounds every year during adulthood. Add up these pounds and you will see how this slow and steady weight gain can result in 10–20 pounds per decade. That's enough extra weight to push a person at risk of type 2 diabetes to pre-diabetes or even type 2 and/or other chronic diseases. Because people are becoming overweight earlier in life, we are seeing more children, adolescents, and young adults are developing pre- and type 2 diabetes than ever before.

Improving Glucose Levels With Weight Loss and Medication

The point at which a small amount of weight loss (5 to 10%) is most likely to improve your blood glucose is when you first learn you have type 2 diabetes (as long as it is early enough in the process) or even more so, if/when you are diagnosed with pre-diabetes.

Losing weight early on helps your body become less insulin-resistant and more sensitive to the insulin your body still makes. In fact, blood glucose can plummet with only a few pounds lost. Over time, as type 2 diabetes progresses and you lose your ability to make sufficient insulin, weight loss and physical activity alone will not be enough to control your blood glucose. You will likely need one or more blood glucose–lowering medications.

Research shows that you and your health care providers can observe whether your healthier eating habits and weight loss are working to help you lose weight anywhere from six weeks to three months. You can do this by tracking your blood glucose levels and observing if you are hitting your desired targets [also check out *Chapter 2*, page 23].

If you have been diligent with healthy eating and physical activity, and your blood glucose levels have not reached your targets, then it is likely that you'll need to start taking a blood glucose–lowering medication NOW. Don't think of this as failure, and don't resist going on a blood glucose–lowering medication.

The more time your blood glucose levels are elevated, the more damage there is to your organs and tissues from high blood glucose. Don't avoid certain foods, such as those that contain carbohydrate, which raises blood glucose, as a means of avoiding the initiation of blood glucose–lowering medication. Research in both people with pre-diabetes and type 2 diabetes shows that because the loss of insulin production is so great even in pre-diabetes, blood glucose–lowering medications (one or more) are needed early on [also check out *Chapter 1*, page 5].

This is also true for insulin when other blood glucose–lowering medications no longer help you hit your targets. Too many people with type 2 diabetes and their health care providers spend too much time putting off the inevitable insulin injections. A word to the wise: If your health care provider suggests it, don't resist! You will likely feel better once you have adjusted to being on it.

Any progress you have made with weight loss and leading a healthier lifestyle is beneficial to your health. Keep up your new habits. Healthier eating and being active will always help you manage your diabetes. It simply means that your type 2 diabetes is progressing and that you are either not making enough insulin and/or have too much insulin resistance to manage these situations without medication to address these issues.

Myth

Once you are on blood glucose–lowering medication, you can't get off even if you lose weight

Fact

Your glucose might be high enough when you are diagnosed to make it necessary for you to take a blood glucose–lowering medication, but because blood glucose can plummet with a few pounds lost, you may be able to lower your medication dose or get off the medication for a time. If you are on a blood glucose–lowering medication that can make your blood glucose too low [also check out *Chapter 8*, page 101] and are experiencing low blood glucose, talk to your health care provider immediately. Ask about taking less or discontinuing the medication. Keep in mind that, as the years go on, your insulin reserve will likely dwindle, and you'll need to take medication [also check out *Chapter 1*, page 5].

Eating to Lose Weight

The latest nutrition recommendations from the ADA suggest that there is no one combination of nutrients or a specific amount of the calorie-containing nutrients (carbohydrate, protein, and fat) that have been shown to be superior in helping people with diabetes lose weight and keep it off more successfully. In fact, ADA suggests that either a low carbohydrate (under 130 grams/day) or low-fat (under 30% of calories/day) eating plan may be effective for short-term weight loss (for up to one year). Obviously, you'll be fighting this battle way longer than one year!

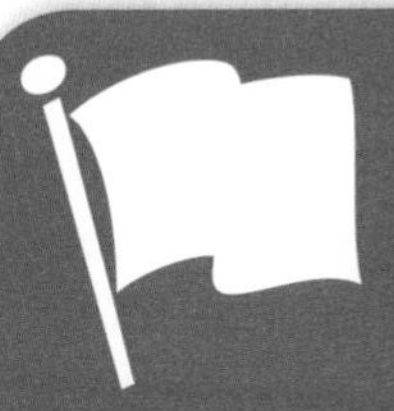

RED FLAG

Set Weight Loss Expectations Straight

You may have grandiose expectations about how much weight you want to lose each week. That's understandable when you watch TV shows and read advertisements that promise amounts of weight loss that are unrealistic for most people unless you are exercising hours a day or eating very few calories—neither which is healthy long term or realistic for most. It's important to set your expectations for weight loss straight right off the bat. Learn to be satisfied with about 1 pound of weight loss a week on average. Don't get on the scale more than once a week. Use the same scale and weigh at about the same time.

Also, don't put all your energy into the number on the scale. Find other positive results that are happening with your body to feel good about and positively reinforce your efforts, such as clothes fitting less snuggly, using a tighter notch on your belt, people noticing your weight loss, being able to bend or breath easier, sleeping better, walking further, and having lower glucose levels.

People with diabetes can safely follow a low-carbohydrate eating plan for a year (the longest time for which a study is available), and these diets do help with weight loss. Additionally, they can improve blood lipids; however, the long-term data (from six months and beyond), which track weight loss and maintenance on low-carbohydrate diets, don't show that people are able to follow these programs and maintain weight loss long-term. By one year, research shows that a lot of people drop out of studies and can't follow the plan, even when they get a lot of support from researchers. Another problem with following low carb diets over the long term is that you may miss eating the amounts of fruits, vegetables, and whole grains that provide your body with essential energy and nutrients—vitamins, minerals, and fiber.

What will work best for you is a healthy eating plan that meshes well with your lifestyle and that you can follow day in and day out, now and for years to come. That's not a diet, that's an eating plan that is part of a real-life diabetes care plan.

Determine how many calories you need to eat each day to maintain your weight or lose weight [also check out *Chapter 5*, page 59]. In general, you need 500–1,000 fewer calories to lose weight than you estimate you need to maintain your weight. If you carefully estimate portions and are faithful to eating fewer calories, you can lose 1–2 pounds per week.

Calories Here and There Add Up

The trick to losing weight and keeping it off comes down to whether you unintentionally eat a few more calories here and there that you aren't keeping track of. Think about it: You may overeat by 200, 300, or 400 calories each day without even realizing it. If you grab a piece of fresh fruit that is large rather than small, if you have an extra 1/3 cup of pasta, or if you eat two extra ounces of chicken, you could be eating several hundred calories that you aren't counting. Extra calories here and there add up and can be enough calories to stunt your weight-loss progress.

Interestingly, research shows that people underestimate what they eat by about 500 calories a day. The best advice to follow is to practice portion control. Use your measuring equipment and put the portion-control tips and tactics into practice [also check out *Chapter 6*, page 75].

Meal Replacements May Offer Assistance

Meal replacements are typically portion- and calorie-controlled foods or drinks that supply about 100 to 300 calories to replace a meal or snack in the form of shakes, soups, snack bars, or packaged and portioned entrées. People and programs that use meal replacements typically replace one to two meals a day. Meal replacements can help you minimize your food choices and decisions about food, control your calories, and offer structure and convenience.

Recent research in people with pre-diabetes and those with type 2 diabetes who need to

Myth

All blood glucose–lowering medicines pack on the pounds

Fact

Review the blood glucose–lowering medicines [also check out *Chapter 8*, page 101]. You will note that some of these medicines may cause weight gain and others can help you lose weight. The difference is how they work in your body. One reason for weight gain can simply be better control of blood glucose. Sound strange? This is because when blood glucose is high, your body can't use your calories properly. You literally pee out calories in your urine. Once your blood glucose improves, your body is able to use the calories for energy.

The best defense against weight gain from blood glucose–lowering medication is a good offense. When your health care provider wants to put you on a blood glucose–lowering medicine, ask about the weight gain vs. loss side effects. Let them know that this is important to you. If weight gain is a side effect, yet it is the best medicine for you, work to prevent weight gain by being even more vigilant with portions, and up the amount of physical activity you do. If you experience excessive weight gain, report this to your health care provider immediately.

lose weight, shows that they have lost more weight and improved other risk factors using meal replacements as part of their weight loss and maintenance plan compared to a usual calorie-controlled eating plan. In order to be able to use meal replacements long-term, you'll need to find products that you enjoy and are easy to carry and prepare on the run.

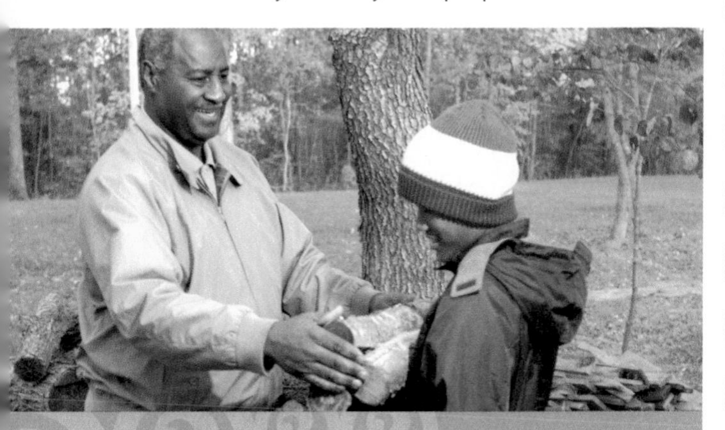

Wonder?

Is being physically active more important during weight loss or maintenance?

Physical activity is an important element of a weight-loss plan in addition to calorie control. Being physically active without restricting calories improves insulin sensitivity and decreases insulin resistance, which lowers blood glucose; however, it only has a modest effect on weight loss. The two elements need to be used in tandem to succeed with weight loss. Interestingly, physical activity along with calorie control seems to play an even more essential role in weight maintenance.

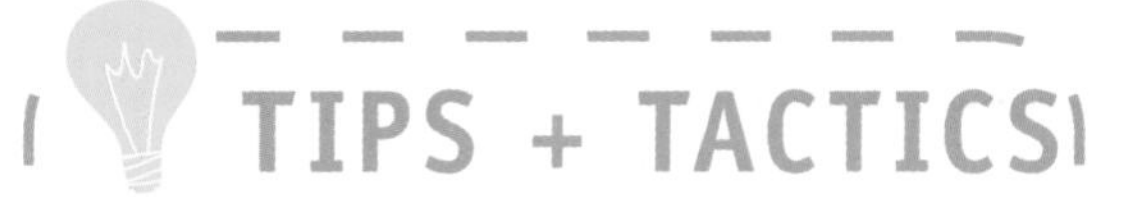

How to Control Calories

- *Be vigilant about portion control.*
- *Carefully monitor the amount of fat you eat.*
- *Eat restaurant foods less frequently (if you eat them more than a few times a week), and be careful with portions and fat when you do.*
- *Keep your "danger" foods out of the house (if possible). If there are foods you just can't stand to have around because they tempt you to overeat, keep them out of your house (as long as others in your household are willing). If your list is long, try to narrow it down to your worst offenders.*
- *Put the plate method of meal planning into practice to help you eat the lower-calorie foods, like fruits and vegetables, and limit portions of starches and meats.*
- *Use smaller plates to limit portions.*
- *Use shorter glasses for beverages that contain calories to limit portions.*
- *Consider using meal replacements to control and structure your calorie intake.*
- *Don't let yourself get very hungry. If you do better with one or two snacks during the day, plan them and carry the healthy foods you'll need.*

Research Brief

CONFIDENTIAL

The LookAHEAD Study in Type 2

The Look AHEAD (Action for Health in Diabetes) study is a multi-center randomized clinical trial that is examining the effects of healthy lifestyle changes (decreased caloric intake and physical activity) to achieve weight loss and maintenance as a means to prevent heart attacks and strokes and provide other health benefits. The study will be completed in 2012. More than 5,000 overweight and obese people with type 2 diabetes between the ages of 45–74 have been assigned randomly to one of two groups. The intensive lifestyle intervention (ILI) group has regular group and individual meetings with behavioral counselors. The other group receives standard diabetes support and education (DSE), which means they receive much less support and assistance in achieving their weight loss goals.

One-year results of the study were reported in 2007. They showed that people in the ILI group lost an average of 8.6% of their initial weight vs. 0.7% in DSE group. The fitness level of the ILI group increased. A greater proportion of ILI participants reduced their blood glucose, blood pressure, and lipid-lowering medicines and dropped their mean A1C from ILI 7.3 to 6.6% vs. DSE 7.3 to 7.2%. Blood pressure, lipids, and kidney function improved more in the ILI vs. DSE groups.

The outcome of this study shows that healthy eating (which includes eating less fat and more fiber), weight loss, and increasing physical activity makes BIG health impacts. The question is whether the LookAHEAD study will demonstrate whether people in the two groups can maintain the healthy lifestyle changes and their weight loss over time and whether these changes help reduce heart attacks, strokes, and other diabetes-related heart and blood vessel diseases. More will be known when the trial ends in 2012. Learn more about LookAHEAD at *www.niddk.nih.gov/patient/SHOW/lookahead.htm.*

If I Only Knew . . .

Keep trigger foods out of the house . . .

I can bypass the cookies and ignore the candy bars, but my downfalls are roasted nuts and ice cream. After many failed attempts at keeping my hand out of the peanut jar, or my spoon out of the ice cream container, I admitted that I was human and asked that no one bring these items into our house. I can't eat just a couple of roasted nuts, nor can I eat just one spoonful of ice cream. If it's in the house, I'll devour it, and that makes me feel like a failure. My husband was willing to grant me this request. Now, when I do eat ice cream, it is a special treat, and I eat it out. I order the junior or kid's size dish or cone, and I don't feel guilty. If I buy nuts for a party, I store the remainders in the basement, where I can't see them so I'll forget about them. Finding simple solutions is what works for me.

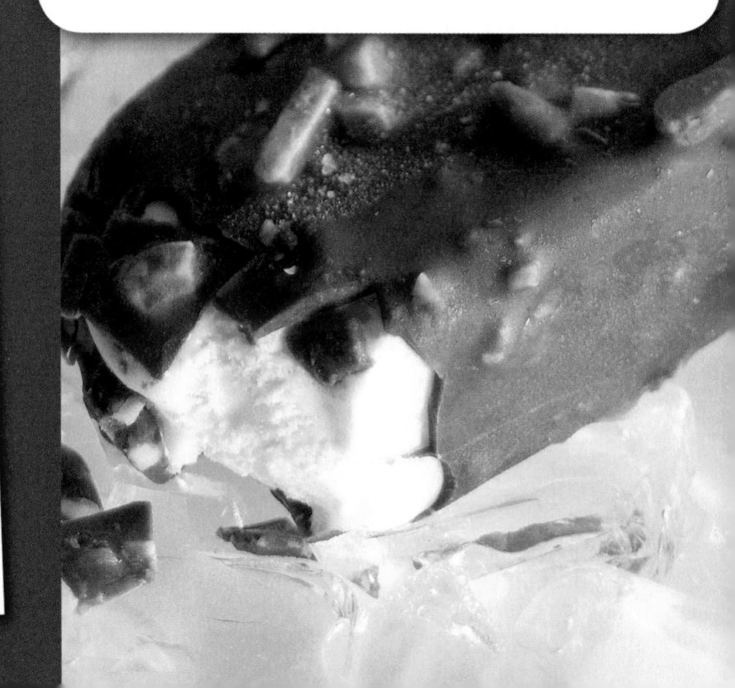

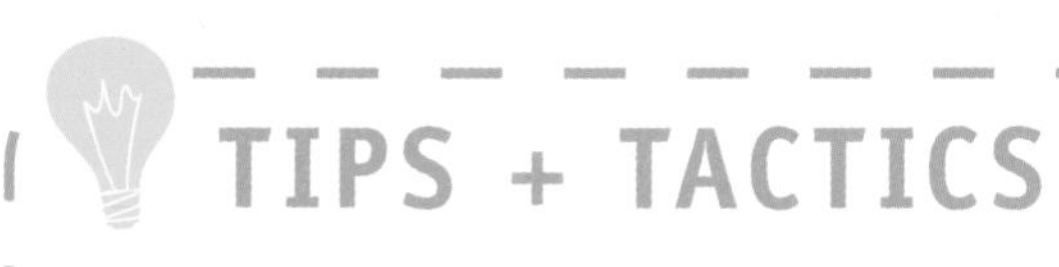

Keep the Weight Off

- *Slowly change your food and activity habits.*
- *Make sure that you want to lose weight for YOU, that YOU are ready to do this, and that YOU can commit to this being a long-term process.*
- *Have a realistic and achievable weight-loss goal in mind, and take the long view of this effort.*
- *Read up on your options, and mix and match strategies to put together a plan that works for your life and lifestyle.*
- *Maintain ongoing contact with a health care provider, behavioral counselor, or other supporters.*
- *Manage your environment and food cues.*
- *Eat between 25 and 30% of calories from fat and no more.*
- *Eat more high-fiber foods.*
- *Eat breakfast every day.*
- *Weigh yourself at least once a week, and if weight starts to increase, react by getting back to basics.*
- *Watch less than 10 hours of TV per week.*
- *Keep records of various aspects of your plan. Keep records of different elements as needed.*
- *Get and stay physically active (the most common form of activity is walking) at least 30 minutes a day and closer to an hour a day for weight maintenance.*

Keeping the Weight Off

Unfortunately, research is leaning toward the conclusion that there are physiological reasons why keeping weight off once you are overweight is so tough. When weight gain occurs, the body seems to reset the many mechanisms (brain, hormones, thyroid gland, and others) that have to do with weight control. The body adapts to the new, higher weight.

Research in this area has and will continue to explore the impact of hormones and nutrients in the gut and fat tissue (adipose), which help or hinder weight control. When you try to lose weight, the body resists this effort and wants to get back to the higher weight. This just adds to the challenge of keeping weight off. It also underscores the importance of preventing weight gain in the first place or immediately working to take off those few added pounds before the weight gain is into double digits.

Mounting research and resources provide insight into the elements you need to put and keep in place in order to take weight off and keep it off for years to come. Though you may think barely anyone is successful at this effort, the number of people who are successful is rising, and the lessons from their experiences sew common threads. For example, members of the National Weight Control Registry (*www.nwcr.ws*) have lost an average of 66 pounds and kept it off for nearly 6 years. Now that's success!

Find and Stay Connected to Support

A common thread for weight-control success from research and successful losers, is to find

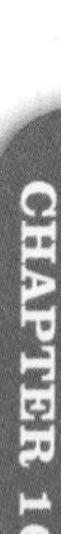

and stay connected to support. (This is true for helping you manage your diabetes as well.) Support can be provided individually or in a group with a health care provider, such as a diabetes educator, dietitian, behavioral counselor, or mental health provider. Your health plan may or may not cover these services. Support may come in the form of attending a local weight-control program, such as Weight Watchers, a community-based weight-control program, or partnering with a few neighbors.

Another option that the technology age has birthed is online weight-control programs. There are both free and fee-based alternatives. In our hurried lives, they offer benefits such as 24/7 access, no travel time (or gas usage), lots of options to communicate, tracking tools, and more. Search and you shall find.

Online Weight-Control Sites

Free online weight-control sites:

- FitDay (*www.fitday.com*)
- MyPyramid (*www.mypyramid.com*)—U.S. Government resource
- Calories Count (*wwwcaloriescount.com*)
- SparkPeople (*www.sparkpeople.com*)

Fee-based online weight-control sites:

- MyFoodDiary (*www.myfooddiary.com*)
- Weight Watchers (*www.weightwatchers.com*)
- e-diets (*www.ediets.com*)
- diet.com (*www.diet.com*)
- Calorie King (*www.calorieking.com*)

Weight Loss Medications

Currently there are two FDA-approved prescription weight-loss medications: sibutramine (Meridia) and orlistat (Xenical). There are also two over-the-counter medications: a lower dose (60 mg) of orlistat was approved by the FDA in 2007 and is called Alli, and phentermine, which is available as several brand names.

Sibutramine works by increasing the level of serotonin, which provides a feeling of fullness and decreases food intake. Orlistat works in the digestive system to block an enzyme that breaks down fat from food, thereby allowing less fat to be absorbed. The prescription dose is 120 mg taken with meals. Phentermine increases norepinephrine, which speeds up metabolism.

DEFINITION:

serotonin: a neurotransmitter that is involved in sleep, depression, memory, and other neurological processes.

norepinephrine: a neurotransmitter released by the brain that has such effects as constricting blood vessels, raising blood pressure, and dilating bronchi.

By no means have these weight-loss medications been found to be miracle cures for weight control, and like all drugs, they have side effects. Expect weight loss with any of the currently available weight-loss medications to be less than 10% of your starting body weight. According to the ADA, they may be considered as part of a weight-loss plan and can help people lose weight when they are partnered with a calorie-controlled eating plan and physical activity.

Be prepared to see many more weight-loss medications in the future. Most large drug companies have one or more of these in their new-drug pipeline due to the epidemic of obesity and a greater understanding of the biochemistry of obesity. Before you opt to take a weight-loss drug, educate yourself about their pros and cons, and discuss these with your health care provider.

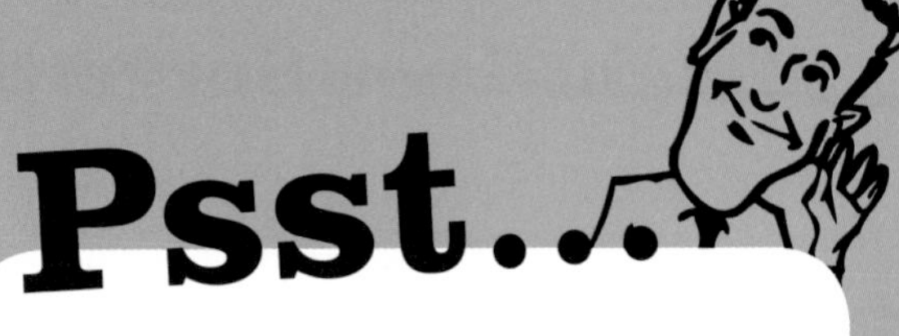

Could You Have an Under-Active Thyroid?

If you feel that you have pulled out all the stops in your weight loss efforts and you can't budge that scale downwards, or you have been gaining weight for no good reason, you could have an under-active thyroid. Read up on how common thyroid problems are in people with diabetes [also check out *Chapter 9*, page 121] and discuss this with your health care provider.

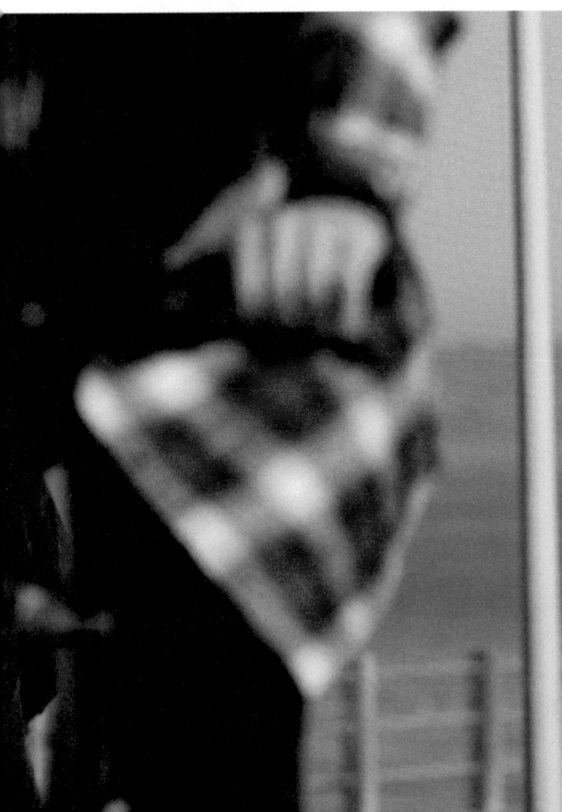

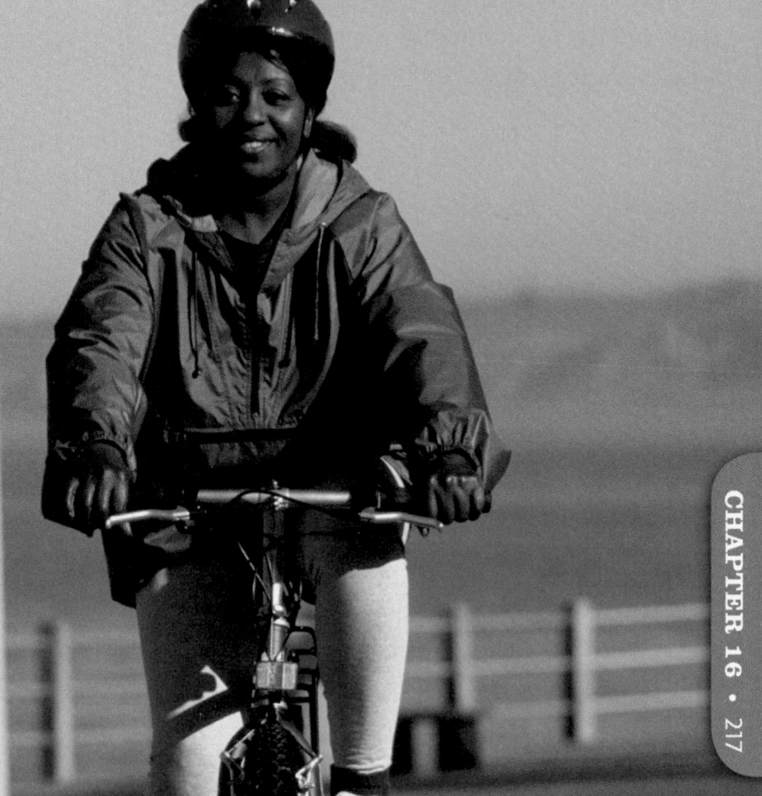

Weight-Loss Surgery

More research, and of course sensational headlines, have spawned interest in weight-loss surgery as a means to prevent, delay, or "cure" type 2 diabetes. Several types of surgery have been explored, from the less-invasive and less restrictive laproscopic adjustable gastric band procedure, where a band is placed around the upper part of the stomach. The more invasive and restrictive gastric bypass surgery is the Roux-en-Y gastric bypass.

Large weight losses, about 30–35% of total weight, have been observed with both procedures, with the gastric bypass procedure yielding greater weight loss. Weight loss occurs because of a lower calorie intake, as well as changes in the biochemistry of the brain and hormones, which have to do with the physiology of obesity. More success with reversing type 2 is seen when surgery is done early in the progression of type 2 [also check out *Chapter 1*, page 5]. Additionally, people on blood glucose–lowering medications are able to significantly decrease or stop taking them. Weight-loss surgery is not usually considered unless your BMI is over 40, or is between 35 and 40 and you have other health risks, such as type 2 diabetes.

There's no doubt that losing weight and keeping it off require changing many lifestyle behaviors for good. There's also no doubt that it's hard work, but losing weight frequently improves pre-diabetes and type 2 diabetes and medical conditions related to insulin resistance, such as high blood pressure. Weight loss can also help you decrease the amount and types of medicines you need to manage these conditions and benefit you in many other ways.

Give some thought to how you can change for good. Review how to make these changes, and learn how to set SMART goals for change [also check out *Chapter 4*, page 49].

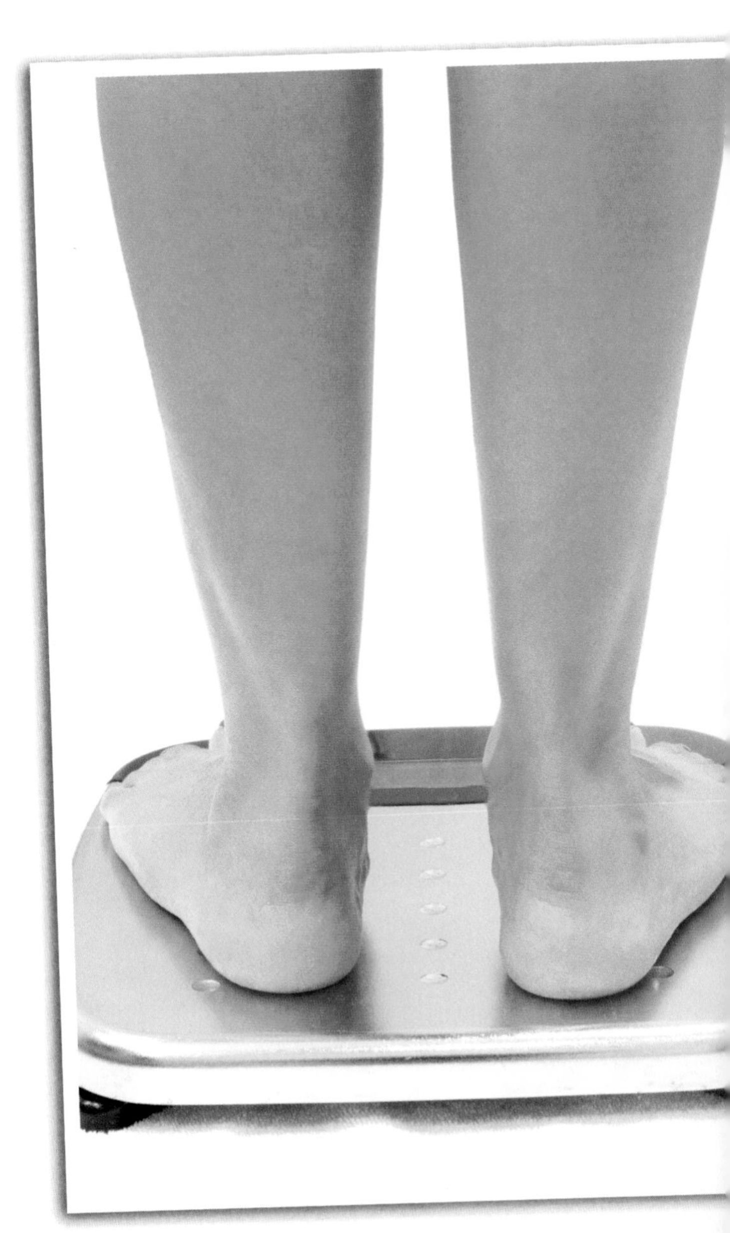

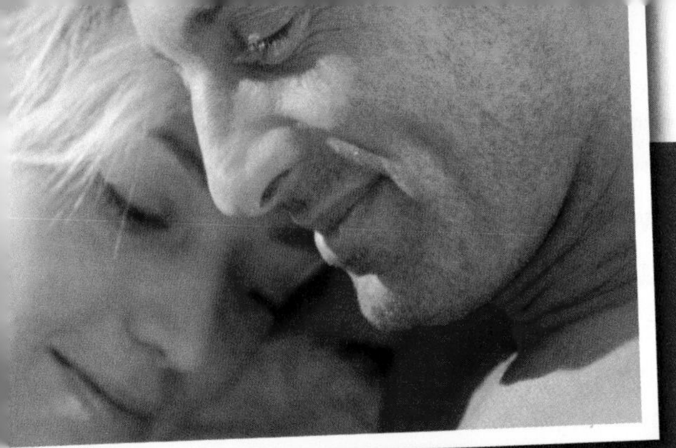

CHAPTER 17

Your Sexual Health

Sex is an important part of life and relationships. Diabetes can affect your sex life, whether you are a man or a woman, but it affects men and women differently. Having diabetes won't necessarily hamper your sex life, but it's good to know that if it does, there are steps you can take and treatments you can use to resolve the problems. You may also discover ways to improve your sex life even if you didn't think you were having problems.

Some people equate the word sex with the act of sexual intercourse. Others equate it with intimacy. To some, it means love or lovemaking. Others think of it as any sexual act. Some think of it as the distinction of gender between males and females. And the list goes on. For our purposes, Anna Freud said it well when she said, "Sex is something you do, and sexuality is something you are."

What You'll Learn:

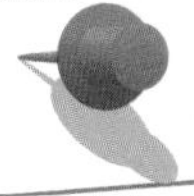

- How diabetes can affect your sex life
- How to identify aspects of your diabetes management that may affect your sex life
- The impact of diabetes on a woman's sexual health
- The impact of diabetes on a man's sexual health
- Treatment options for diabetes related sexual problems

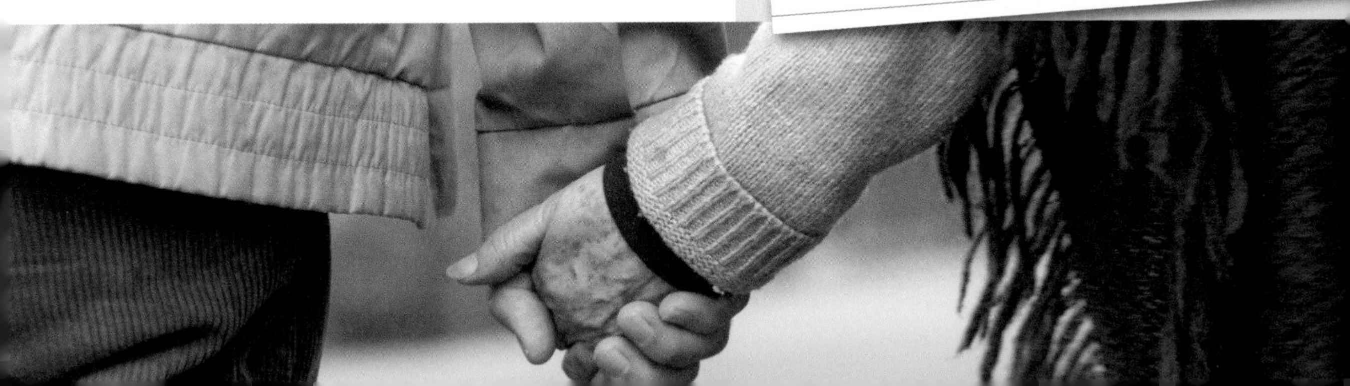

Sex and Diabetes

Both type 1 and type 2 diabetes can affect sex and sexuality in different ways. The fact that you have diabetes may not affect it in any way, or it can affect you emotionally and/or physically, which can ultimately affect how you experience having sex and your sexuality. If you are stressed or depressed as a result of having diabetes, you might not feel good enough emotionally to even think about having sex. On the other hand, if the nerves in your body that impact your sexual organs have been affected, you may want to have sex, but your body might not respond the way you would like it to.

In their book *Sex and Diabetes*, Janis Roszler RD, CDE, LDN and Donna Rice, MBA, BSN, RN, CDE talk about the two types of intimacy and how these play an important role in love and in sex. The two types of intimacy are physical intimacy and emotional intimacy.

Physical intimacy is all about touch and involves sexual attraction, holding, touching, caressing, and intimate actions. It is what many of us yearn for when we are alone and what we feel we need to connect with someone in a physical way.

Emotional intimacy is what happens in our heads. This is the non-physical sharing of two people who care deeply about one another. Emotional intimacy between two people grows through sharing experiences together and learning to understand and trust each other. Many sexuality experts think the brain is the sexiest of all organs because when an emotional relationship exists between two individuals that is built on mutual respect and caring, the relationship becomes far more precious. Physical intimacy is enjoyable on its own, but when combined with emotional intimacy, the passion that develops is special indeed.

If your thoughts are keeping you from enjoying sex like you did before you were diagnosed with diabetes, there are things you can do. Use the information in this book to learn more about diabetes. You'll learn that you can live a healthy life with diabetes. You'll learn healthier ways to eat, to move, to sleep, to lose weight and more. Making some changes in your life can make you feel better about yourself than you have for a long time. Another important way to deal with your feelings is to talk with your partner. Ask your

Psst...

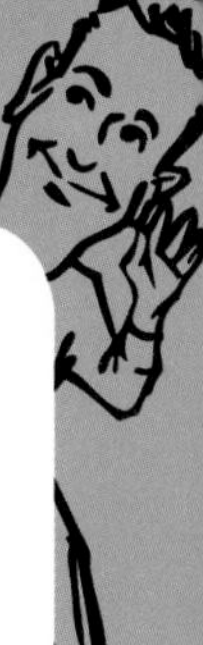

How Diabetes May Affect You Sexually

- You may not be comfortable with the fact that you have diabetes and/or your being overweight. If you feel this way about yourself, you may think others, including your partner, see you as not sexual [also check out *Chapter 1*, page 5].
- You may blame yourself and feel guilty that you have diabetes or you may feel like you're imposing on your partner because of your self-care needs.
- You may not have the sex drive you used to have because you're trying to figure out your diabetes, or you are stressed, and/or depressed, or under financial duress [also check out *Chapter 1*, page 5 and *Chapter 12*, page 149].

partner whether your diabetes has gotten in the way of your relationship. If you think you need to talk about it with your health care provider or a relationship counselor, do so.

Diabetes and Men's Sexual Health

The most common sexual side effect in men is erectile dysfunction (ED). At some point in their lives, most men will have some difficulty getting or keeping an erection, so it's not a serious concern until the man is having trouble in at least half of his attempts at sexual intercourse. If you have diabetes, the blood vessels and nerves in the penis can become damaged over time and lead to ED. ED is not a normal part of getting older and doesn't happen to all men who have diabetes. Diabetes is not the only cause of ED; it can develop after prostate or bladder surgery, can be caused by emotional problems, or can develop as a side effect of certain medications.

If you have ED or some other sexual problem, it's normal to feel embarrassed or upset. You may blame yourself or your partner. Some men feel guilty and angry, while others feel like there's no hope. These feelings can make it hard to talk openly with your partner or your health care provider, but talking to someone is an important first step on your way to getting help. If you have a problem with ED, think about whom you may feel comfortable talking to. It's important to know that there are many methods on the market for treating ED. Talk to your health care provider about whether you should start to use a treatment option and which one is right for you.

By the Numbers

Although erectile dysfunction is not usually locker room talk, you need to know you are not alone. ED can be a total inability to achieve erection, an inconsistent ability to do so, or a tendency to sustain only brief erections and not be able to complete sexual intercourse. These variations make defining ED and estimating its incidence difficult. Estimates range from 15 million to 30 million men affected, depending on the definition used. ED increases with age. It is estimated that 9% of men from 20 to 29 years of age have ED whereas 95% of men over 70 years old have some ED. More than 50% of men who have had diabetes for more than 10 year notice some ED.

Treatments for Erectile Dysfuction

One of the greatest things about living in our world today is scientific advancement, and there has been a lot of advancement in the treatment of ED with both medications and devices. Thanks to modern medicine, erectile dysfunction is no longer an untreatable condition. There are several oral medications on the market, along with other options like injections, suppositories, and a number of treatment devices like constriction rings worn around the base of the penis, vacuum pumps, and penile support sleeves. This wide variety of treatment options makes it easier than ever for you to find a treatment that's right for you.

Before you pick a treatment option, make an

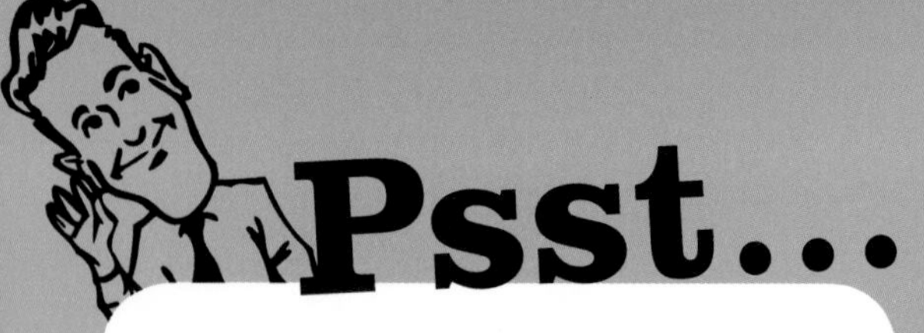

Causes of Erectile Dysfunction

- Damage to your nerves, arteries, smooth muscles, and fibrous tissues, often as a result of a disease.
- Diseases—such as diabetes, kidney disease, chronic alcoholism, multiple sclerosis, atherosclerosis, vascular disease, and neurologic disease—account for about 70% of ED cases.
- Smoking, being overweight, and avoiding exercise.
- Surgery (especially radical prostate and bladder surgery for cancer) can injure your nerves and arteries near your penis. Injury to your penis, spinal cord, prostate, bladder, and pelvis can lead to ED by harming nerves, smooth muscles, arteries, and fibrous tissues in your penis.
- Use of many common medicines—blood pressure drugs, antihistamines, antidepressants, tranquilizers, appetite suppressants, and cimetidine (an ulcer drug)—can produce ED as a side effect.
- Psychological factors such as stress, anxiety, guilt, depression, low self-esteem, and fear of sexual failure cause 10 to 20% of ED cases.

appointment with your health care provider, endocrinologist, or urologist to talk about the problems you are experiencing. Through an examination of your medical and sexual history, a physical examination, and lab tests, your health care provider should be able to determine the cause of your ED and the best treatments.

A medical history can disclose diseases that lead to ED, while a simple recounting of sexual activity might distinguish problems with sexual desire, erection, ejaculation, or orgasm. Using certain prescription or illegal drugs can suggest a chemical cause because drug effects account for 25% of ED cases. Cutting back on or substituting certain medications can often alleviate the problem.

A physical examination can give clues to problems in other systems of your body. For example, if your penis is not sensitive to touching, a problem in the nervous system may be the cause. It is common to find that, in addition to ED, the person with diabetes also has evidence of nerve loss in other parts of their body, such as the legs or feet. Abnormal secondary sex characteristics, such as hair pattern or breast enlargement, can point to hormonal problems, which would mean that your endocrine system is involved. The examiner might discover a circulatory problem by observing decreased pulses in your wrist or ankles. And unusual characteristics of the penis itself could suggest the source of the problem. For example, a penis that bends or curves when erect could be the result of Peyronie's disease.

Laboratory tests can help diagnose ED. Tests for systemic diseases include blood counts, urinalysis, lipid profile, and measurements of creatinine and liver enzymes. Measuring the amount of free testosterone in the blood can yield information about problems with your endocrine system and is indicated especially if you have a decrease in sexual desire.

Low Testosterone

If you are having problems maintaining an erection and have tried one of the medications without success, you may have a low testosterone level, known as low T. Men who have diabetes are twice as likely to have low T as men who do not. There is also a high incidence of low T in men who are obese and or have high blood pressure. It is estimated that 13 million American men 45 years old and older have low T, yet fewer than 10% seek treatment. low T can be easily treated. Those who have low T may experience decreased sex drive, erectile dysfunction, or depression.

If you have the symptoms of low T, ask your health care provider to take a blood test

RED FLAG

There Are No Guarantees

Regardless of which option you and your health care provider decide upon for treatment—oral medications, injections, insertion of pellets, or surgery—there is no guarantee that the treatment will work. There is the possibility of side effects to every medication, as well as the possibility of complications from surgery. Learn all you can about these treatment options, and make sure you work with your health care provider to make the best decision for you for any of these options.

DEFINITION:

testosterone: a hormone that promotes hair growth, muscle development, bone health, and sperm production and helps you maintain a healthy sexual appetite.

Psst...

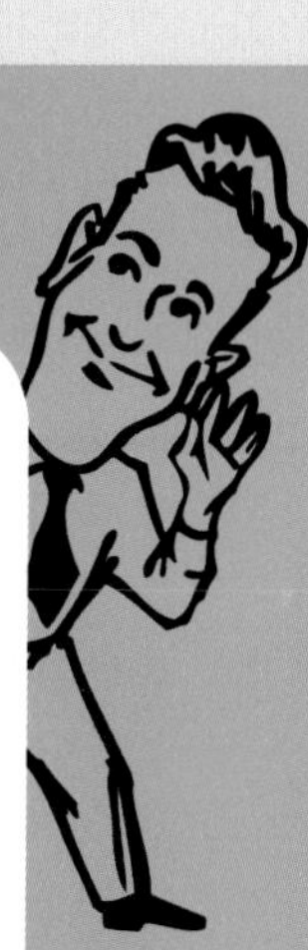

Symptoms of Low T

- Decreased sex drive
- ED
- Depression
- Fatigue
- Weight gain
- Drop in bone mineral density
- Reduced strength and muscle mass

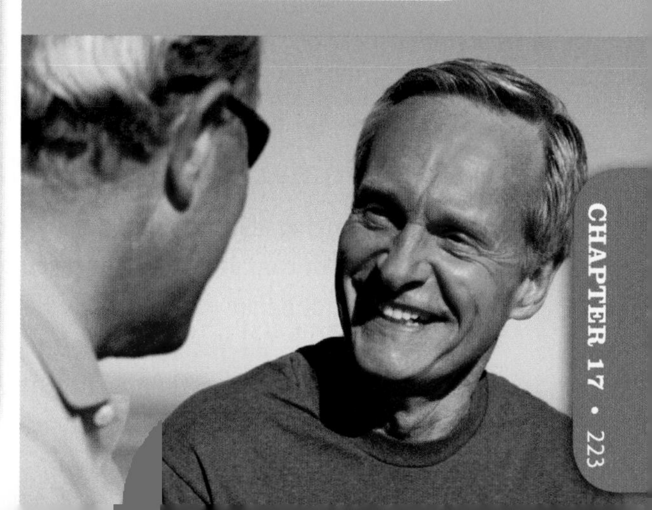

early in the morning that measures your testosterone levels. Testosterone levels usually peak in the morning, so this test is usually run at this time. If your levels are low, there are some very effective treatments.

Like erectile dysfunction, there are several very effective treatments for low T. Talk with your health care provider to find out what treatment is best for you. Testosterone gels are one of the most popular treatments and are easy to use. You simply rub the prescribed amount of gel into your skin. Patches are another easy treatment method and work for a full 24 hours. You place the patch with a prescribed amount of testosterone on your shoulders, abdomen, or upper arms.

The two other types of low T treatments are injections and oral (buccal) tablets. There are several different types of testosterone injections that you can take. Your health care provider can give you this injection every 7-21 days, depending on the type of injection you are using. While testosterone pills are generally not effective or safe to swallow, oral (buccal) tablets can be placed on the inside of your cheek and can be left there for a 12-hour period, slowly administering the testosterone to your system.

Diabetes and Women's Sexual Health

People don't often think of diabetes causing sexual complications in women; however, research in recent years has started to show that diabetes can have an impact on several areas of sexual health for women.

It's not unusual for a woman to find out she has diabetes when she tells her health care provider she is experiencing painful sex or itching or burning when urinating. A check-up may then reveal a yeast infection or a urinary tract infection that won't heal. Further blood tests uncover the underlying cause; she has diabetes.

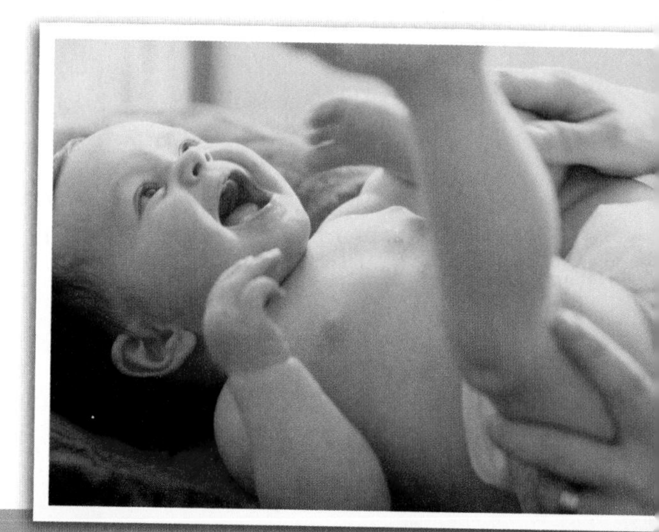

Wonder?

I am a woman and I have diabetes. Can I have a baby?

If you are thinking about having a baby and have either type 1 or 2 diabetes, start working with your health care provider before you get pregnant to get your blood glucose levels under excellent control before you conceive. Have your A1C, blood pressure, heart, kidneys, nerves, and eyes checked. Talk with your health care provider about how being pregnant will affect both your short- and long-term health. If you have type 2 diabetes and take oral or injectable medications (other than insulin), you may need to switch to insulin to protect the baby.

RED FLAG

Type 2 is Different From Gestational During Pregnancy

Because women are getting type 2 diabetes at younger ages and are more overweight and older when they get pregnant, more woman today are finding out that they have type 2 diabetes once they get pregnant or during their pregnancy. This is not gestational diabetes (diabetes during pregnancy). It is type 2 diabetes that will not resolve once the pregnancy is over. You may be referred to a special diabetes and pregnancy team. You will help keep yourself and your baby healthy and safe if you get your blood glucose in your target range before you get pregnant and until the baby arrives. That will lower your chances of having a premature baby or a baby who's larger than normal. You'll also lower the risk of having a baby with birth defects by keeping your blood glucose close to normal in the first few weeks of pregnancy. Today, more women with diabetes are able to have healthy babies. With planning and hard work, you can, too.

There are a numerous ways that diabetes can adversely affect a woman's interest in sex. Lack of interest in sex can often be caused by high or low glucose levels. If you're tired all the time, you may not be interested in sex. If you're taking medications that lower your blood glucose, you may experience a low blood glucose reaction during or after sex, which can decrease your spontaneity, or your desire for sex in the future.

Pain during sex and the inability to reach orgasm are two other common problems that women with diabetes experience. Pain during sex can be due to a decrease in lubrication or a yeast or urinary tract infection. Diabetes can also have an effect on the blood vessels and nerves that cause you to have an orgasm. If your nerves or blood vessels have been affected by diabetes, it may take longer and may not be possible for you to reach a climax, or the climax you do have may not be as enjoyable as it once was.

Treating Women's Sexual Problems Associated with Diabetes

With the variety of sexual complications women may experience, there are also a number of solutions. If poor diabetes management is causing your problem, your first step will be to better manage your diabetes. Use the information in this book to learn more about diabetes and how to get your ABCs under control.

Some medications for high blood pressure and depression can cause changes in your sexual response. Talk with your health care provider to see whether you are taking any of these medications. If so and if possible, ask to be switched to another kind that does not have this side effect [also check out *Chapter 9*, page 121, and *Chapter 12*, page 149].

High blood glucose levels can sometimes contribute to yeast or urinary tract infections and make sex painful. If you are experiencing painful sex because of an infection, work on managing your diabetes, as well as getting treatment for your infection.

One of the best solutions for sexually related complications is communication with your partner. Ask your partner whether your diabetes has gotten in his or her way of your relationship. Don't give up. If you find that you don't enjoy sex anymore, it's normal to feel upset. You may blame yourself, or your partner or feel angry or depressed. These feelings can make it hard for you to talk openly with your partner, so if you can't, find someone—either a friend or member of your health care team—to talk with [also check out *Chapter 3*, page 35].

Women and Hormones

Many women feel that hormones direct their lives. Whether it's the time before your period, during your period, during pregnancy, post-partum, during perimenopause, and even during menopause, your hormones affect your body (and mind) and can hinder your diabetes management as well.

Some women find it hard to keep their blood glucose on track the weeks before and during their menstrual period. Your blood glucose levels may go up and down because of changes in hormone levels. Make a note in your blood glucose records of the days when you're having your period. Look for patterns, and then talk with your health care provider about ways you can adjust your care plan before, during, or after your period to keep your blood glucose levels on target. Managing blood glucose levels at this time is particularly challenging if you take insulin. You may need to develop several insulin plans to manage your blood glucose during the phases of your menstrual cycle.

Perimenopause is also called menopause transition because it usually begins several years before menopause. It is the period of time when your ovaries produce less estrogen. It usually starts in your 40s, but some women enter this stage in their 30s, and it lasts through your first year of menopause. Your periods can become irregular during this time. Menopause is the term used for any of the changes you experience either just before or after you stop menstruating, which marks the end of your reproductive period.

If you are going through menopause, you may also experience changes in your blood glucose. Talk with your health care provider about whether hormone replacements or other options are right for you. You may also need to make a change in your diabetes

Wonder?

Can I take birth control pills if I have diabetes?

If you don't want to get pregnant, you'll need to use some kind of birth control. Even if you don't have regular periods but are still menstruating, you can still get pregnant. Most birth control methods are safe for women with diabetes. Talk with your health care provider about your options. If you do start a method of birth control, check your blood glucose more often than usual early on to see how it affects your blood glucose.

treatment, which includes your eating, your physical activity, your sleep, and your medications [also check out *Chapter 5*, page 59, *Chapter 7*, page 89, *Chapter 11*, page 141, and *Chapter 16*, page 207].

As mentioned earlier, sex is something you do, and sexuality is something you are. Just because a man has ED, or a woman experiences vaginal dryness, does not mean two consenting adults cannot still have sex and feel sexy. There are a lot of alternative options that work. Take care of yourself, and manage your diabetes to feel healthy. Put some time and energy into looking the best you can. When you look better, you feel better about yourself, reviving not only your self-esteem, but your sex life as well.

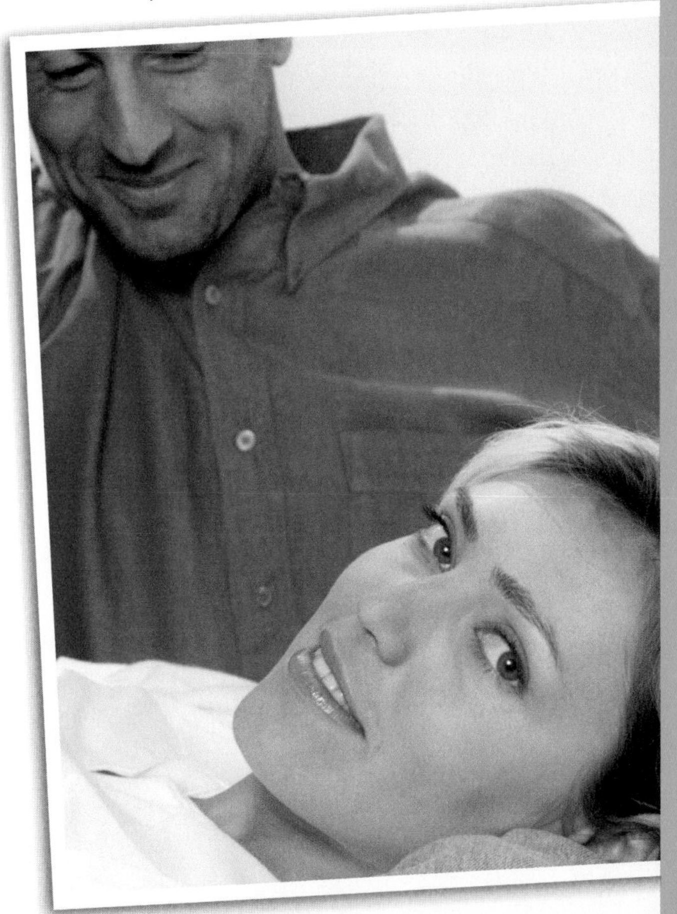

Psst...

Symptoms of Menopause

Symptoms you may experience during peri-menopause and menopause are:

- Hot flashes or night sweats
- Bouts of rapid heartbeat
- Chills or periods of extreme warmth
- Depression
- Fluctuations in sexual desire and sexual response
- Frequent urination and urinary leaking during coughing, sneezing, or orgasm
- Menstrual changes
- Migraine headaches
- Mood swings
- Painful intercourse
- Sleep problems and unusual dreams
- Tingling in hands
- Vaginal dryness or infections
- Weight changes

Some of these symptoms are the same as symptoms of low and or high blood glucose levels. Check your blood glucose often to help you differentiate whether the cause of your symptoms is related to your glucose level or your raging or dwindling female hormones.

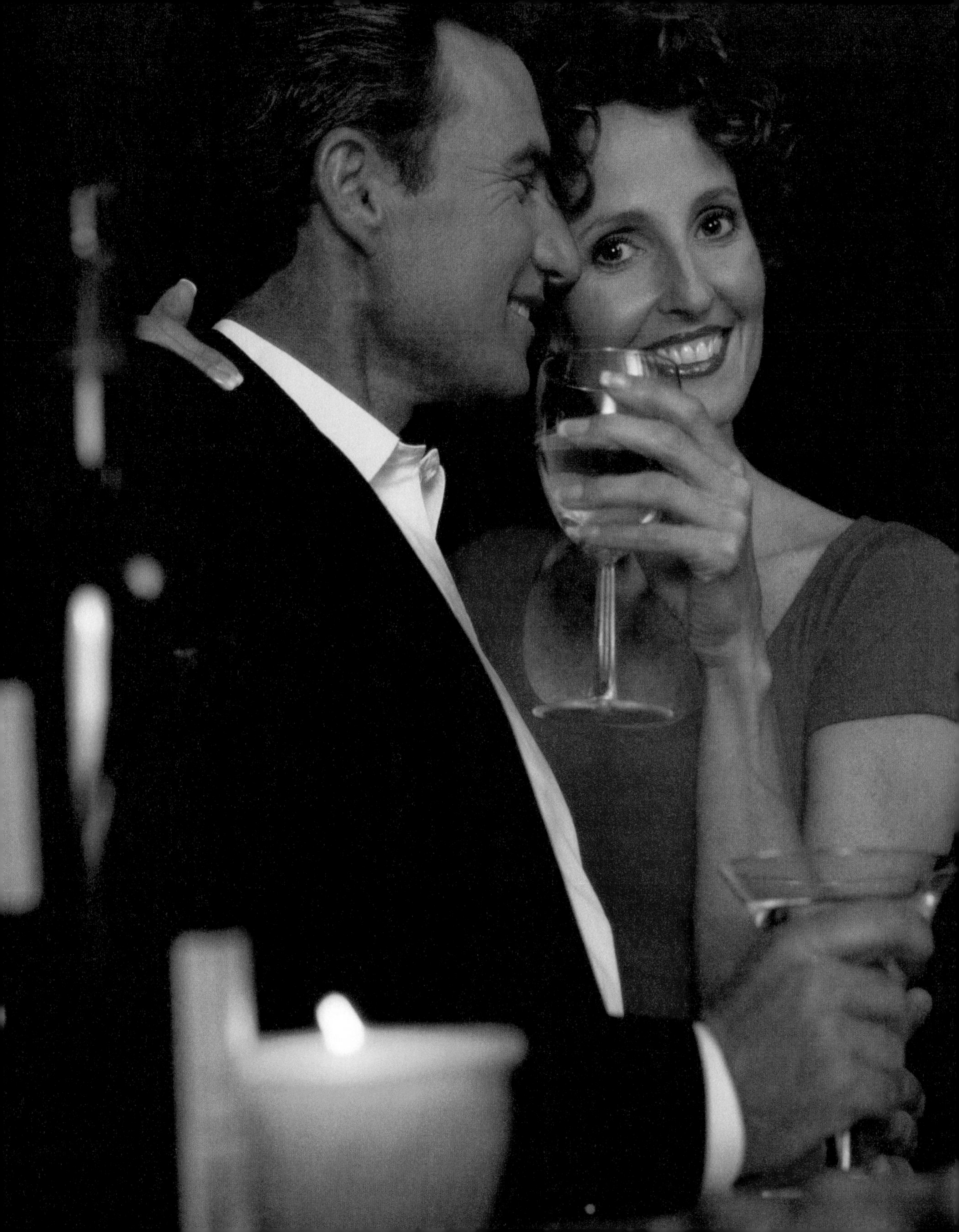

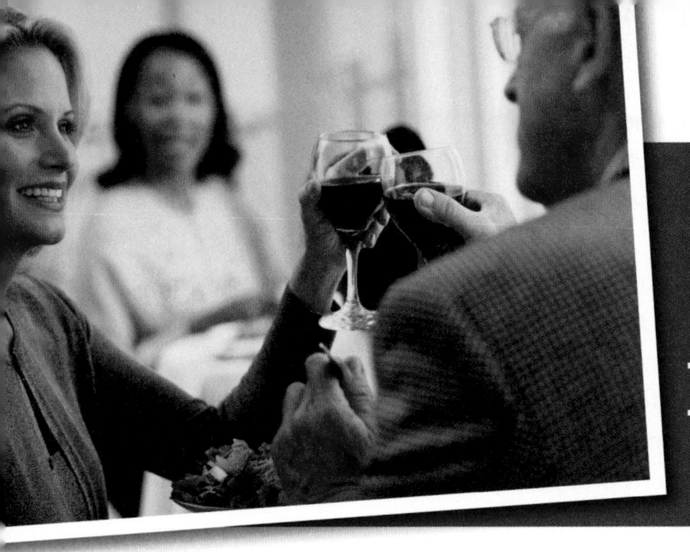

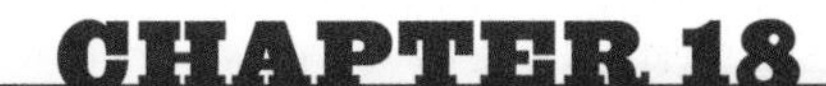

CHAPTER 18

Tobacco and Alcohol: How They Mix with Diabetes

Alcohol and tobacco are commonly used substances. You may use neither, one, or both.

When it comes to tobacco, there are virtually no benefits for your diabetes or health. If you currently smoke, quitting is the healthiest solution. When it comes to alcohol, there are actually a few health benefits from moderate use. If you choose to, and are able to drink moderately, you can learn to drink safely with diabetes.

If you use one or both of these, it's time to evaluate your habits. It might be time to decrease or eliminate the use of them entirely. Knowledge is power, so read on and learn about the health risks of smoking tobacco, and gather tips for drinking alcohol wisely.

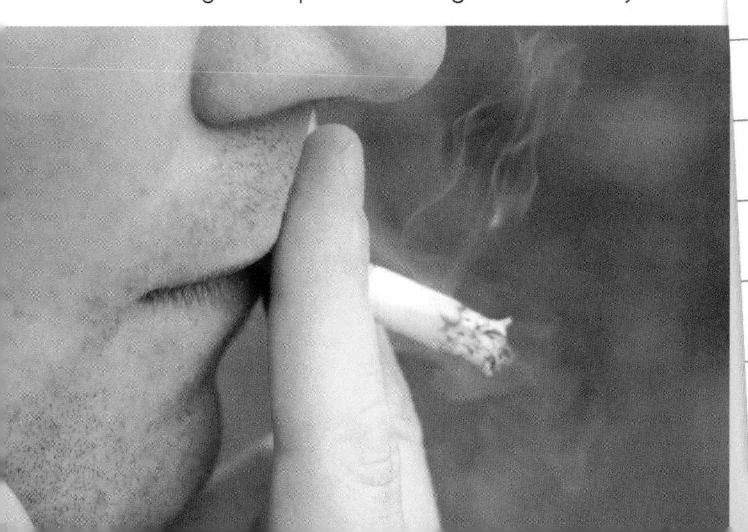

What You'll Learn:

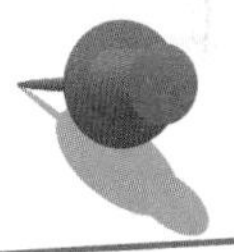

- The negative effects of tobacco (cigarette smoking) on your diabetes and health
- Treatment options available to quit smoking
- What it takes to quit smoking for good
- Ways to work with your health care provider to help you quit smoking
- How alcohol impacts blood glucose and diabetes care
- The benefits of moderate alcohol consumption
- How alcohol can negatively effect your diabetes and health
- How to drink alcohol safely and healthfully

The Dangers of Smoking

No doubt about it, smoking cigarettes is dangerous to your health, and that's true even without diabetes. Add diabetes into the picture, and the danger to your health escalates. If you have diabetes and you smoke, you should do everything you can to quit. In fact, quitting tobacco use may be one of the most important lifestyle changes you make to get and stay healthy.

By the Numbers

Tobacco Smoking

- Every year in the U.S., over 438,000 people (one in five deaths from all causes) die from tobacco-related disease, making it the leading cause of preventable disease and death.
- Each day, more than 1,000 children become regular, daily smokers, and one in two will eventually die as a result of their addiction.
- The cost to the U.S economy is over $167 million in yearly health care costs and lost productivity.
- In 2004, nearly 21% of people 18 years of age and older (44.5 million people) were smokers.
- The overall prevalence of smoking in the U.S. decreased 40% between 1965 and 1990 but has remained level since then.
- Smoking rates among people aged 18-24 years has increased.

Source: American Lung Association: www.lungusa.org.

It's not an easy task to quit smoking, because nicotine, the drug in tobacco, is one of the most addictive substances known. Besides the physical addiction, many smokers also become psychologically hooked on tobacco. Smoking-cessation experts agree that you may have to make several attempts to quit before you are able to quit for good. You can increase your chances for success with a multi-pronged approach, such as counseling and a medication treatment.

The good news is that quitting smoking greatly reduces your risk of having a heart attack. One year after quitting, the risk drops to about half that of current smokers and gradually returns to normal in people without heart disease. Even among people with heart disease, the risk of a heart attack drops sharply one year after you stop smoking, and it continues to decline over time; however, the risk never returns to normal.

The most common health effects of smoking are:

- Can cause lung cancer and cancer of the mouth, throat, lung, and bladder.
- Causes constriction of the blood vessels, and can damage your blood vessels, increase your blood pressure, and cut the amount of oxygen reaching your tissues. This decrease in oxygen can lead to a heart attack, stroke, miscarriage, or stillbirth.
- Can increase cholesterol levels and the levels of some other blood fats that raise the risk of a heart attack.
- Can increase your frequency of colds and respiratory infections.

- Can cause erectile dysfunction [also check out *Chapter 17*, page 219].

The Impact of Smoking on Diabetes

Smoking can lead to numerous health problems that only multiply when you combine smoking with diabetes. Interestingly, some research suggests that smoking can even increase the risk of type 2 diabetes [also check out *Research Brief: Can Smoking Cause Type 2 Diabetes?*, right]. When you smoke and have diabetes, you not only encounter the general health risks of smoking, but smoking can also raise your blood glucose; increase your risk of heart and blood vessel diseases; increase your risk of blood vessel diseases in your legs and feet, which may lead to amputation; and increase your risk of small blood vessel diseases, such as kidney disease, eye disease, and nerve diseases [also check out *Chapter 21*, page 257].

Be upfront and honest with your health care provider about your tobacco use. Research shows there's a 50/50 chance your health care provider will not ask you if you smoke, so it's up to you to be proactive. Let them know you smoke cigarettes and how often you smoke. Let them in on what treatment strategies you have tried to quit. They may be able to offer you other solutions [also check out *Quit with a Multi-Pronged Approach*, page 232]. Be clear when telling them about your readiness or reservations about quitting. You've got to be ready to take action and make a change in your life or it won't happen [also check out *Chapter 4*, page 49].

CONFIDENTIAL

Research Brief

Can Smoking Cause Type 2 Diabetes?

Researchers in Switzerland conducted a review and analysis of 25 previously done studies completed between 1992 and 2006. These reviewed the link between both former and active smokers and their incidence of pre-diabetes and type 2 diabetes.

A total of 45,844 new cases of diabetes were reported during the range of follow-up from 5 to 30 years. Analysis showed that active smokers had a 44% increased risk of developing type 2 diabetes, compared with non-smokers. Former smokers had an increased risk (23%) of pre-diabetes or type 2 diabetes. Another analysis suggested that the more someone smoked, the more likely they were to develop type 2 diabetes.

Though not definitive, the researchers concluded that there was an association between smoking (even a history of smoking) and the development of type 2 diabetes.

Source: *Journal of the American Medical Association*, December 12, 2007.

Quit with a Multi-Pronged Approach

Experts in smoking cessation believe that a multi-pronged approach works best if you want to quit smoking successfully. Here are some tips: First, set the date when you are going to quit, and set up your environment so you can successfully implement your plan. If you have cigarettes in your house, get rid of them before that date. Inform your family and friends that you are quitting, and let them know your quit date. Ask them for their support during what's going to be a difficult time for you. If you don't have support of family or friends or if you just think you may need additional support, consider getting support from an individual or group counseling service or online support. Choose the type of support you think will work best for you. A few good websites for online support are *www.lungusa.org*, *www.smokefree.gov*, and *www.quitnet.com*.

Cost may be a factor as well as what's accessible. The good news is that when it comes to smoking cessation, there are a few free programs. Whatever option you choose, make sure you have your support system set up before your quit date. There are quite a few medications on the market today to help you stop smoking. Some of these are available over the counter, and others are prescription drugs. Talk to your health care provider, and find out what options might work best for you.

Keep in mind that the toughest period is the first three months after you quit. If you can get through this time, you are more likely to successfully quit this time. If not try, try again!

Wonder?

What are the medication options to help you quit smoking?

Currently, there are seven available treatments approved by the FDA for smoking cessation. Five of these are in the category of nicotine-replacement therapy, and two are in the non-nicotine treatment category.

Nicotine-replacement therapy comes in several forms: nicotine patches, gums, and lozenges, which are available without prescription. Nicotine nasal sprays and inhalers are available by prescription. You will have to stop smoking completely before starting any of these treatments to increase your success. The antidepressant nortriptyline has also been shown to be effective in smoking cessation. There are currently two non-nicotine treatments. Bupropion SR is the first non-nicotine treatment approved by the FDA for smoking cessation and is only available with a prescription. The second prescription medication is called Varenicline.

Talk to your health care provider about which medication option is best suited to your needs and smoking habits.

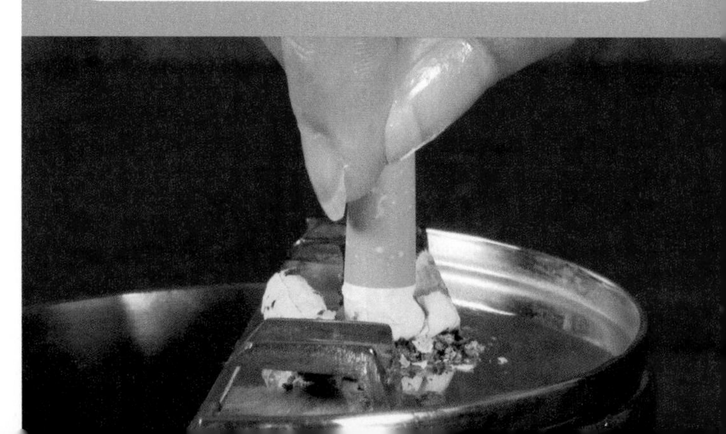

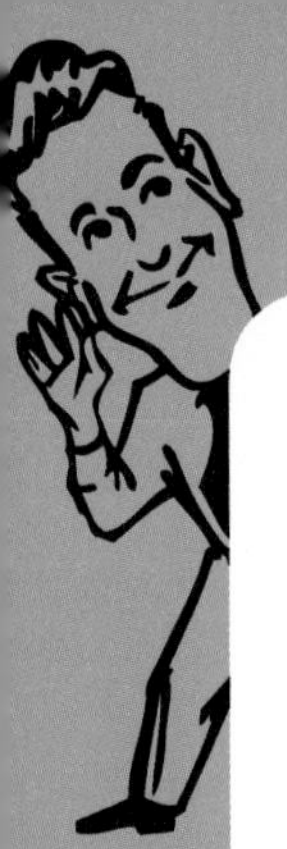

Psst...

A Serving of Alcohol

The ADA concurs with the Dietary Guidelines for Americans and recommends that women limit their intake of alcohol to one drink (or less per day), or two drinks or less per day for men.

A serving of alcohol is considered:

- 12 oz of beer
- 5 oz of wine
- 1.5 oz of distilled spirits

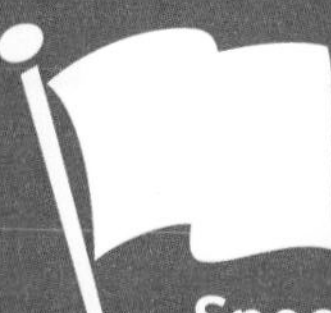

RED FLAG

Special Caution with Metformin

While alcohol decreases the liver's ability to make new glucose, it also decreases the amount of lactate cleared by the liver. This increases the amount of lactate in the blood. One concern in general with metformin, though rarely seen, is a potential side effect called lactic acidosis. If you are a binge drinker or regularly drink more than a few drinks, and you take metformin, or your health care provider wants you to start taking it, alert them about your alcohol use. It may not be the right medication for you, or you may be motivated to decrease or omit your use of alcohol.

Alcohol and Your Blood Glucose

For most people, alcohol is fine in moderation and is often consumed socially at the holidays, with friends, or at celebrations like weddings. Moderate alcohol intake is defined by the Dietary Guidelines for Americans as one drink per day or less for women and two drinks per day or less for men on average. Keep in mind that research has shown that, as people age, the same amount of alcohol can have greater negative effects on you physically and mentally. Believe it or not, there are even some beneficial health effects associated with drinking alcohol in moderation [also check out *Alcohol's Health Benefits*, page 236]. Be in the know! Learn the impact of alcohol on blood glucose and gather a few tips to sip by.

The negative component of alcohol comes when it is consumed excessively. Alcohol can slow you down physically, impair your judgment, and cause long-term health problems like liver disease. When you combine alcohol with diabetes, the risk of hypoglycemia is your biggest concern, particularly if you take a blood glucose–lowering medication(s) [also check out *Chapter 8*, page 101].

DEFINITION:

lactic acidosis: a serious and possibly fatal condition caused by the build-up of lactic acid in the body, which is produced when cells burn glucose for energy without enough oxygen; signs are deep and rapid breathing, vomiting, and abdominal pain.

Research Brief

Is it better for your health to drink more, less frequently or drink less, more often?

A population of 44,000 people initially surveyed in 1988 and then again in 2002 about their alcohol intake reveals interesting data from researchers at the National Cancer Institute. In 1988, almost half of the 44,000 people surveyed identified themselves as drinkers who had at least 12 drinks of alcohol during the previous year. By the end of 2002, more than 2,500 of these individuals had died.

The researchers found that, in men, alcohol frequency and quantity had opposite effects on death from heart and blood vessel diseases. The greater the amount of alcohol that men consumed, the greater their risk for death from heart and blood vessel diseases. For example, men who had five or more drinks on the days they drank had a 30% greater risk for death than men who had just one drink per drinking day.

On the other hand, men who reported drinking smaller amounts of alcohol 120 to 365 days per year, compared to men who drank more but just one to 36 days per year experienced a 20% lower risk for death from heart and blood vessel diseases.

Among women, frequent drinking was associated with a significantly increased risk of cancer, while an increased amount of alcohol was associated with risk for death from all causes.

This study points out that drinking moderately over many days a year may be more beneficial to your health than drinking a lot a few times a year. Researchers point out that this detail is often obscured when studies average a person's alcohol intake.

Source: March, 2008 issue of *Alcoholism: Clinical and Experimental Research*. National Institute on Alcohol Abuse and Alcoholism (NIAAA), part of the NIH. *http://www.nih.gov/news/health/mar2008/niaaa-04.htm*.

Alcohol tends to speed up the effects of these blood glucose–lowering medicines while also slowing down the liver's ability to make new glucose to raise your blood glucose. (That's because the liver is working to rid the alcohol from the body.) Hypoglycemia from too much alcohol can happen in a delayed fashion and up to 24 hours later with significant alcohol intake (if you are taking blood glucose–lowering medications that can cause blood glucose to get too low [also check out *Chapter 15*, page 195].

Consider the fact that most alcohol is consumed in the evening hours. Alcohol decreases the body's normal output of growth hormones and reduces the normal rise of blood glucose in the early-morning hours. Keep in mind that the effect of alcohol on blood glucose depends on the amount of alcohol you drink at one time and whether you eat when you drink. Alcohol can also slow down your physical and mental reaction time and can impair your good judgment, which can affect your ability to recognize hypoglycemia and appropriately manage your blood glucose.

Alcohol does not raise blood glucose on its own, but when alcohol is consumed along with carbohydrate, such as within a mixed drink or as part of a carbohydrate-containing meal, blood glucose may rise, and it may also drop later. Alcohol consumption can worsen some diabetes complications, such as diabetic neuropathy (nerve damage) and retinopathy [also check out *Chapter 21*, page 257].

Fitting Alcohol Into Your Eating Plan

The ADA recommends that you factor alcoholic beverages into your eating plan. When you choose to fit alcohol into your eating plan, be aware of its calories and nutritional contributions—or lack thereof. Alcohol contains 7 calories per gram, mostly from carbohydrate, protein, and fat. This can add up. Think about having two 5 oz glasses of wine at dinner, which adds up to 200 calories. If you are trying to eat 1,400 to 1,600 calories a day, 200 calories are nearly 15% of your calories.

Alcohol contributes nearly no nutritional value. If you use up 200 calories on alcohol, you'll be even more hard-pressed to get all the nutrients you need. Also, alcohol can relax your fortitude to stay on course with your healthy eating plan. Consider your priorities, and make your choices wisely.

Do not cut calories from your eating plan to make room for the calories from alcohol if you take a blood glucose–lowering medication that puts you at risk of hypoglycemia [also check out *Chapter 8*, page 101].

RED FLAG

Stay Away From Alcohol If You...

- *have abused alcohol in the past or have challenges managing to drink only moderate amounts*
- *are thinking of becoming pregnant*
- *are pregnant or breastfeeding*
- *have pancreatitis (an inflamed pancreas)*
- *have very high triglyceride levels (over 500)*

By the Numbers

Calories in Alcohol

Alcoholic Drink	Serving	Calories	Carbohydrate (g)
Regular Beer	12 oz	155	13
Light Beer	12 oz	105	6
Wine (any type other than dessert wine)	5 oz	125	4
Distilled Spirits, 80-proof	1 1/2 oz	95	0

Source: USDA Nutrient Database Version 20, www.nal.usda.gov/fnic/foodcomp/.

Alcohol's Health Benefits

Alcohol in moderation has been shown to offer health benefits, compared to minimal or zero consumption. Research shows that health benefits of moderate alcohol center on the health of your heart and blood vessels. It can raise HDL cholesterol (the healthy kind) and lower LDL (the bad kind), lower triglycerides, and decrease blood pressure. In people with type 2 diabetes, some research shows that moderate alcohol intake can lower insulin resistance, and improve blood glucose and overall A1C. Research also shows that middle-aged and older people gain the most benefits from moderate alcohol intake.

There's been hype about the health benefits of red wine, both related to the French way of life and the presence of a component of red wine called resveratrol, which has been linked to reducing cancer risk; however, at this time there has been no human research done to verify this benefit.

With the research to date in hand, the bottom line is that any type of alcohol can benefit your heart and blood vessels as long as it's consumed in moderate amounts. When it comes to calories, the differences between types of alcohol are minimal.

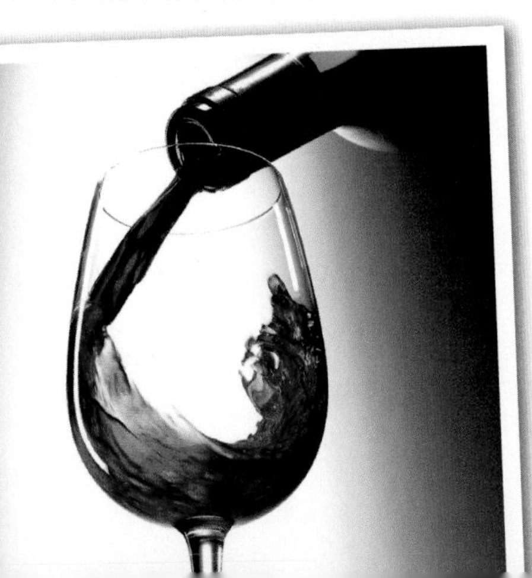

TIPS + TACTICS

Sip Alcohol Safely and Healthfully

- *Don't drink when your blood glucose is too low.*
- *If you take insulin or other blood glucose–lowering diabetes medications that can cause low blood glucose, always consume some food that contains carbohydrate when you drink.*
- *Wear medical ID. This is always a wise idea, but particularly wise when you drink alcohol. If you happen to become hypoglycemic, it can prevent you from being mistaken for being drunk [also check out* Chapter 15, *page 195]*.
- *Check your blood glucose levels more often when you drink alcohol. These checks will help you learn more about the effect of alcohol on your body and help you prevent or manage hypoglycemia.*
- *Don't drink and drive. If you drive several hours after drinking alcohol, make sure your blood glucose is in a safe range and that you feel your judgment is not impaired.*
- *Sip a drink slowly to make it last. Have a no-calorie beverage, like water, club soda, or diet soda on the side to quench your thirst.*
- *Make a glass of wine last longer by making it a "spritzer." Mix the wine with sparkling water or club soda or diet ginger ale.*
- *Choose light beer over regular beer if you want to save a few calories.*

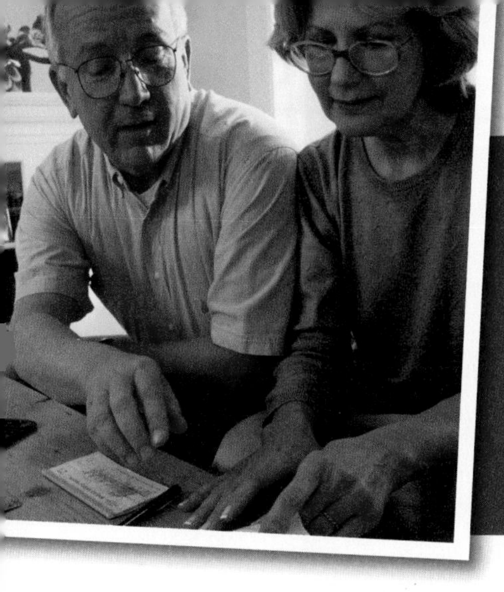

CHAPTER 19

Health Care Plans and Money Matters

When it comes to managing your diabetes, you and your health care providers will focus a lot of energy on your diabetes care plan. It's important not to overlook how having diabetes for the rest of your life will impact the health care coverage you have now and will need to have for the future. Caring for your diabetes and getting insurance coverage when you have diabetes can be expensive. Unfortunately, having diabetes will impact your ability to get these insurances if you don't currently have them independently or through your employer.

The good news is that thinking about how having diabetes impacts your health care plan and other insurance will help you both health-wise and financiallyThere is one small word with three letters that can help you navigate this sometimes challenging maze. That word is "ask." Since no two plans or policies are the same and since there are so many out there, consider this chapter a place to start, a resource to point you in the right direction. Remember, when it comes to health care, what you read today may change tomorrow. Continue asking questions so you're always up to date on the information you need to care for yourself better.

What You'll Learn:

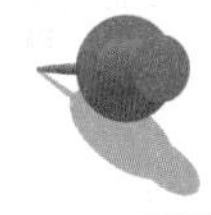

- Common options for health plans
- How to find out what is covered and what is not covered by your health plan
- Finding health care coverage if you are uninsured or underinsured
- Tips to find deals on diabetes supplies
- How health care is likely to be reformed or changed?
- Tips to find other insurances (life, disability)
- How the ADA can help

Health Care Coverage: Am I Covered?

This question comes up frequently. Unfortunately, there's no simple or single answer for all health plans—from Medicare to Medicaid to private health insurance plans. The answer depends on your health coverage and the state or federal regulations that apply to your plan. Today, many people who have health insurance can get coverage and reimbursement for diabetes supplies and education.

Coverage for diabetes education has improved over the last decade for two reasons. The first is that federal law now requires Medicare to cover diabetes self-management education (DSME) and medical nutrition therapy (MNT) for people diagnosed with diabetes. (Note: Unfortunately, if you have pre-diabetes, DSME is not currently covered. In the near future, due to the passage of Medicare legislation in 2008, Medicare beneficiaries with pre-diabetes may be able to get some coverage for MNT.

The second reason that coverage of diabetes supplies has improved is that 46 states have laws requiring coverage of diabetes supplies and DSME for health plans that are mandated by state laws (which are about one-third of plans) to cover at least some of these services. In the case of the individual and small group markets, these laws can change at any time. This is another reason why it is good for you to be well informed and active by being an advocate. Learn more at ADA's Action Center at *www.advocacy.diabetes.org/site/PageServer?pagename=AC_homepage* and sign up to become a diabetes advocate today.

By the Numbers

Study Reveals Costs Have Climbed 32% Since 2002

Early in 2008, the ADA put out a press release about a study it had commissioned, *The Economic Costs of Diabetes in the U.S. in 2007*. According to the study, diabetes costs Americans $174 billion annually, a figure that has increased by 32% since 2002!

- Direct and indirect medical costs of diabetes were estimated at $174 billion annually, including $116 billion in excess medical expenditures and $58 billion in reduced national productivity.
- Medical costs to care directly for diabetes are estimated at $27 billion with about 50% of this total for inpatient care.
- About $58 billion is estimated to treat diabetes-related chronic complications.
- People with diabetes spend over half of their medical expenditures caring for their diabetes (total $11,744; $6,649 on diabetes).

Source: Diabetes Care, *March 2008.*

DEFINITION:

diabetes self-management education (DSME): the ongoing process of managing diabetes by the patient in collaboration with a health care team, including meal planning, planned physical activity, blood glucose monitoring, taking diabetes medications, handling episodes of illness, and more.

If you have health insurance, the best way to find out whether your supplies are covered is for you to either contact your insurance company, or ask your health care provider to refer you to a DSME program or diabetes educator who may be able to guide you. If your plan covers DSME or MNT, you will most likely need a referral from your health care provider for the services. Give the DSME program or diabetes educator the name of your health plan. They may be able to tell you whether their services are covered.

You can also get details about this coverage from your health plan by calling the toll-free number on your health plan card or by using the plan's website. Ask what services and how many visits are covered, whether you have to go to a particular person or program, and whether you need a referral for the service from your diabetes care provider. If you feel you should be covered for DSME and/or MNT, but your health plan is denying this coverage, ask questions and demand answers. Plead your case! You may not get coverage at the time, but this is a chance for you to start advocating for yourself and for others who have diabetes.

Wonder?

Can I be turned down for health insurance because of my diabetes?

Employer-sponsored group health insurance plans are not allowed to turn you down for health coverage based on your health status. Some employers require newly hired employees to take and pass a physical exam (or to fill out a health questionnaire) before enrolling in health coverage.

Individual health insurance policies are not subject to the same consumer protections. The individual health insurance market in most states is characterized by medical underwriting. That is, insurers in this market decide whether to sell coverage (and if so, what benefits to offer and what premium to charge) based on your health status, prior medical history, age, gender, and other characteristics. Diabetes is a condition for which most medical underwriters will automatically deny coverage; however, this is not true in all states.

In a few states, medical underwriting is illegal. In others, only certain residents must be sold individual health insurance policies. Still other states designate one or more insurance companies (usually Blue Cross Blue Shield) as "insurers of last resort" that may not turn you down for coverage based on your health status. For more information on individual policies in your state, visit the Georgetown University Health Policy Institute's website at *www.healthinsuranceinfo.net* for a health insurance consumer guide for your state.

In most states, all private insurers in the individual market may medically underwrite coverage at least some of the time. Many (though not all) of these states establish high-risk pools that offer coverage to certain "uninsurable" individuals whom private insurers turn down.

With regard to large group and special policies, employers have the option to cover specific needs within a policy. Since every policy is different, you need to check with your particular provider to see what is actually covered. When you make contact, be specific. If it is blood glucose–monitoring strips you want to know about, ask how many are covered during what period of time. Ask what the amount of the co-pay will be.

Most laws regulating health insurance are developed and implemented by the 50 state governments. As a result, the health insurance options that exist in one state do not necessarily exist in another. A few laws, such as COBRA and HIPAA, were developed by the federal government and are available in every state.

COBRA stands for the Consolidated Omnibus Budget Reconciliation Act, a federal law that has been in effect since 1986. COBRA permits many employees and their dependents, in some circumstances, to continue on an employer's group health plan even after coverage would otherwise end. For example, if for some reason you lose your job, ask about COBRA. Although you will have to pay for COBRA yourself, at least you will have health insurance. This will give you some time to look into another plan. While on COBRA, learn all you can about it and about transferring to another type of insurance before canceling it. Once you cancel COBRA, it may be difficult for you to get insurance without employment.

HIPAA stands for the Health Insurance Portability and Accountability Act of 1996. HIPAA established special protections for certain people—called federally eligible individuals or HIPAA-eligible individuals—when they lose group health coverage. Once people become HIPAA-eligible, they are guaranteed an offer of at least two health insurance policies that do not impose pre-existing condition–exclusion periods. A pre-existing condition–exclusion period means that if you have a health problem that existed prior to or at the time you apply for your health insurance, the company may accept you, but not cover any costs related to that particular health condition for a certain period of time, which they determine.

Psst...

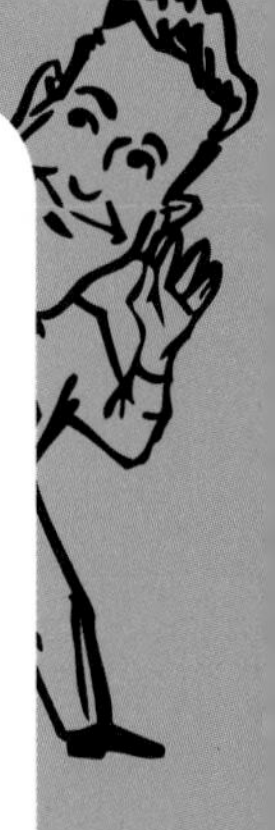

Understanding the Confusing Co-pay

A co-pay can be associated with your health care provider visit, any procedure you may have, hospitalization, your medications, and your supplies. Understanding your policy's co-pay is important. If you don't understand it, it can cost you a lot of money over the years. If you do, it can save you money. For example, you may know your plan covers blood glucose strips. But what you may not know is that the brand of strips you purchase may have different co-pays. Your co-pay can be $10, $25, or $50 for the same amount of strips. Ask your plan if they have a preferred brand (the brand you have to pay the least co-pay for). If you're concerned about accuracy, keep in mind that meters and strips have to be approval by the FDA to be sold. The major brands of blood glucose monitors available are considered accurate [also check out *Chapter 13*, page 163].

Wonder?

Will Medicare cover my insulin pump and the supplies I need for my pump?

Medicare now covers insulin pumps, single and multiple use medical supplies for use with a pump, and insulin for insulin pump users; however, there are several restrictions. Medicare restricts coverage for insulin pumps and related supplies to enrollees who use insulin to manage their diabetes. Medicare limits coverage for a pump and the supplies to people who have C-peptide test results within a range that shows they produce very little insulin. You must obtain a prescription from their health care provider for the pump and its supplies and must also go through a diabetes training program in order for Medicare to cover the pump and its related supplies.

Medicare and Diabetes

Medicare provides health insurance benefits to persons 65 and older, persons under 65 who are disabled, and individuals with end-stage kidney disease. Medicare includes:

- **Part A (Hospital Insurance)**: helps cover your inpatient care in hospitals, skilled nursing facilities, hospice care, and some home health care if you meet certain conditions.
- **Part B (Medical Insurance)**: helps cover medically necessary services like doctors' services that Part A doesn't cover (like physical and occupational therapists) and some home health care. Also helps cover some preventative services to help maintain your health and to keep certain illnesses from getting worse.
- **Part C (Medicare Advantage Plans)**: private insurers like HMOs and PPOs provide Part A, Part B, and, sometimes, Part D coverage to people who enroll.
- **Part D (Medicare prescription drug coverage)**: helps cover prescription costs.

Learn more about Medicare coverage for diabetes at *www.medicare.gov/Health/diabetes.asp.*

All American citizens over age 65, the disabled, and individuals with end-stage kidney disease who purchase Medicare Part B coverage and/or Medicare managed care policies are eligible for the following:

Blood glucose testing supplies, such as:

- Blood glucose monitors
- Blood glucose test strips
- Lancets
- Spring-loaded lancet devices
- Glucose control solution for calibrating meters

Some limitations apply, including:

- All people with diabetes are entitled, upon receipt of a health care provider's prescription, to a blood glucose monitor for the life of the monitor.
- If you take insulin (whether you have type 1 or 2), you are eligible for 100 blood glucose test strips and 100 lancets per month.
- If you do not take insulin, you are eligible for up to 100 test strips and 100 lancets every three months.
- If you need more than the number you are entitled to, your health care provider

may prescribe more test strips, but they must document in writing why you need additional testing supplies. This documentation must be renewed every six months.

In order for you to receive coverage for blood glucose test strips and related supplies, a prescription must be written by your health care provider. This prescription must meet the following guidelines:

- Your prescription must be renewed every six months.
- Your prescription must clearly document the number of strips and lancets to dispense.
- Your prescription must document whether or not you use insulin to manage your diabetes.
- The frequency with which you should monitor your blood glucose level or use the supplies must be clearly identified. (Note: This point is extremely important as Medicare will not accept prescriptions stating that supplies should be used or monitoring should occur "as needed.")

Health Care for People with Low Income and Limited Resources

Medicaid is a program that provides health care for certain individuals and families with low incomes and resources. This program became law in 1965 and is jointly funded by federal and state governments (including the District of Columbia and U.S. Territories). This funding allows states to provide health care to people who meet certain eligibility criteria.

Medicaid covers many groups of people. Even within these groups, certain requirements must be met. Criteria for Medicaid eligibility may include your age, whether you are pregnant, disabled, blind, or aged; your income and resources; and whether you are a U.S. citizen or a lawfully admitted immigrant. The rules for counting your income and resources vary among states and groups. There are special rules for those who live in nursing homes and for disabled children living at home.

You should apply for Medicaid if your income is low and you are one of the following:

- Pregnant
- 65 years or older and eligible for Medicare, but have extremely low income and limited resources
- Blind
- Disabled

If you are not sure whether you qualify for Medicaid, you should apply for Medicaid and have a qualified caseworker in your state evaluate the situation. To find a qualified caseworker, contact your state's division of social or family services.

As for coverage of diabetes education and supplies, since Medicaid is a state-administered program, each state sets its own guidelines regarding eligibility and services. Learn more at *www.diabetes.org/advocacy-and-legalresources/healthcare/healthinsurance/medicaid.jsp* and *www.cms.hhs.gov/home/medicaid.asp.*

State Children's Health Insurance Program (S-CHIP) provides health insurance coverage to children whose families may have too much income to qualify for Medicaid. It is a low-cost, private health insurance plan that provides health insurance coverage to eligible children until the age of 19.

By the Numbers

Medicare Co-pays and Deductibles

Deductibles and co-pays for an enrollee's Medicare Part B policy will often apply to the described benefits. The deductibles generally require an enrollee to pay for the first $100 of care purchased in a calendar year. After reaching the deductible, a Medicare enrollee is typically required to pay 20% of all charges for items and services while Medicare pays the remaining 80%. Patients with Medigap, other forms of supplemental insurance, including Medicaid, or those enrolling in a Medicare HMO are generally not responsible for these deductibles and co-pays. Supplemental policies like these typically cover the usual Medicare Part B deductibles and co-pays within the parameters of the supplemental policy's insurance program.

DEFINITION:

Medigap: Medigap policies are available to Medicare-eligible individuals. They can be purchased from private health insurance carriers and provide benefits that are otherwise not included in Medicare Part A or B. For more in-depth information on Medigap coverage, go to www.medicare.gov/medigap/.

Wonder?

What is a prescription-assistance program?

Most pharmaceutical companies offer financial-assistance programs to persons who are uninsured. This assistance is available to help cover the cost of medications and supplies when they cannot be paid for out-of-pocket. Each pharmaceutical company has specific criteria that need to be satisfied in order for an individual to be considered eligible for a financial-assistance program. If you are taking brand-name medications, contact the company to find out if you are eligible.

Users of some blood glucose meters may be eligible for reduced-priced meters and test strips. Contact Together RX Access at *www.togetherrxaccess.com/Tx/jsp/home*.jsp for more information, or call 1-800-444-4106. Some diabetes medications are also available at a reduced rate through this program. Other manufacturers of blood glucose meters and test strips may have established patient-assistance programs for people who are unable to purchase testing supplies out-of-pocket. To find out who these companies are, check with your health care provider, look on the Internet, or contact testing supply companies directly.

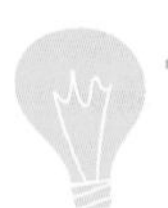

TIPS + TACTICS

Diabetes Deals

With or without insurance, it's always nice to save a little money. While very little is free in this world, you will see deals advertising free or discounted medical supplies. Know the facts and which deals are just going to cost you more in the long run.

- ***Free Blood Glucose Monitor Offers.*** *You may receive an offer for a free blood glucose meter. Once you have a meter, you need to use the brand of strips that go with the meter. The blood glucose monitor companies want to give you a meter because they make their money on the strips—not the meters. You need to know that it's no bargain for you to get a free meter and have to pay more for your strips. You'll be buying a lot of strips over time. Always check with your plan first before taking a free meter. It will save you money, and it will also save the environment from wasted meters.*
- ***Mail-Order-Companies.*** *Many people order from mail-order-companies for the convenience and money-saving offers. Many times, your local pharmacies and/or medical supply companies can offer you the same services. For example, the offer may be that you don't have to pay upfront if you have Medicare and a secondary insurance. It is most likely that your local pharmacy works the same way and will deliver your supplies if you would like. It is important for you to have a relationship with the company you buy from* *[also check out* Chapter 8, *page 101]*.

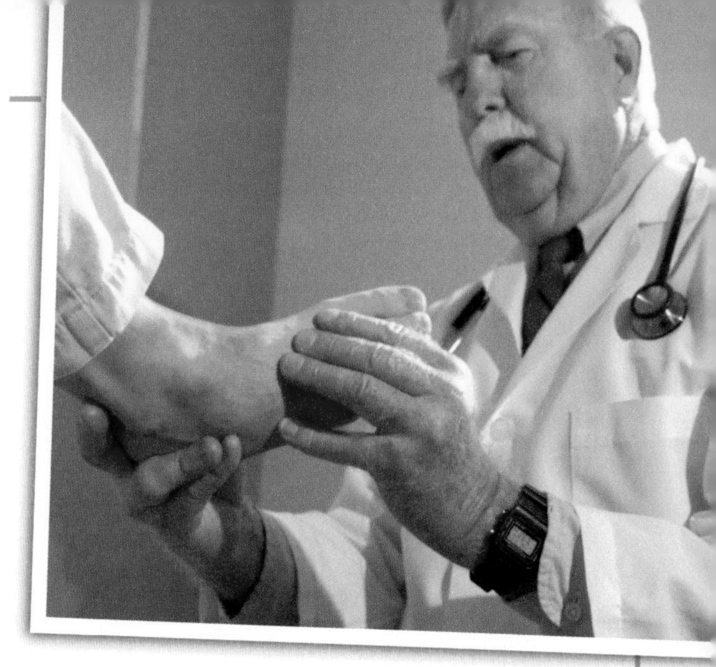

- ***Diabetic Shoes.*** *Your feet are important* *[also check out* Chapter 21, *page 257]**. Just because you have diabetes doesn't mean you need "diabetic shoes." Your feet are so important that you should see a podiatrist at least once, or on a regular basis if you have problems with your feet. If you are truly in need of a custom fit shoe, make sure your advice comes from a professional, such as a podiatrist, an orthopedic surgeon, or a certified pedorthist. Medicare will cover some therapeutic shoes and inserts. There has been some Medicare fraud with these items.*
- ***Lotions, Creams, Ointments, and Some Foods.*** *Many lotions or creams will work well for your skin. Some companies use the same formulary for their lotions and creams, then add the word diabetes, or diabetic, to the label or brand. Many times having these terms on the label increases the price. Unless recommended by your health care provider, stick with the products that don't say diabetes on the label.*

Health Care for Disabled Persons

There are several options of health care available if you are disabled and have a low income. Supplemental Security Income (SSI) and Social Security Disability Insurance (SSDI) provide benefits to low-income individuals and persons with disabilities.

SSI pays monthly cash benefits to people who are age 65 or older, those who are blind, or those who have a disability, and who do not own much or have a lot of income. SSI is not just for adults. Monthly benefits can go to disabled and blind children, too. The cash benefits you can receive depends on the state in which you live. The basic SSI amount is the same nationwide; however, many states add money to the basic benefit. Call the Social Security Administration at 800-772-1213 to find out the benefit amount for your state.

SSDI pays monthly cash benefits to people who are unable to work for a year or more because of a disability. After a 24-month waiting period, SSDI eligibility allows you to receive Medicare benefits even if you are under age 65.

Life Insurance Policies

Once you are diagnosed with diabetes, life insurance policies sold in the U.S. can become unaffordable or unavailable. This is because life insurance policies are allowed by state and federal law to rate, or charge, a premium based upon an applicant's health status. In addition, a plan can choose to not provide a policy, based upon an applicant's health status.

Even so, it is possible for many people with diabetes to find affordable life insurance policies in the U.S. Certain life insurance companies, or carriers, specialize in selling policies to people with chronic health conditions like diabetes.

To find the best life insurance policy for you, consider the following:

- A major factor in the cost of life insurance policies for people with diabetes is how well they manage their diabetes. If you have a lower A1C and good blood glucose control, lead a healthy lifestyle, and do not have complications from diabetes, chances are your rate will be more reasonable, too.
- Find an insurance agent that is experienced in obtaining policies for individuals with "impaired risk." A good agent will know which carriers may offer you a policy and which may not.
- Apply for a policy with a life insurance carrier that uses "clinical underwriting," a process that looks at your total health, not just what health conditions you may have.
- Shop around—on the Internet, by phone, or through referrals from family and friends. Becoming your own advocate will help you to find a life insurance policy that best fits your needs.
- Never take no for an answer! Just because one company declines your application does not mean that another company will not look at you more favorably.
- Each state has a department of insurance. Before you sign up for any plan, contact your state department of insurance. They will give you information about every insurance company and more.

Short-Term Disability Insurance

Since Social Security pays for only total disability, no benefits are payable for partial disability or for short-term disability (STD). STD requires you to pay a percentage of your salary if you become temporarily disabled, which means you are not able to work for a short period of time due to illness or injury. This excludes on-the-job injuries that are covered by workers' compensation insurance. A typical STD policy provides you with a weekly portion of your salary, usually 50, 60, or 66 2/3% for 13 to 26 weeks. Most STD policies have a cap, meaning you receive a maximum benefit amount per month.

Some people have an option for STD through their employer, or you can purchase your own STD directly from an insurance agent. Remember to always contact your state's department of insurance to make sure you have a good plan.

Psst...

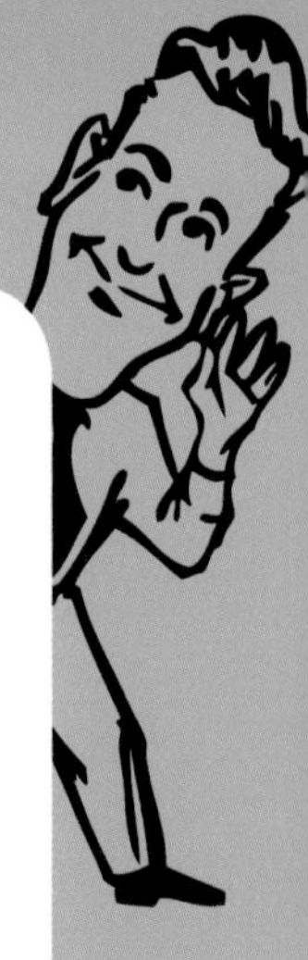

Long-Term Care Insurance Usually Covers or Helps Cover These Costs

- Assisted living services that are provided in a special residential setting other than your own home. These services may include meals, health monitoring, and help with daily activities.
- Community programs, such as adult day care.
- Help in your home with daily activities like bathing, dressing, eating, and cleaning.
- Visiting nurses.
- Care in a nursing home.

Long-term care insurance

With people living longer and longer, the risk of you having serious health problems that can cost you all of your remaining life savings rises. About 60% of people over age 65 will require at least some type of long-term care during their lifetime.

Ordinary health insurance policies and Medicare usually do not pay for long-term care expenses. Medicaid will only pay for long-term care if you've already spent most of your savings or other assets.

Long-term care insurance is an insurance option that helps you pay for many services beyond medical and nursing care if you have a long-term disability or a chronic illness that you need care for. This type of care can be very expensive. A long-term care policy allows you to make your own choices about what long-term care services you receive and where you receive them.

Long-term care insurance is something you should think about before you need it. If you wait until your 70s or 80s, your costs will go up. Do your homework. Talk with an insurance agent you can trust, and call your state department of insurance to make sure you have a good plan.

Health Care Reform For the Future

There's been a lot of talk about health care reform over the years. The goal for reforming our health care system is to provide quality health care to all people. How this can happen is a daunting task and has not yet been agreed upon. There are a lot of questions, but fewer answers about how to:

- Ensure that all people are covered by health insurance
- Increase the number and type of health care professionals one can choose from
- Improve access to health care
- Decrease the cost of health care
- Improve the quality of health care

With a new president and new administration in the White House, and health care costs steadily rising, we may very well see some changes. President Barack Obama has said, "Providing quality affordable health care for all Americans is one of my top priorities for this country because our long-term fiscal prospects will have a hard time improving as long as sky-rocketing health care costs are holding us all down."

Keep up to date by watching the news and getting involved. Learn more about the ADA's Health Reform Priorities at *www.diabetes.org/advocacy-and-legalresources/HRP-executive-summary.jsp.*

Navigating insurance and paying for diabetes is complicated and expensive. Visit ADA's Government Affairs and Advocacy website for more comprehensive information, or call ADA at 1-800-DIABETES (1-800-342-2383), and ask to speak with someone in Advocacy or Health Insurance. They have been working hard to advocate for you. Don't forget to sign up to be an advocate for yourself and other people by visiting *www.advocacy.diabetes.org/site/PageServer?pagename=AC_homepage*. ADA listens to you, works hard to make changes, and has been behind many of the positive changes made thus far.

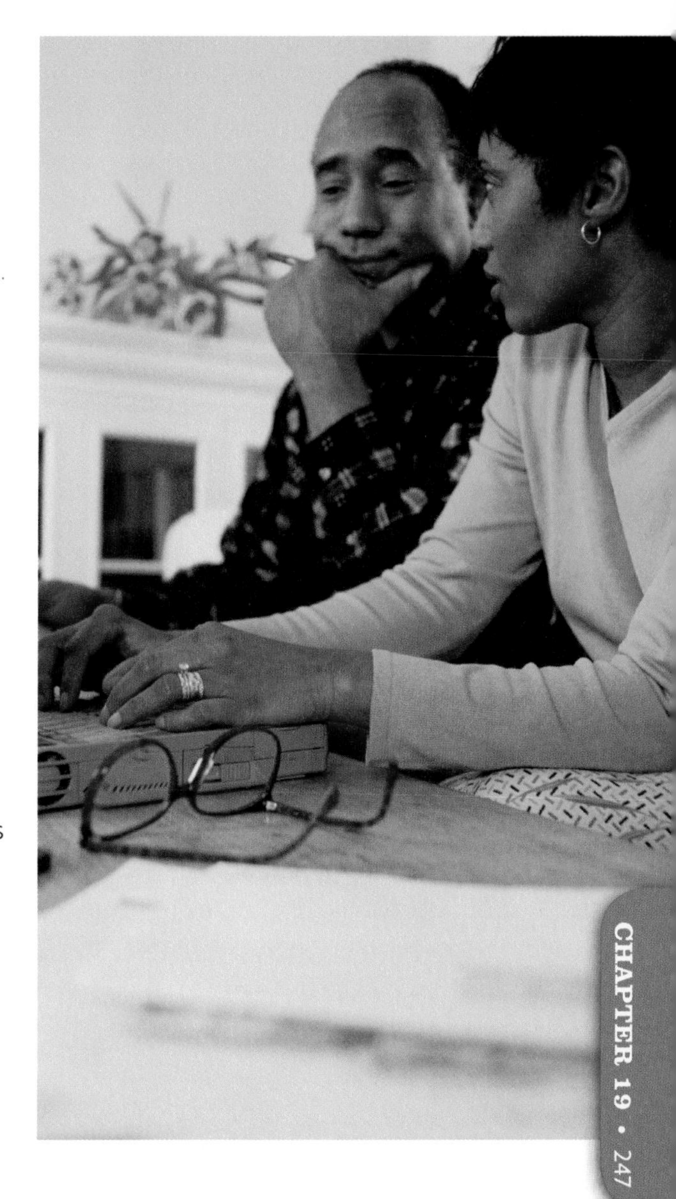

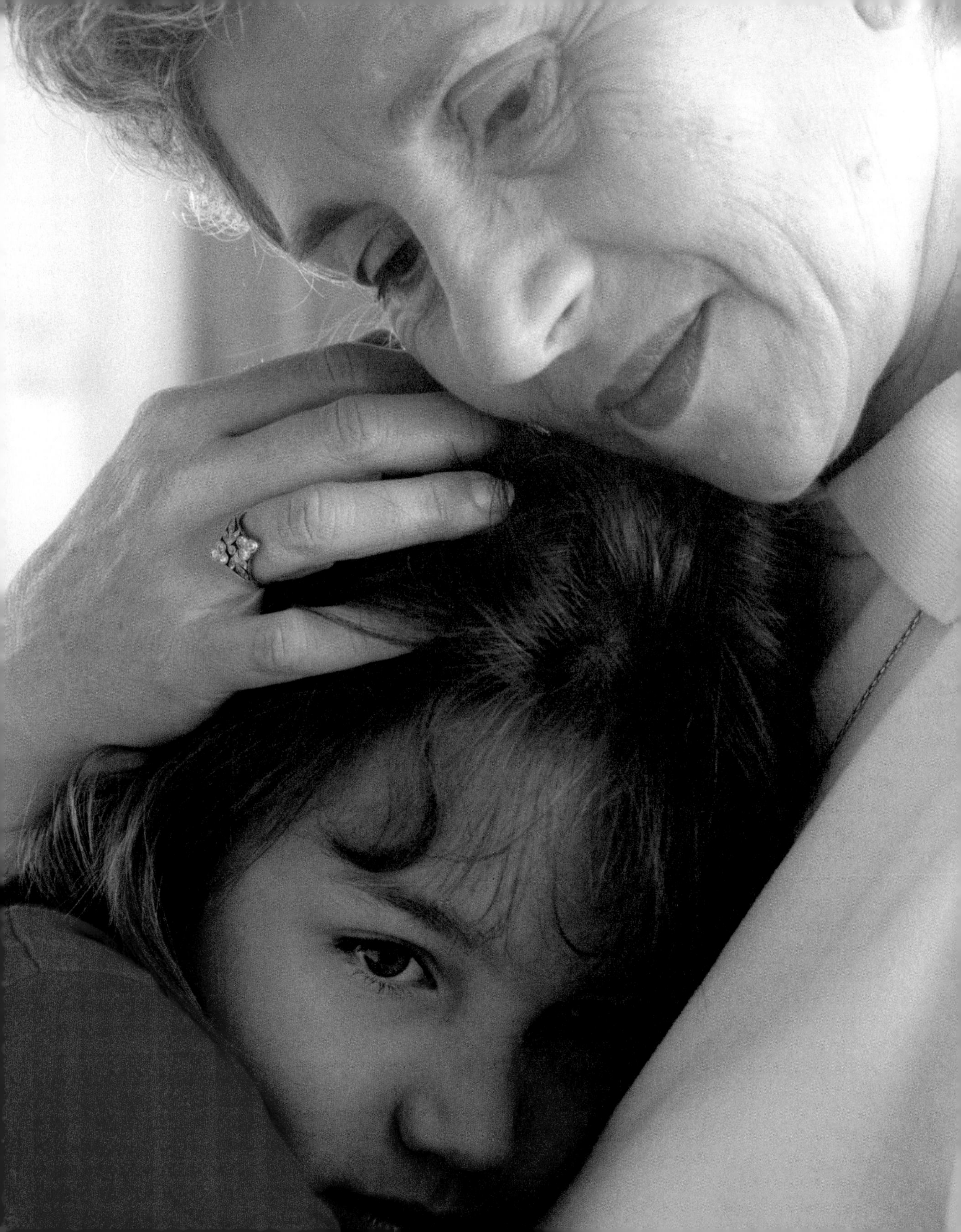

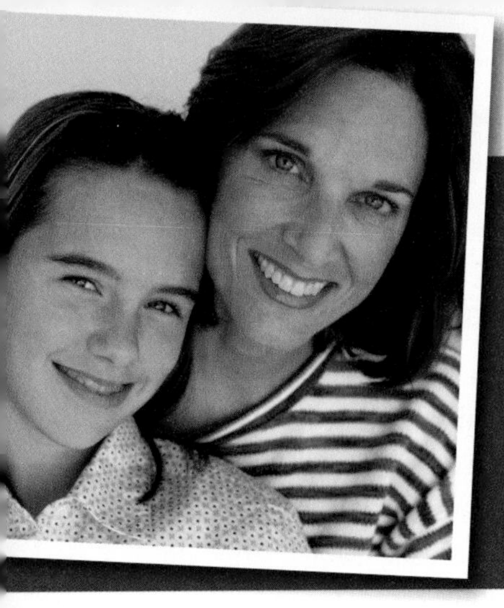

CHAPTER 20

Know Your Rights, Don't Be Wronged

Just like people who don't have diabetes, you want to be able to get and hold on to the job you want (and need), be able to go and do the activities you choose. If you are a parent of a child with diabetes, you want your child to receive a quality education and be safe while at school. Diabetes shouldn't stand in your way. It is important to understand your rights and the laws that may protect you, and how to use the ADA's 4-step approach to ending discrimination: educate, negotiate, litigate, and legislate. Keep in mind that if you stand up for your rights and educate people around you about managing diabetes in the 21st century, you'll help everyone with diabetes now and tomorrow.

Consider yourself an educator. Recognize that many people don't have up-to-date knowledge about diabetes and how it is managed and controlled today. These myths and misconceptions are perpetuated by stories in the media, profiles in movies or TV shows, and more. When you have the opportunity and/or the need, educate people around you about diabetes. This may happen in your workplace, at a social event, or elsewhere. Together we can bring the knowledge of diabetes and its management into the 21st century.

What You'll Learn:

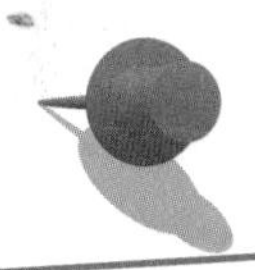

- ADA's four-step process to protect your rights: educate, negotiate, litigate, and legislate
- How ADA has and continues to fight against discrimination
- Your rights in the workplace and the laws that protect you against discrimination
- Your rights in places of "public accommodation" (such as restaurants and community centers) and the laws that protect you against discrimination
- The rights of children to receive a proper education and maintain safety in school and the laws that protect them
- What resources are available from ADA to help protect your rights

Ending Discrimination Against Diabetes

The ADA has developed an extensive legal advocacy program to help end discrimination against people with diabetes, which is based on the four-step approach detailed below. The goal is to resolve the discrimination issue at the earliest step possible.

Step 1 is to educate. People with diabetes often face discrimination by employers, schools, and others in decision-making capacities because of a lack of understanding about diabetes and current methods of diabetes management and about the requirements of federal and state laws. Therefore, step one is to educate decision makers to prevent or stop ongoing discrimination.

Step 2 is to negotiate. If you experience discrimination, contact ADA. You can speak with a legal advocate who can provide case-specific information and resources to help you negotiate with your employer, school, or other entity causing the discrimination.

Step 3 is to litigate. When efforts to educate and negotiate fail, litigation may be necessary to protect your rights. The ADA has a network of lawyers and school advocates who work to help people facing discrimination because of diabetes.

Step 4 is to legislate. Sometimes the most appropriate tool is to work to change the laws or policies that lead to discrimination. ADA has worked to ensure that students with diabetes are safe at school by advocating for school-diabetes-care legislation in states. In late 2008, ADA successfully lobbied with many other organizations for important amendments (changes) to the existing Americans with Disabilities Act to ensure that people with diabetes are protected from discrimination.

Wonder?

What do I do if I feel like I'm being discriminated against?

If you feel you are being discriminated against because you have diabetes contact ADA by calling 1-800-DIABETES. You'll be sent written materials and, if need be, given the opportunity to speak to a legal advocate about your specific situation.

Federal Anti-Discrimination Laws Protect You in the Workplace

Two major federal laws that help ensure fairness in the workplace for individuals with diabetes are the Americans with Disabilities Act and the Family Medical Leave Act (FMLA). The Americans with Disabilities Act prohibits discrimination in the workplace based upon a disability such as diabetes, and the FMLA allows workers to take medical leave from a job in order to care for their own or a family member's serious health condition.

In order to be protected by the federal anti-discrimination laws, a worker must show that he or she is a "qualified individual with a disability." The first step is to establish that the worker has a disability or "a record of" a

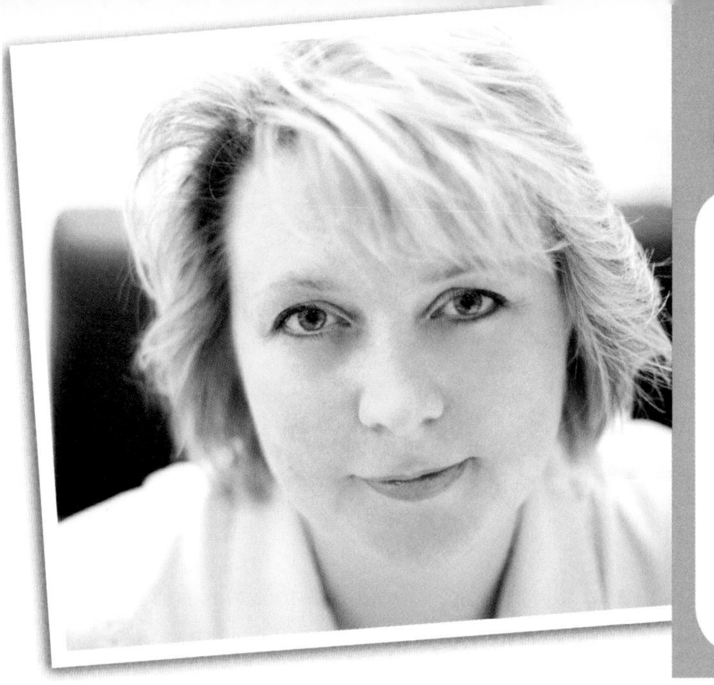

Wonder?

Are there any jobs that a person with diabetes who takes insulin can't hold?

The only job for which the answer is a blanket YES is being a commercial pilot, such as for an airline (though you can get a private pilot's license). Thanks to the ADA, fewer jobs are off limits to people who take insulin.

disability or is "regarded as having" a disability. A disability is defined in these laws as a mental or physical impairment that substantially limits one or more major life activities—such as eating, walking, seeing, or caring for oneself, or a major bodily function such as endocrine function. In the case of a person with diabetes, all you have to prove is that your body doesn't function properly without insulin or blood glucose–lowering medications.

Americans with Disabilities Act

The Americans with Disabilities Act of 1990 was amended by the Americans with Disabilities Act of 2008. This act prohibits discrimination (in hiring, firing, promotion, pay, and all other terms and conditions) in employment against qualified individuals with disabilities. The Americans with Disabilities Act applies to private employers, labor unions, and employment agencies with 15 or more employees and to state and local government.

Although Congress intended for people with diabetes to be covered by the Americans with Disabilities Act when it passed the law in 1990, as a result of several Supreme Court decisions over the past decade that narrowed the scope of the law, many people with diabetes were unable to prove that their diabetes qualified as a disability under the Act. Prior to the 2008 amendment, it was perfectly legal to fire a person from his or her job because of his or her diabetes. This put people with diabetes in a catch-22: The better the person managed his or her diabetes, the less likely he or she would be protected from discrimination. People with diabetes were told that they managed their condition so well with the use of certain mitigating measures, like insulin or oral blood glucose–lowering medications, that their diabetes did not substantially limit any major life activities. Instead of proving to a court that what happened to them constituted illegal discrimination, people with diabetes were forced to provide detailed information

Wonder?

Can I be restricted from joining the military, or can I be discharged if I have diabetes?

Generally speaking, having diabetes will restrict you from military service in all branches, and if you are diagnosed with diabetes while serving, you may be discharged. However, there have been exceptions handled on a case-by-case basis, and such an assessment depends on many factors including the job you do and your diabetes management.

about the severity of their diabetes just to prove they were eligible for the law's protections—while also proving that they remained qualified to do the job in question.

Congress passed the Americans with Disabilities Act Amendments Act (ADAAA) in 2008 specifically to address this catch-22. The ADA fought hard to make sure that people with diabetes are not kicked out of court on the issue of whether they have a disability. This new law is a great victory for people with diabetes and people with other chronic medical conditions. ADAAA still requires a person to prove that he or she has a disability, but it makes it clear that one way to do so is to prove that he or she has a substantial limitation on a major bodily function (like the endocrine system) and that a person with diabetes should be assessed as that person would be without mitigating measures such as the use of insulin.

Two other laws that have made an impact on the rights of those with disabilities are the Rehabilitation Act of 1973 and the Congressional Accountability Act. The Rehabilitation Act applies to most federal employees and contractors. The Congressional Accountability Act applies to employees of Congress. The law covers a "qualified person with a disability" who is someone who can perform the essential functions of the position, with or without reasonable accommodation. To qualify, a person must have either:

- a physical or mental impairment that substantially limits one or more of an individual's major life activities; or
- a record of such an impairment, or being regarded as having such an impairment.

The Family Medical Leave Act (FMLA)

The Family Medical Leave Act (FMLA) allows employees to take leave because of their own or an immediate family member's (child's, spouse's, or parent's) serious health condition, such as diabetes. FMLA covers private employers with over 50 employees and public employers (including local, state, and federal). This leave can be taken in small blocks of time to deal with such things as short-term problems

Wonder?

What about state anti-discrimination laws?

All states have their own anti-discrimination laws and agencies responsible for enforcing these laws. Some state anti-discrimination laws provide more comprehensive protection than federal laws.

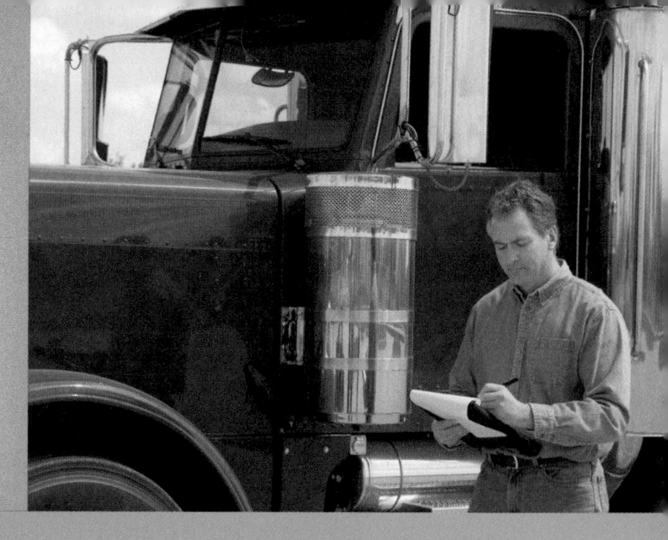

Myth

People who take insulin can't get a license to drive trucks, buses, or other commercial vehicles across state lines (interstate).

Fact

There used to be a blanket ban on interstate commercial driving by anyone with diabetes taking insulin (both type 1 and 2 diabetes). This ban was based on outdated science and medicine and did not reflect current diabetes-management therapies. It applied to all interstate commercial drivers. Interstate driving is involved whenever a driver carries goods or passengers from one state to another one, regardless of whether the driver him/herself actually crosses state lines. The good news is that the blanket ban is no more! After much work by ADA, including two acts of Congress, the U.S. Department of Transportation, Federal Motor Carrier Safety Administration (FMCSA) instituted a system of individual assessment—where each potential driver is evaluated based on how diabetes affected him or her. The FMSCA Diabetes Exemption, instated in 2003 and amended in 2005 to make it easier for people with diabetes to obtain an exemption, allows people who take insulin to obtain a commercial driver's license and to drive in interstate commerce.

Many states have medical waiver programs that allow a person who takes insulin and who meets the state's criteria, to operate intrastate (driving within a state) commercial vehicles including trucks and buses. Drivers who wish to continue driving intrastate only, and who are licensed by their state to do so, may continue driving as normal and do not need to apply for a diabetes exemption. To find out more information, go to *www.diabetes.org/advocacy-and-legalresources/discrimination/drivers/pvt*.

caused by managing blood glucose levels or for appointments with health care providers.

To gain the benefits of the FMLA, a worker must have a "serious health condition"—which diabetes has been found to be—or must be providing care for an immediate family member's serious health condition. FMLA entitles the worker to 12 weeks of unpaid leave and requires that employers return the worker to his or her job or a similar job at the conclusion of the leave. The leave can be taken intermittently or in longer periods of time, and often allows workers with diabetes the time they need to attend medical appointments, have surgery, or treat an illness.

The Role of Insulin and Hypoglycemia in Discrimination Cases

Insulin can play a large role in many discrimination situations and cases. This includes carrying the necessary equipment, eating meals and snacks, and the possibility of hypoglycemia. The discrimination is often due to lack of understanding about current diabetes management and the person's ability to keep their glucose under good control.

There remains a fear factor with insulin and hypoglycemia among people who don't understand diabetes. As a person with diabetes, take on the task of bringing people up to speed about how diabetes management has evolved and the realities of taking insulin today. Then, if you take insulin, let your actions speak more loudly than words, and try to manage your diabetes well.

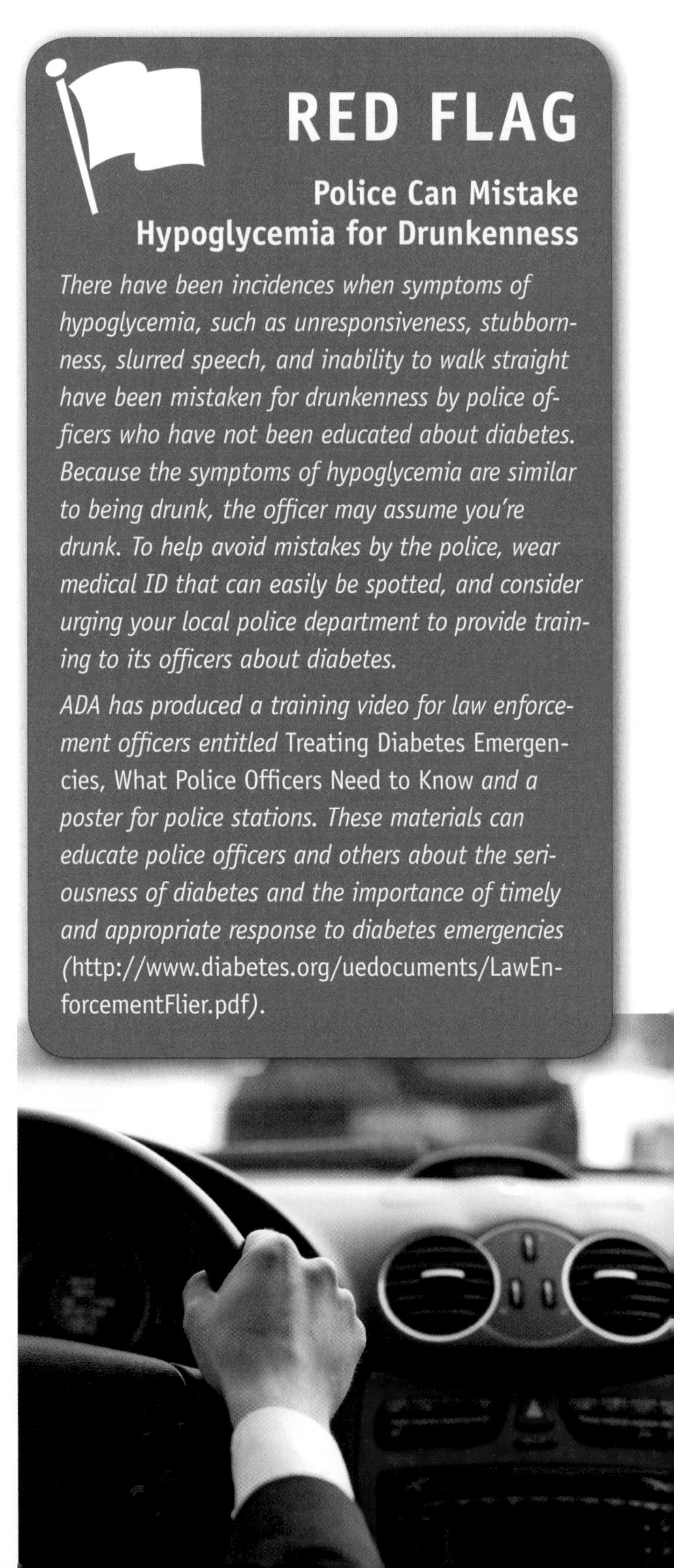

RED FLAG

Police Can Mistake Hypoglycemia for Drunkenness

There have been incidences when symptoms of hypoglycemia, such as unresponsiveness, stubbornness, slurred speech, and inability to walk straight have been mistaken for drunkenness by police officers who have not been educated about diabetes. Because the symptoms of hypoglycemia are similar to being drunk, the officer may assume you're drunk. To help avoid mistakes by the police, wear medical ID that can easily be spotted, and consider urging your local police department to provide training to its officers about diabetes.

ADA has produced a training video for law enforcement officers entitled Treating Diabetes Emergencies, What Police Officers Need to Know *and a poster for police stations. These materials can educate police officers and others about the seriousness of diabetes and the importance of timely and appropriate response to diabetes emergencies (*http://www.diabetes.org/uedocuments/LawEnforcementFlier.pdf*).*

Your Rights in Places of Public Accommodation

Beyond your workplace, your hobbies, interests, family activities, and other activities take you to various places during your life. You may travel on commercial airplanes; attend concerts, plays, movies, and sporting events; go to restaurants; and more. You may choose to exercise at a gym or community center. While you are in these "places of public accommodation," you want your rights as a person with diabetes to be protected. This means that in addition to simply being at any facility you choose to visit, you are allowed to take care of your diabetes as need be, such as taking your insulin, carrying your supplies, and wearing and using your insulin pump.

With security having tightened over the last several years, people must pass through more security gates than ever—whether you are going to a concert, into a state or federal building, or onto a plane. Most of the time you will have no problem carrying your diabetes supplies into these locations, but there have been instances where these rights have been challenged.

One example is a case that was settled by the U.S. Department of Justice (DOJ) with a large concert promoter. Prior to the settlement, the company had prohibited people with diabetes from keeping their lancets for blood glucose testing or insulin syringes with them at its venues. This was a problem for concert-goers with diabetes who needed to have these supplies with them in order to manage their diabetes and enjoy the concert. The settlement allows people with diabetes to keep their medical supplies and food with them at concert venues. It's important to realize that every time a case like this has a positive outcome, it makes it easier for the next person down the road to get a similarly positive result.

Airports are another public place where security has tightened. The ADA and Transportation Security Administration have worked together to develop airport security checkpoint guidelines and protocols to ensure that passengers with diabetes are able to board planes with their necessary diabetes supplies and equipment [also check out *Chapter 14*, page 181].

Your Child's Rights at School

Families of children with diabetes know that diabetes must be managed around the clock and that diabetes does not take a break when a child enters the classroom. You and your child have the right to a "free, appropriate public education" without discrimination. This means your child has a right to be medically safe in school and have the same access to education as other students.

The following federal laws protect you and your child in schools: Section 504 of the Rehabilitation Act of 1973 protects individuals with disabilities against discrimination in any program or activity receiving federal financial assistance. This includes all public schools and day-care centers and those private schools and centers that receive federal funds.

To qualify for protection under Section 504, a child must have a physical or mental impairment that substantially limits one or more

Wonder?

How will my child's needs be met at school? What should I expect?

Schools and day-care centers are required by federal and some state laws to meet the needs of children who qualify for services under these laws. Parents/guardians should document accommodations in either a Section 504 plan, an IEP, or as written accommodations under the Americans with Disabilities Act. The document should specifically state the child's disability, needs, and accommodations and how these accommodations will be delivered. As the parent or legal guardian of a child with diabetes, you have the right to:

- Ensure that a school nurse or other trained staff member is always available to monitor your child's blood glucose levels, recognize and treat hypoglycemia and hyperglycemia, and administer insulin and glucagon at school, on field trips, and at school-sponsored activities.
- Allow your child to provide self-care in the classroom and in other locations, including allowing your child to promptly treat hypoglycemia and hyperglycemia.
- Ensure full participation in all sports, extracurricular activities, and field trips, with the necessary assistance and/or supervision provided.
- Eat whenever and wherever necessary, including eating lunch at an appropriate time with enough time to finish eating.
- Take extra trips to the bathroom or water fountain.
- Permit extra absences for medical appointments and illness due to diabetes when necessary.

major life activities (such as eating, caring for oneself, learning, or a major bodily function such as endocrine function), have a record of such an impairment, or be regarded as having such an impairment. In making this determination, a person with diabetes is viewed as he or she would be without the help of mitigating measures such as insulin. Students with diabetes have been found to meet this standard. Parents of qualifying children should work with their child's school to develop a Section 504 plan. Schools can lose federal funding if they do not comply with this law.

The Americans with Disabilities Act prohibits all schools and day-care centers, except those run by religious organizations, from discriminating against children with disabilities. The standard to qualify for protection is the same as under the Rehabilitation Act.

The Individuals with Disabilities Education Act (IDEA) states that the federal government provides financial assistance to state and local education agencies in order for these agencies to provide a "free, appropriate public education" to qualifying children with disabilities. In order to be covered by IDEA, a child with diabetes must show that the disease adversely affects his or her educational performance. Once shown, parents and school officials develop an Individualized Education Program (IEP).

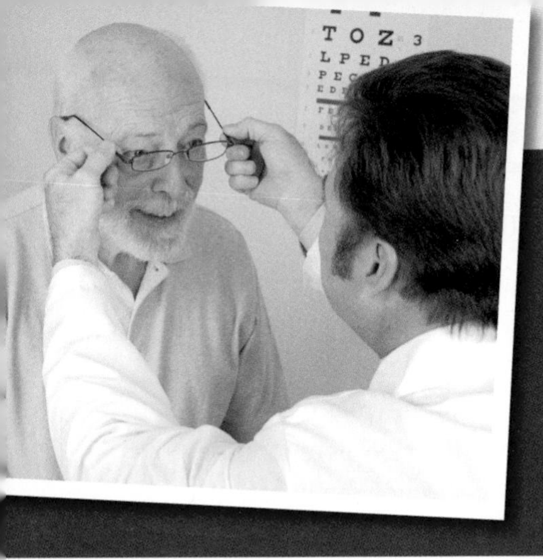

CHAPTER 21

Prevent and Delay Long-Term Diabetes Problems

When it comes to discussing the long term complications of diabetes, a historical perspective is enlightening. Prior to 1922, when insulin was isolated and first given to humans, the chief goal in managing diabetes was to keep people's blood glucose from being either dangerously high or low, which would only really prevent acute (immediate) complications—the only complications known at the time. The chronic (long-term) complications of diabetes were still unknown, and there was not yet a distinction between type 1 and 2 [also check out *Chapter 15*, page 195]. In the 1930s, health care providers began to observe that people with diabetes developed complications related to both small vessel (microvascular) and large vessel (macrovascular) problems. Medical experts hypothesized that the common denominator to these complications was chronic high glucose levels; however, there still wasn't a consensus on why.

For years, arguments ensued about whether glucose control could prevent or delay

What You'll Learn:

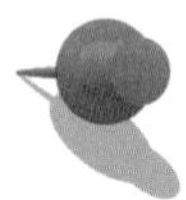

- The two categories of common long-term health problems associated with diabetes
- Current theories about why complications happen and when
- How to prevent or delay complications with measures and early detection
- The self-care steps you need to take to prevent problems
- Tests and checks to get done every three to six months or annually to prevent and/or detect and treat complications early
- Tips to track the results of your tests and checks

Psst...

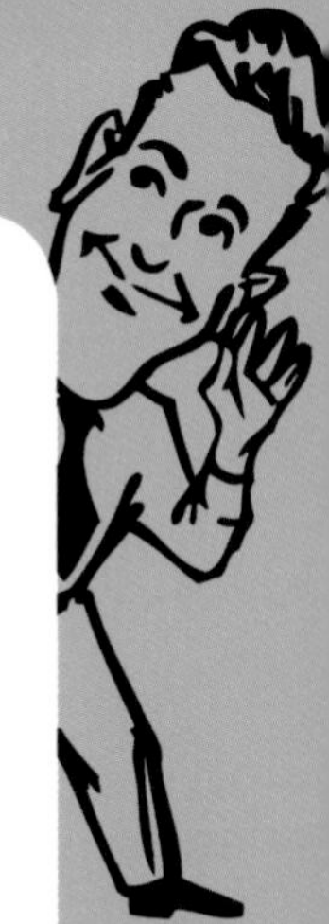

Fears About Complications Are Perfectly Normal

It's no wonder you fear the possible complications associated with diabetes. When you hear about diabetes in the media and public service campaigns, you may hear about amputations, kidney disease, blindness, and other devastating complications. When you talk with your health care providers, they may try to scare you into taking action to control your diabetes. You may have watched a relative or other loved one have to deal with the slow deterioration from one or more diabetes complications. It's perfectly normal to be fearful of complications, but try not to let these fears overwhelm you and your efforts to take care of yourself. Learn about your real risks for complications. Are you likely to develop kidney disease, or are you more likely to have a stroke? Learn the actions you need to take to minimize the complications you are most likely to be at risk for. With good diabetes self-care and a plan with your health care provider, you can successfully reduce or prevent complications.

complications. The Diabetes Complications and Control Trial (DCCT), the United Kingdom Prospective Diabetes Study (UKPDS), the ACCORD and ADVANCE trials, and the follow-up studies to DCCT and UKDPS put this argument to rest [also check out *Chapter 2*, page 23]. Today, research and experts support the premise that glucose control over time can help prevent or delay complications; however, research to determine all of the causes of diabetes and its complications continues.

Numerous studies also show that regularly doing diabetes self-care behaviors, such as healthy eating; being active; taking prescribed medications to control glucose, lipids, and blood pressure; and working with your health care provider to get the tests and checks that monitor and detect complications early, can greatly help you stay healthy over the years. The challenge is learning what preventive steps to take and make sure they get done.

If I Only Knew . . .

To put fears of complications in perspective . . .

What are my biggest fears about complications? Losing my eyesight and kidney failure! When I check my blood glucose and get a high number, my mind wonders what the toll will be on my body. Recently, I asked my health care provider to tell me which complications he thought I am most at risk for. His response: "I'm not worried about kidney disease or eye problems for you. I want to place our focus on preventing heart disease and a stroke." That put some of my worst fears to rest! If I only had known to ask that question a few years ago, I could have saved myself a lot of sweat and tears. Try posing this question to your health care providers.

How Complications Develop

Since awareness about diabetes complications only became a reality over the last several decades, various theories about why they develop have been proposed and studied. It is now clear that high blood glucose levels, high blood pressure, and abnormal blood lipids over time all play a role in diabetes complications [also check out *Chapter 2*, page 23].

A few other theories are detailed below. Some of the theories play a bigger role in the development of microvascular complications, whereas others play a bigger role in the development of macrovascular complications. It is likely that the causes of the various complications are due to a combination of these theories.

Glycemic variability. The excursion of blood glucose from low to high and back again or vice versa. Both the amount of rise (magnitude) and the length of time the rise lasts (duration) contribute to blood vessel damage. Blood glucose levels after meals (post-prandial levels) are seen to be the leading contributor to these large rises in blood glucose. Glycemic variability has been shown to cause oxidative stress.

Oxidative stress. High glucose levels cause oxidative stress and stimulate the production of free radicals. Frequent high blood glucose levels during times of fasting and wide swings of blood glucose from high to low and vice versa are both associated with oxidative stress and free radical production. The use of antioxidants, such as vitamins A, C, and E to prevent oxidative stress, have been studied, but treatment has not proven beneficial. Oxidative stress is more associated with microvascular complications [also check out *Chapter 10*, page 133].

Advanced glycation end products (AGEs). High glucose levels promote the formation of

Myth

For people with type 2 diabetes it takes many years to develop any of the complications of diabetes

Fact

Recent studies, including the Diabetes Prevention Program (DPP) [also check out *Chapter 1*, page 5], point out that people with both pre-diabetes and type 2 diabetes can have existing diabetes complications—both microvascular and macrovascular disease—at diagnosis. Research concludes that higher-than-normal levels of glucose and blood pressure and abnormal blood lipids over time combine their forces to cause the varied diabetes complications. These findings just reinforce the importance of controlling glucose, blood pressure, and blood lipids before abnormalities are discovered—no need to even wait for the diagnosis of type 2 diabetes.

molecules that are a combination of glucose and protein—glycoproteins—which form advanced glycosylated end products, abbreviated as AGEs. AGEs accumulate when blood glucose is higher than normal.

Polyol pathway. The polyol pathway is the pathway the body normally uses to convert glucose in the body into sorbitol (a glucose alcohol). High glucose levels increase the amount of glucose molecules that go through this pathway and cause the build-up of sorbitol in cells. The polyol pathway is more associated with microvascular complications. (Note: This has nothing to do with eating sorbitol in sugar-free foods.)

Two Groups of Complications: Macrovascular and Microvascular

Diabetes complications fit into two main groups—either problems related to small vessels (microvascular) or large vessels (macrovascular). To prevent and/or delay all complications, your first line of defense is to get and keep your ABCs in the target zones [also check out *Chapter 2*, page 23]. To hit your ABC targets, it's important to implement your daily diabetes self-care plan.

There are other tests and checks to get done at appointments with your health care provider (every 3–6 months), and several should be done annually. These tests and checks focus on the early detection of any problems from complications. If problems are detected, it's critical to get them dealt with quickly.

By the Numbers

Cost of Treating Complications

Of the total estimated direct and indirect cost of diabetes in the U.S. in 2007, $58 billion was used to treat diabetes-related complications.

Source: Economic Costs of Diabetes Care–2007. Diabetes Care, *2008.*

Meeting ADA Standards of Care

Though ADA publishes standards of care for diabetes each year in January, data from the National Health and Nutrition Examination Survey (NHANES), a nationally representative survey of people with diabetes conducted by the National Center for Health Statistics from CDC, noted that only:

- 37% of people surveyed are achieving ADA's goal for A1C (7% or less) with slightly less than 30% having had an A1C check
- 36% met the blood pressure goal of 130/80 mm Hg
- 52% had total cholesterol levels above 200 mg/dl
- 63% had a dilated eye exam within the previous year
- 55% had a foot exam within the previous year

Learn more about the major macrovascular (large vessel) and microvascular (small vessel complications) in the pages ahead. You'll learn what can happen to an organ or system and why. You'll gather the self-care steps to take to help prevent or detect each problem. The chart on page 273 helps you learn the tests or checks to have ordered or done by your health care provider to prevent or treat these problems early.

Research studies tell the tale. The earlier you detect a diabetes problem, whether it's an eye, foot, kidney, or common circulatory problem, early detection and aggressive treatment slow the progression of all of these complications. Take an eye problem, for example. According to the Centers for Disease Control and Prevention (CDC), finding early damage to one or both retinas from a dilated exam, along with quick action with laser therapy, can reduce the development of severe vision loss by an estimated 50 to 60%.

Macrovascular (Large Vessel) Problems

Macrovascular (or large blood vessel) problems involve complications with the blood vessels of your heart and circulatory system, including coronary (heart) artery disease, cerebrovascular (blood vessels in your brain) disease, and peripheral vascular disease (blood vessels in your extremities). Large vessel diseases are covered first because they are the most common complications of diabetes. This is due in part to high blood glucose, high blood pressure, and abnormal lipid levels.

Wonder?

Which complication is most common?

When people hear the words "diabetes complications," they often think of kidney failure, amputation, and blindness. These are understandably the feared complications; however, the most serious and common complication is heart disease, which can result in heart attacks or strokes. Studies show that many people with diabetes don't make the connection between diabetes and heart disease. You are two to four times more likely than people without diabetes to have heart disease or a stroke. Your chance of having a heart attack is the same as someone who has already had one. Having a heart attack or stroke makes it more likely that you will have another. The good news: Controlling your ABCs can prevent or delay heart and blood vessel diseases.

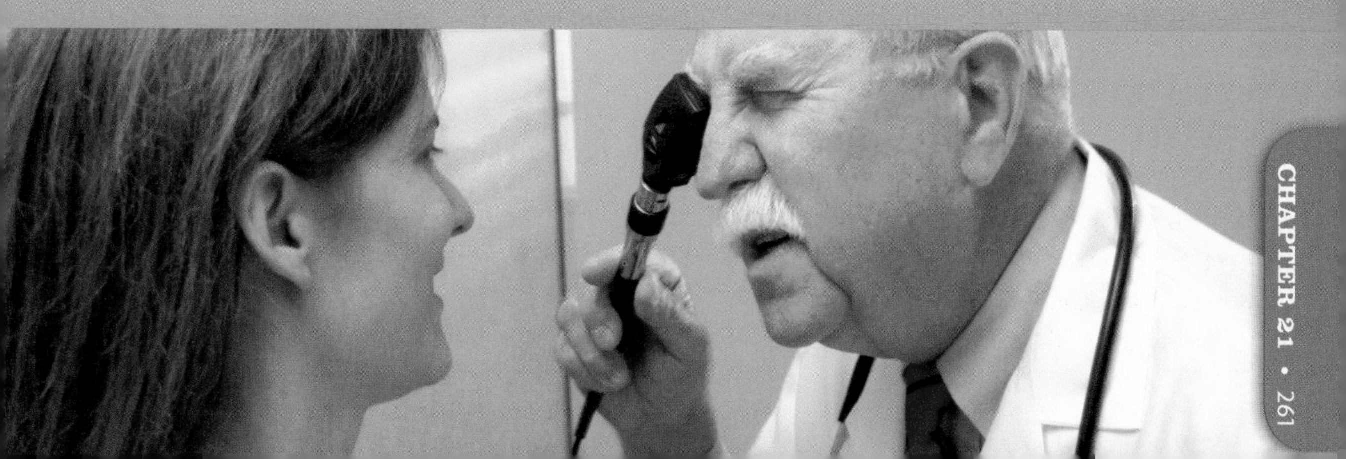

Heart and Circulatory Problems: What Can Happen?

- People with diabetes are more likely to have heart disease or a stroke and tend to develop these problems at an earlier age.
- People with pre-diabetes and type 2 often have risk factors for heart disease and/or high blood pressure and abnormal lipid levels when they are diagnosed with diabetes.
- If you are middle-aged and have type 2 diabetes, your chance of having a heart attack is as high as someone without diabetes who has already had one heart attack.
- People with diabetes who have already had one heart attack run an even greater risk of having a second one.
- Women who are pre-menopausal are not as protected from heart disease as women without diabetes.

By the Numbers

Heart Disease and Stroke

- Heart disease and stroke account for about 68% of deaths in people with diabetes (as recorded on death certificates).
- Adults with diabetes have heart disease death rates about 2 to 4 times higher than adults without diabetes.
- Risk for a stroke is 2 to 4 times higher among people with diabetes.

DEFINITION:

cardiomyopathy: a heart disease in which the heart is weakened and does not function properly.

Coronary artery disease is caused by a hardening or thickening of the walls of the heart's blood vessels, which narrows the opening for blood to flow through. Plaque or fatty deposits on artery walls can break off and get lodged in artery walls, which can reduce or cut off blood supply and result in a heart attack. If the blood flow to your heart isn't restored quickly, the section of your heart muscle that was without blood flow becomes damaged from the lack of oxygen and begins to die. Heart attacks can take place in different vessels of your heart and can vary in their severity.

Heart failure is caused when your heart cannot pump blood properly. It develops over several years, and symptoms can get worse over time. People with diabetes have at least twice the risk of heart failure as people who don't have diabetes. One type of heart failure is congestive heart failure, in which fluid builds up inside the body's tissues.

Blockage of the blood vessels and high blood glucose levels can also damage heart muscle and cause abnormal heartbeats. If you have cardiomyopathy, you may have no symptoms in the early stages, but later you may experience weakness, shortness of breath, a severe cough, fatigue, and swelling of your legs and feet. Diabetes can also interfere with pain signals normally carried by your nerves, explaining why you may not experience the typical warning signs of a heart attack. Having diabetes increases your risk for atrial fibrillation, a type of irregular heartbeat that increases your risk for having a stroke.

Cerebral vascular disease occurs when the blood vessels in your brain become narrowed or hardened because of plaque buildup and can cause a stroke or transient ischemic attack (TIA). A stroke cuts off blood supply to an area of brain. It deprives your brain cells of oxygen and causes cell death. Strokes can vary in intensity and have various physical or mental repercussions based on the location of the stroke. A stroke may also be caused by an aneurysm—a blood vessel that bleeds in the brain. TIAs are caused by a temporary blockage of a blood vessel to the brain that causes a sudden change in brain function, such as temporary numbness or weakness on one side of the body. Most symptoms disappear quickly, and permanent damage is unlikely. TIAs are alerts about the increased risk for having a stroke. If you are having TIAs, talk with your health care professional about more aggressive ways for you to prevent a stroke.

The peripheral system refers to your legs, feet, arms, and hands. If you have diabetes and high blood pressure, you are at increased risk for peripheral vascular disease, in which case the blood vessels in your legs are narrowed or blocked by calcium and fatty deposits, which decreases the blood flow to your legs and feet. This can lead to poor circulation and can make foot problems challenging to heal.

RED FLAG

Symptoms of a Heart Attack

When you are having a heart attack, you may have one or more of these symptoms:

- *chest pain or discomfort*
- *pain or discomfort in your arms, back, jaw, neck, or stomach*
- *shortness of breath*
- *sweating*
- *nausea*
- *light-headedness*

People with diabetes may have more subtle or no symptoms of a heart attack because of a neuropathy *that affects the heart rate and your senses that detect pain. Women might not have chest pain but might have shortness of breath, nausea, or back and jaw pain when having a heart attack. If you have symptoms of a heart attack, call 911 right away. Treatment is most effective if given within an hour of a heart attack. Early treatment can prevent permanent damage to the heart.*

DEFINITION:

neuropathy: disease of the nervous system; a complication of diabetes.

By the Numbers

Vision problems

- Diabetes is the leading cause of blindness among 20–74 year olds, with complications from diabetic retinopathy being a leading cause.
- Diabetic retinopathy causes blindness in 12,000 to 24,000 people in the U.S. each year.

Kidney disease

- Diabetes is the leading cause of kidney failure, accounting for nearly half of new cases.
- Nearly 50,000 people begin treatment for end-stage kidney disease each year.
- African Americans, American Indians, and Hispanics/Latinos develop diabetes and kidney failure at rates higher than Caucasians.

Nerve damage

- About 60–70% of people with diabetes have damage to one or more parts of their nervous system.

Foot problems

- Almost 30% of people with diabetes who are older than 40 have impaired sensations in their feet.
- More than 60% of nontraumatic lower-limb amputations occur in people with diabetes. In 2004, 71,000 of these amputations in the U.S. were done in people with diabetes.

Dental problems

- Almost one-third of people with diabetes have severe periodontal (gum) disease.

Source: CDC National Diabetes Fact Sheet (*www.cdc.gov/diabetes/pubs/factsheet.htm*).

Microvascular (Small Vessel) problems

Microvascular (small blood vessel) problems center on complications with the eyes, kidneys, nervous system, feet, or teeth and gums. Microvascular disease occurs when the blood vessel walls become abnormally thick, but weak, which causes them to bleed, leak protein, and slow the flow of blood to the cells. This weakening of the small blood vessels can cause serious damage to your body over time.

Eye Problems: What Can Happen?

Diabetic retinopathy (damage to the retina of the eyes) is the most common eye problem. Retinopathy develops slowly, but people with pre-diabetes and type 2 may have evidence of it at diagnosis.

The retina is the lining at the back of each eye. It senses light coming into your eye. Research shows that, over time, high blood glucose and high blood pressure can damage the tiny blood vessels in the retina. Research also shows that other actions happen to cause the damage. Initially, the vessels can swell and weaken. They can leak blood and form fatty deposits or small aneurysms (dilation of small vessels). These changes are referred to as background or non-proliferative retinopathy.

You might not have any vision loss from these problems. If these vision problems aren't detected and treated, they can progress to proliferative retinopathy, in which new blood vessels form on the surface of the retina. This

TIPS + TACTICS

Steps Specific to Eye Problems

- *Ask to be referred to an eye doctor when you are diagnosed for an initial eye exam. If you have just been diagnosed with diabetes, let the eye doctor know you have diabetes. Make sure the exam includes a dilated retinal eye exam.*
- *Adults and children age 10 and older should have an annual eye exam. (If you have an eye problem, you may need more frequent visits.) Make sure they do a dilated retinal exam and check for signs of cataracts and glaucoma.*
- *Check with your health care plan about what eye services your plan covers and who must provide the service.*
- *If you experience an eye problem, contact your health care provider or eye doctor immediately.*
- *If you are pregnant and have diabetes, get an eye exam during your first 3 months of pregnancy.*

can cause a hemorrhage in the eye's vitreous humor (the jelly-like fluid that fills the back of your eye) through a detachment of the retina from the back of your eye. You may or may not have these signs of damage to your retinas: blurry or double vision; rings, flashing lights, or blank spots; dark or floating spots; pain or pressure in one or both of your eyes; or trouble seeing things out of the corners of your eyes.

Laser therapy, done by a trained opthalmologist, is commonly used to treat these leaking blood vessels. The laser beam closes off leaking blood vessels and may stop blood and fluid from leaking into your vitreous in an effort to slow your vision loss. If a lot of blood has leaked into your vitreous humor, an ophthalmologist may perform a surgery called a vitrectomy. This removes blood and fluids from the vitreous humor of your eye and replaces clean fluid into your vitreous to improve vision.

While cataracts and glaucoma are not unique to people with diabetes, you can get them more frequently and at a younger age. A cataract is like a cloud over the lens of an eye. The lenses focus light onto your retina. Your vision becomes cloudy as cataracts form. This is often a slow process, and the decision to have surgery is made over time. Surgery is needed to remove the cataract. Today, the lens is taken out and replaced with a plastic lens that is permanent. Glaucoma starts from pressure building up in the eye. The pressure, over time, can damage the optic nerve—the eye's main nerve. Today, glaucoma is usually treated with drops, prescribed by your eye doctor, that reduce the pressure in your eyes.

Psst...

A Dilated Retinal Eye Exam?

This test should be done when you are diagnosed with diabetes (unless you are a child with type 1 under 10 years old), and then annually or as often as your eye care professional recommends. The eye doctor will put drops in your eyes to make your pupils larger (or dilated). This allows your eye doctor to see the back of your eye and check for problems. Your vision will be blurred so you should not drive until your vision clears. This can take several hours. Make sure you have someone to drive you home after the exam. Bring sunglasses to wear after the exam, since a dilated eye allows a lot of light into your eyes. This can be uncomfortable and disorienting.

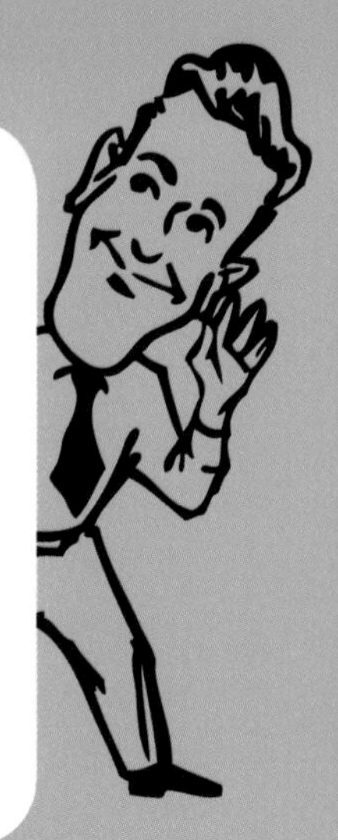

Wonder?

I was recently diagnosed with diabetes. My vision is blurred. I was told to wait until my blood glucose is stabilized before I get my vision checked. Why?

Your diabetes eye exam and your vision exam are two different exams. When your blood glucose is elevated, this causes fluid balance changes in your eyes. This affects your vision. Once your blood glucose is closer to normal and stabilized for a few weeks, your vision usually clears. You may need to buy some over-the-counter glasses until your vision improves. You should get your vision checked if you feel you need a new prescription for glasses or contact lenses.

Kidney Damage: What Can Happen?

Kidney disease is scary; however, it is good to know that most people with diabetes do not develop kidney disease severe enough to cause kidney failure. Diabetes is a leading cause of kidney failure. Kidney damage is a slow process and can take years to develop. Out-of-control blood glucose and blood pressure can cause kidney damage, along with other changes.

Over the years, small amounts of albumin, a protein in blood, begins to leak into the urine. This is called microalbuminuria (or small amounts of albumin in the urine). If this progresses and large amounts of protein leak into your urine, it's defined as macroalbuminia (large amounts). With macroalbuminuria, your kidney's ability to filter waste product from your body begins to fail. As kidney damage develops, your blood pressure often rises. If you already have high blood pressure, it quickens the progression of kidney disease.

The key to preventing kidney disease or slowing its progression is for you to work to manage your blood pressure and blood glucose [also check out *Chapter 13*, page 163]. A blood pressure medication from one of two categories—an ACE inhibitor or an ARB—is recommended by the ADA for initial use [also check out *Chapter 9*, page 121]. If you have kidney damage, you may need to pay attention to other elements in your eating plan, such as protein, sodium, potassium, and phosphorus. Consider meeting with a registered dietitian who specializes in, and works with, people who have kidney disease as well as diabetes [also check out *Chapter 5*, page 59].

If you develop what's called end-stage kidney disease, you will need either dialysis or a kidney transplant. Even if you are able to get a kidney transplant, you are usually placed on dialysis for at least a while. Obtaining a kidney transplant can be challenging [also check out *Myth/Fact: People with diabetes can't get kidney transplants*, this page].

Myth

People with diabetes can't get kidney transplants

Fact

Years ago, people with diabetes were not thought to be good candidates for transplants, but they are successfully being done today. In a small number of instances, people who are receiving a kidney transplant may be able to have a pancreas transplant as well. In most instances, the kidney and pancreas are from a cadaver (deceased donor), but there are instances where the kidney is from a living donor and the pancreas is from a cadaver.

Categories of Kidney Damage

Category	Amount of Albuminuria (protein in urine)
Normal	< 30 micrograms (mcg) per milligram (mg) of creatinine or per 24 hours
Microalbuminuria	30–299 mcg/mg or per 24 hours
Macroalbuminuria	> 300 mcg/mg or per 24 hours

Note: Screening for kidney damage can be through a 24-hour urine collection or a spot urine test. Spot measurements are more convenient and easy to do and have become the more commonly done test. Another test used to assess kidney damage is the estimated glomerular filtration rate (GFR).

DEFINITION:

albumin: a protein found in animal tissues, manufactured by the liver and circulated in human blood.

glomerular filatration rate (GFR): GFR can be calculated from the results of a blood creatinine test. GFR determines the amount of kidney damage and the stage of kidney failure.

TIPS + TACTICS

Steps Specific to Kidney Problems

- *If you have type 2 diabetes, ask your health care provider to get a measurement of your urine albumin excretion level initially at diagnosis and each year after. People with type 1 who have had diabetes for five years or more should also have this test done.*
- *Get and keep your blood pressure in control and take medications as prescribed. You may need more than one blood pressure medication to achieve normal blood pressure [also check out* Chapter 13, *page 163]*.
- *Eat healthy:*
  - *Lighten up on sodium and salt [also check out* Chapter 5, *page 59]*.
  - *Meet with a registered dietitian who specializes in kidney problems to learn more and to design an individualized meal plan with you[also check out* Chapter 5, *page 59]*.

Nerve Damage: What Can Happen?

Nerve damage can occur at any time; however, it is more common as you age and the longer you have diabetes. Nerve problems are also more common if your ABCs are not under control.

Because the different neuropathies impact various organs and systems, the options to treat these vary as well. Neuropathies can be challenging to manage because there are few therapies available that totally alleviate most of the problems. In general, getting and keeping blood glucose under control can improve neuropathies. In addition, you may be advised to decrease alcohol use and quit smoking. A variety of pain relievers can be used alone or in combination to lessen symptoms. Other medications and therapies are available for certain diabetic neuropathies.

Peripheral neuropathy (most common type) affects the parts of the body that are on the periphery of your body—your arms, hands, feet, and legs. Problems are most common in your legs and feet. If you start having problems in this area, it's usually starts first in your toes and then progresses up your feet. The symptoms may include: a tingling, burning, or prickling sensation; numbness or insensitivity to pain or temperature; sharp pains or cramps; extreme sensitivity to touch, even light touch; or loss of balance and coordination. The symptoms may be worse at night.

Autonomic neuropathy affects organs and systems that control your body functions, such as:

- **Heart and circulatory system:** damage to the nerves can cause problems in keeping your blood pressure and heart rate under control. Your blood pressure can drop quickly when you change positions. Your heart rate can stay high instead of rising and falling normally, and silent heart attacks can occur.
- **Digestive system:** nerve damage can be throughout your digestive system, causing nausea and vomiting, bloating, constipation, and/or uncontrolled diarrhea. Gastroparesis refers to a condition when the stomach empties irregularly, varying

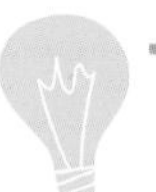

TIPS + TACTICS

Steps Specific to Nerve Damage

- *Alert your health care provider to any problems you are having that you believe may be related to a type of neuropathy.*
- *Make sure your health care provider does a complete foot exam annually to check for problems.*

  A complete foot exam should include four actions by your health care provider:
  1) *test for adequate sensation using a monofilament*
  2) *look at the bone structure and how you walk*
  3) *check for blood flow by checking your pulses and feeling your skin temperature*
  4) *observe the skin for signs of decreased blood flow and feeling*

DEFINITION:

monofilament: A tool used by your health care provider to check your sense of touch on five sites on your feet. Research has shown that if you can't sense pressure from a pinprick or monofilament, you may have lost protective sensation and are at a higher risk for developing foot problems.

between too fast and too slow. This affects how your food is absorbed, which causes challenges with blood glucose control.

- **Sexual organs:** damage can affect your sexual response whether you are a man or woman [also check out *Chapter 17*, page 219].
- **Sweat glands:** damage can cause difficulty controlling sweating, which leads to challenges in regulating body temperature, especially at night or while eating.
- **Lack of sensitivity to feeling low blood glucose:** damage can create an inability to feel the symptoms of hypoglycemia, such as shakiness and sweating [also check out *Chapter 15*, page 195].
- **Eyes:** damage can make the pupils of your eyes less sensitive to changes in light.

Proximal neuropathy can cause pain in the thighs, hips, or buttocks and leads to leg weakness. Focal neuropathy is the sudden weakness of one nerve or a group of nerves throughout your body, causing muscle weakness or pain.

PERIPHERAL NEUROPATHY VERSUS PERIPHERAL VASCULAR DISEASE

A foot problem commonly starts with a sore or blister. For example, if you have lost some sensation in your feet, you may not feel that the shoes you are wearing are too tight and are forming a blister. The blister can open and can become infected. Infection can develop from several reasons, one of which is high blood glucose. Excess glucose provides "food" for bacteria to grow on. The bacteria multiply and create an infection. Diabetes can also

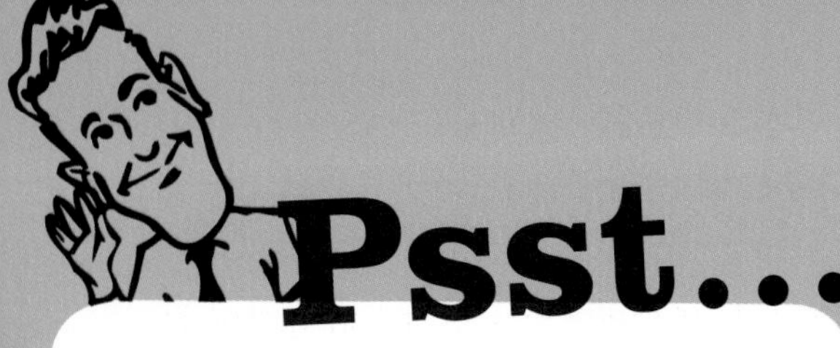

Special Shoes May be Covered by Your Health Care Plan

If you develop certain foot problems, such as a deformity caused by a bone infection, you may be advised to buy a pair of therapeutic shoes (custom molded) and inserts. These shoes are made to fit softly around your sore feet, or if your feet have changed shape due to bunions, a hammertoe, or other problems. They help protect your feet and prevent further problems. Medicare and other health care plans may cover the cost of these shoes if your health care provider completes necessary forms. Not all people with diabetes need these. Make sure you really need them. Get them only under the advice of a podiatrist or orthopedic surgeon.

affect your blood cells that fight against infection, making it more difficult to heal. All of these factors, along with poor circulation and the fact that this area is furthest from your heart, are what adds to the foot problems associated with neuropathy.

If foot injuries are not treated promptly, the infection may spread to the bone and the foot may need to be amputated. Some experts estimate that half of all amputations are preventable if minor problems are caught and treated in time.

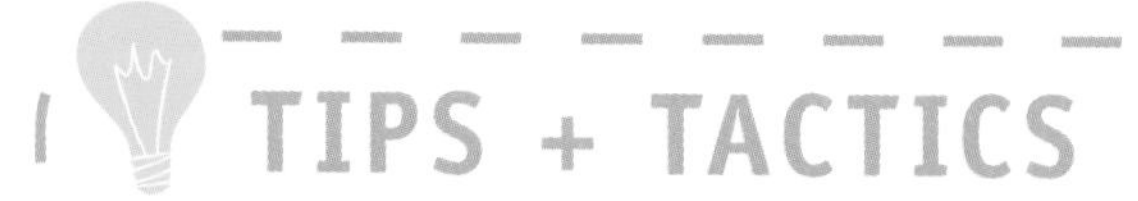

Care for Your Feet

- *Check your feet every day and become familiar with them so you can detect problems early and easily. Check for cuts, blisters, sores, swelling, redness, or sore toenails. If you can't see the bottoms of your feet, use a mirror—laying a mirror on the floor works well—or get help from someone else. If you notice changes, contact your health care provider right away. Don't put it off!*
- *Clean your feet daily, using warm water and a mild soap. Avoid soaking your feet.*
- *Keep your skin soft and supple (not dry and cracked) with a moisturizer, but don't get the moisturizer between your toes as this causes a moist environment that can cause infection.*
- *Clip or file your toenails to the shape of your toes. File corns and calluses gently with a pumice stone, using the kind that is a stone or looks more like sandpaper. Avoid the ones that are metal and look like a grater.*
- *Avoid over-the-counter foot treatments like wart or callous removers, medicated pads, or ointments unless it has been prescribed by your health care provider.*
- *Avoid walking barefoot even at home. Wear comfortable shoes that protect your feet.*
- *Buy and wear shoes that are comfortable (allow your toes to move), are protective, keep your feet warm, and fit you well. When you buy new shoes, break them in slowly. Wear them only a few hours a day at first.*
- *Take brisk walks (if you are able) to increase the blood flow in your feet and get other health benefits.*

Skin Problems: What Can Happen?

Skin problems are not often discussed when it comes to diabetes complications but you should be aware of them. Your body loses fluids with high blood glucose levels. With less fluid in your body, your skin can become dry, which can lead to itchiness, cracks, and/or sores. Scratching these can open sores and allow germs to enter and cause infection. Neuropathy can also decrease your sweat response. Because sweat helps keep your skin soft and moist, less sweat can lead to dry skin.

TIPS + TACTICS

Care for Your Skin

- *After you wash with a mild soap, rinse and pat dry.*
- *Keep your skin moist with a moisturizing cream or lotion. A moisturizer applied to damp skin locks in moisture.*
- *Check your skin for dryness, red marks, or sores that aren't healing. Pay particular attention to your legs, feet, and elbows. They can be the first to become dry, itchy and cracked.*
- *Wear all-cotton underwear. Cotton allows air to move better.*
- *Drink lots of fluids like water, eat healthy, and be physically active to keep your skin moist and healthy.*
- *Report any problems to your health care provider immediately.*

Dental Problems: What Can Happen?

There is a connection between type 2 diabetes and dental problems. That connection is inflammation [also check out *Chapter 1*, page 5]. The relationship is not fully understood at this time. Some experts think the inflammation causes diabetes and dental problems, while others think diabetes causes the dental problem called periodontitis. Periodontal means "around the tooth." Periodontal disease is a chronic infection that affects the gums and bone that supports your teeth. It can affect just one, some, or all of your teeth. You may or may not have symptoms at all. Untreated periodontal disease can increase your blood glucose. This is one reason it is important for you to see your dentist regularly so you can prevent, detect, or treat periodontal disease.

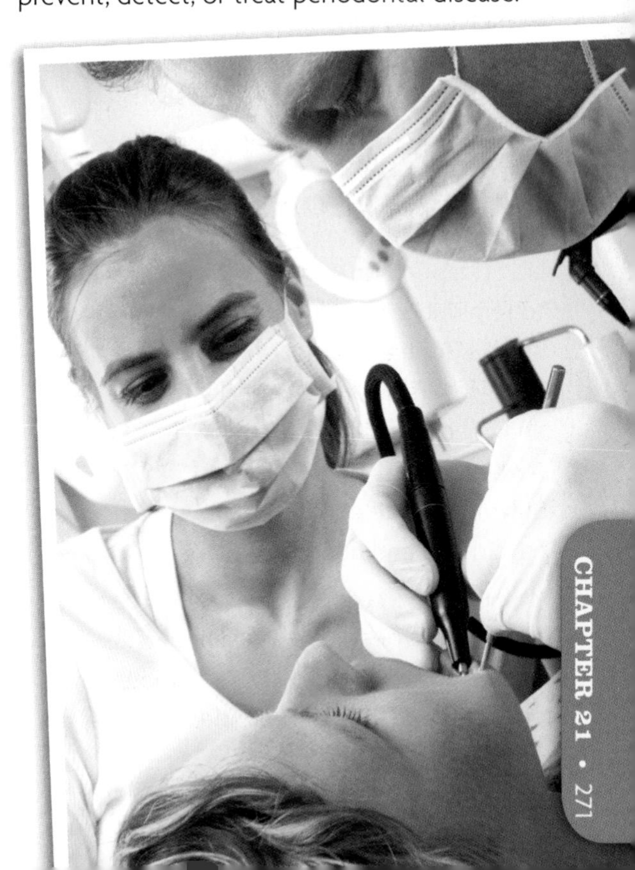

You can also experience more problems with your teeth and gums than people without diabetes if your blood glucose is uncontrolled over time. There may be a time when you do all you can to manage your blood glucose, but it just doesn't come down. You may find that you have a tooth infection, mouth sore(s), or other problems in your mouth that are causing your blood glucose to be elevated. These can then be harder to heal if your blood glucose is elevated.

Both smoking and being over 45 years old also increase your incidence of dental problems. Look out for these problems. They may mean you have a problem: red, sore, or swollen gums; bleeding gums; teeth that look long (because the gums have pulled away); loose or sensitive teeth; bad breath; dentures that are no longer comfortable; and increased blood glucose that you can't associate with other problems.

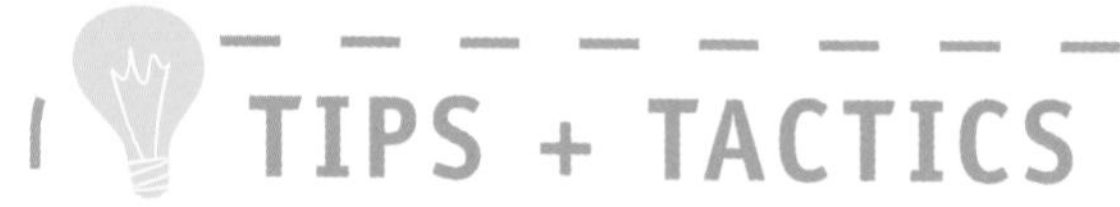

Care for Your Teeth and Gums

- *Brush your teeth at least twice a day and after each time you eat, if possible.*
- *Use a soft toothbrush with small, circular motions or an electric toothbrush. Brush the front, back, top, and gum area of each tooth. Replace your toothbrush every three to four months, or sooner if the bristles are frayed.*
- *Clean between your teeth daily with floss or an interdental cleaner. Decay-causing bacteria linger between teeth where toothbrush bristles can't reach.*
- *Keep your mouth moist. Dry mouth can lead to oral problems.*
- *Keep false teeth clean.*
- *Contact your dental care provider immediately if you have problems.*
- *Get your teeth cleaned and your gums checked twice a year or more often if advised to do so by your dental care provider.*
- *Make sure your dental care provider knows you have diabetes.*

Track Your Tests and Checks Yourself

Don't depend on your health care provider to remember to get your necessary tests and checks done or to record them in an easy-to-review flow sheet. Use the list of tests and checks on page 273 to know what to have done and when to record your results. Stay up to date on which tests and checks to have done, and how often by reviewing the ADA standards of care each January at *www.diabetes.org*, under Clinical Practice Recommendations. Once your tests and checks are complete, get your results from your health care provider and record them.

Observe the tests and checks you need to get at visits to your health care provider. Check whether you can get the lab tests done prior to your visit. Having the results in hand to discuss with your provider can make your visit more productive.

Observe the tests and checks you need annually. Think about when during the year these will be easiest for you to complete. Do you have a lighter schedule during the summer?

Tests and Checks to Prevent and Detect Complications

Get these tests and checks every 3 to 6 months (at appointments with your health care provider).

	Target results	Before and during appointments
Review blood glucose monitoring records	Fasting and before meals: 70–130 mg/dl After meals (1–2 hours after meal start): < 180 mg/dl	• Bring in written, printed, or downloaded records with your markings, observations and questions. • Discuss your targets. • Determine if you need a new meter, check if you are using your meter correctly.
A1C (average blood glucose level over the past 8–12 weeks)	< 7%	• Review your target. • Compare your A1C to your average blood glucose level.
Blood pressure	<130/80mm/Hg	• If your blood pressure is higher than 140/90 ask about blood pressure medication and keep trying to make lifestyle changes. • If you are on blood pressure medication and your blood pressure isn't under control, ask about a change or addition of medications.
Dental Care	Cleaning and exam twice a year or as advised by your dental care professional.	• Follow up on any problems identified by you or your dental provider immediately.
Weight	Modest weight loss (10 to 20 pounds) achieved through changes in eating habits, food choices and increased physical activity.	• Discuss your target weight. • For help and support request a referral to a registered dietitian and/or diabetes self-management education program.
Physical activity	Accumulate at least 30 minutes of moderate intensity activity on, ideally, most days.	• Develop an activity plan that you can implement.
Foot exam	Healthy feet	• Remove your shoes and socks and have your feet ready for your feet to be observed (note a complete foot exam only needs to be done annually. • Draw your provider's attention to any problems.
Daily aspirin use	75–162 mg/day	• If you don't currently take aspirin, ask whether you should.
Cigarette use	No smoking	• If you smoke discuss ways to quit.
Diabetes self-management education (DSME) and medical nutrition therapy (MNT)	Initial and follow up annually	• Request a referral to both DSME and MNT.

Tests and Checks to Prevent and Detect Complications

Get these tests and checks annually.

	Target results	Before and during appointments
Blood lipid profile including: **LDL** **HDL** **Triglycerides**	 <100 mg/dl >50 mg/dl <150 mg/dl	• Get tested more often than once a year if you are starting or changing therapy. • Discuss progress on lifestyle changes. Request help where needed. • If you have heart disease and are over 40 ask about taking a statin medication.
Microalbuminuria (checks kidney function—the amount of protein in urine)	<30 mcg/mg normal	• Discuss your need for a blood pressure medication, such as an ACE inhibitor or ARB.
Comprehensive eye exam with dilation of the retinas	Healthy eyes	• Schedule this to be done by an eye doctor. • Follow up on any identified problems immediately.
Check nerve function in feet and legs (tests may include pinprick sensation, temperature, feeling vibrations, and testing with 10-gram monofilament)	Healthy sensations and circulation	• Remove your shoes and socks and have your feet ready for your feet to be examined.
Flu vaccine	Get the vaccine	• Get a flu shot each year in the fall.
Pneumococcal vaccine	At least one per lifetime	• If you had it when you were under 65, you may need another one. • If you are over 65 and you've never has this you will only need to have it once. • Everyone over 2 years old should get this vaccine.

Do you have some Fridays off? Can you group tests and get them done on one day? Think about scheduling them on a significant day to help you remember—the day you were diagnosed with diabetes, your birthday, anniversary, child or grandchild's birthday.

Check up on your health care providers. Don't depend on them to remember what tests and checks you need and when. Keep track of the results of your tests and checks year after year. This will help you and your provider track your progress over time. You never know when you will have to change providers. Keep these with your important papers and keep a backup copy.

On the Horizon Tomorrow and Beyond

You have learned a lot from the pages of the *Real-Life Guide to Diabetes*. Now put this book on a nearby bookshelf so you'll be able to refer to it as you need—to review a chapter in total, answer a pressing question, or find the link to other print or online resources.

Hopefully, you have also learned that taking care of diabetes, day after day and year after year, is no easy feat. Living a healthy life with diabetes takes ongoing effort, energy, and a long-term commitment. Some days, you'll feel like you have your blood glucose and other elements of your diabetes under control. Others, you'll want to pull the hair out of your head because you just can't figure out why your blood glucose levels are so high. Managing diabetes takes pure guts and determination.

One day in the distant future, diabetes may be just another short entry in medical history books. The hope that a cure will be found is ongoing; however, from today's vantage point, even with many avenues being pursued and millions of research dollars being spent, no sure-fire preventive measures or cures for either type 1 or type 2 are here yet.

Don't hold your breath and delay good day-to-day care waiting for a cure. What's most important for you is to spend time and energy on staying healthy right now and in the future by living a healthy lifestyle and putting the best self-care practices and measures into action to prevent and/or delay complications.

Because the challenges of managing diabetes are constant and overwhelming at times, seek and find the support and coaching you need. Look for this support from your health care providers, diabetes educators, local support groups, online chat rooms, blogs, and diabetes coaching venues [also check out *Psst: Stay Abreast of Research, and Garner Support Online*, next page].

While you work hard to manage your diabetes to the best of your abilities, keep an eye out for new technologies, medications, and management strategies. The epidemic proportion of diabetes means that attention and dollars will be spent on diabetes for many years to come. Read up on these with an understanding of the type of diabetes you have, the reality of how close to the marketplace these solutions are, and how they may help you. Trust ADA and other reliable resources to keep you informed. Another way to meet and connect with people with diabetes, which is so important for both knowledge and support, is to join ADA (*www.diabetes.org*). You can get involved at the local or national level in an area of your expertise or interest.

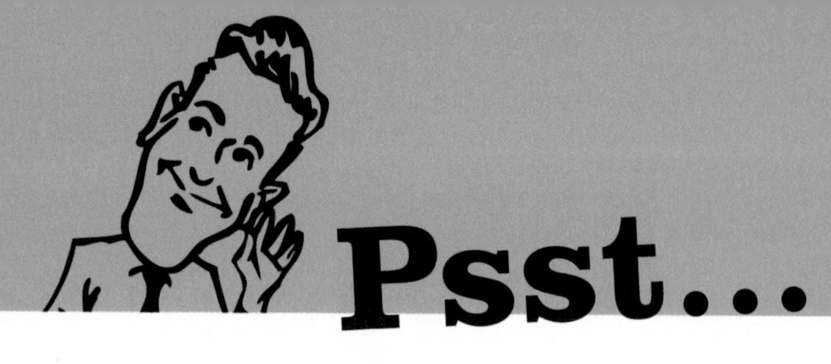

Stay Abreast of Research, and Garner Support Online

Take advantage of the Internet age as you strive to stay abreast of what's happening in diabetes research and seek out regular support.

Routes to diabetes management and research updates:

www.diabetes.org
Sign up to get online updates from *ADA In the News*, Research Summaries, Breaking News, and Tip of the Day.

www.niddk.nih.gov, www.ndep.nih.gov
Learn about large, government-sponsored studies and the latest recommendations for diabetes care from the National Institute of Diabetes, Digestive and Kidney Diseases (NIDDK) at the National Institutes of Health and the National Diabetes Education Program (NDEP).

www.jdrf.org
Juvenile Diabetes Research Foundation, a resource for research about type 1 diabetes and a link to the type 1 community.

www.childrenwithdiabetes.com
Sign up for weekly research updates, check out chats, and more. Particularly good for type 1 diabetes.

www.diabetesmine.com
Award-winning blog of Amy Tenderich, a person with diabetes, filled with up-to-the minute stories about what's happening in the world of diabetes.

Routes to online support:

www.diabetes.org
Join an ADA message board at *www.community.diabetes.org/n/forumIndex.aspx?webtag=adaindex*.

www.behavioraldiabetes.org
An organization developed to tackle the unmet psychological needs of people with diabetes.

www.dlife.com
An online resource for information and community support.

www.diabeticconnect.com
A place to find support and information to help you feel less frustrated about living with diabetes.

www.diabeticlivingonline.com
An online resource for information, recipes, and support.

www.fit4D.com
Obtain one-on-one diabetes coaching with diabetes education experts.

www.mydiabetespartner.org
From the American Association of Diabetes Educators (AADE), this is a partner approach to diabetes self-care, reaching out to people who have diabetes and their partners.

www.diabetesselfmanagement.com
Award-winning, bi-monthly magazine with up-to-date diabetes-related articles.

www.diabeteshealth.com

INDEX

C

D

E

F

G

H

N

O

P

R

S

T

U

V

W

X

Y

Author Biographies

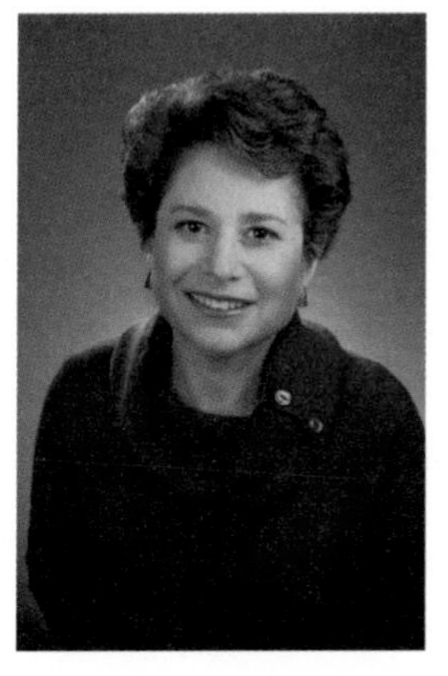

Hope Warshaw, MMSc, RD, CDE, BC-ADM is a nationally recognized dietitian and diabetes educator. She has 30 years of expertise as a book author, freelance writer, media spokesperson, and consultant. Hope has counseled thousands of people individually to make realistic lifestyle changes to improve their diabetes control and health. Hope is currently a contributing editor for *Diabetic Living* (a Better Homes & Gardens magazine). She has authored numerous books published by the American Diabetes Association, including *Diabetes Meal Planning Made Easy*, *Guide to Healthy Restaurant Eating*, and *Complete Guide to Carb Counting*. Hope has been a tireless volunteer in the cause of diabetes and is the recipient of the American Diabetes Association's Outstanding Community Service in Reaching People award and the Distinguished Service award from the American Dietetic Association's Diabetes Care and Education group. Connect with Hope at *www.hopewarshaw.com*.

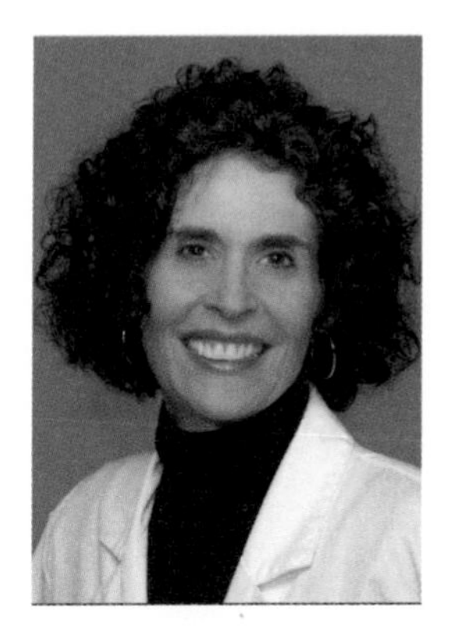

Joy Pape, RN, BSN, CDE, WOCN, CFCN is a nationally recognized certified diabetes nurse educator and certified foot care nurse. Her mission and passion stems from her personal and strong family history of diabetes, obesity, heart disease, depression, and other related problems. Joy has polycystic ovarian syndrome (PCOS) and pre-diabetes. She has lost 60 pounds and has kept it off for 20 years. Joy brings a wealth of knowledge with her lifetime of personal real-life experiences, as well as over 30 years of professional experience with people in nearly every health care setting, from home health, to intensive care units, and everything in between. She understands that knowledge is the beginning of managing health issues, but that it takes spirituality, grit, humor, and love to be able to put it into practice. She is a partner of Laugh It Off!, a health education and comedy team whose mission it is to Educate, Enlighten, and Entertain. Connect with Joy at *www.joypape.com*.

Other Titles from the American Diabetes Association

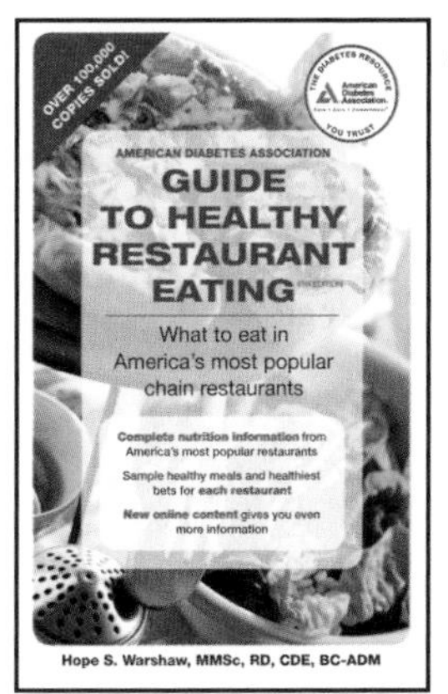

Guide to Healthy Restaurant Eating, 4th Edition
by Hope Warshaw, MMSc, RD, CDE, BC-ADM
Eat smart before you ever sit down! *Guide to Healthy Restaurant Eating* provides essential nutrition information for the nation's most popular restaurants. Get counts for calories, carbohydrate, fat, and protein; know the exchanges/choices and serving sizes for every menu item; and avoid dining disasters and pitfalls. Now you can find a nutritious meal that fits your diabetes meal plan just about anywhere!

Order no. 4819-04; Price $17.95

Ultimate Diabetes Meal Planner
by Jaynie Higgins and David Groetzinger
Fitness and nutrition expert Jaynie Higgins takes the guesswork out of diabetes meal planning and puts everything you need in one amazing collection. With 16 weeks of meal plans and over 300 amazing recipes, this book will guide you toward a healthy, diabetes-friendly lifestyle. You'll find meal plans in four different calorie levels and shopping lists to make grocery shopping a breeze. Take the mystery out of food in just 4 easy steps!

Order no. 4725-01; Price $21.95

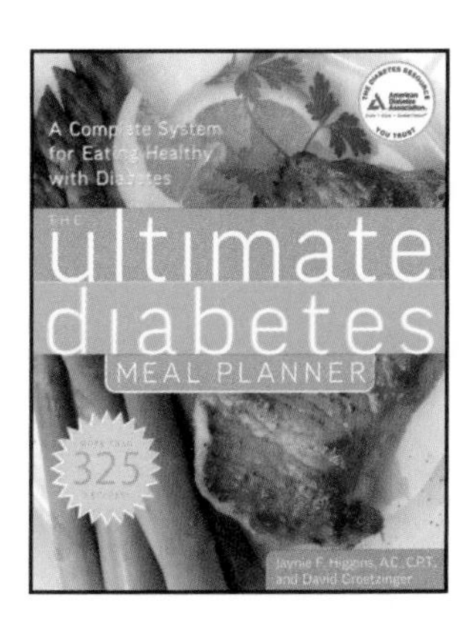

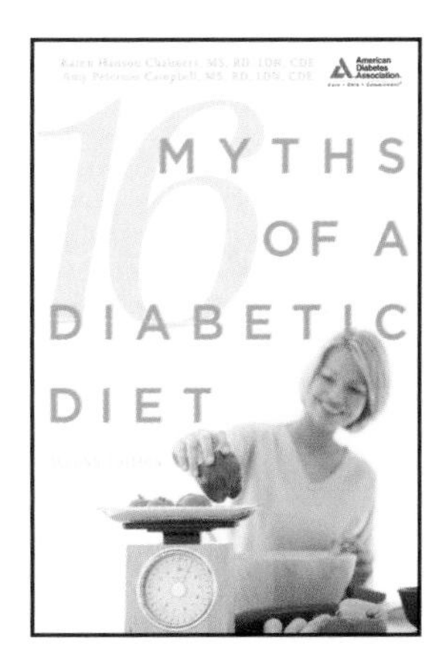

16 Myths of a Diabetic Diet, 2nd Edition
by Karen Hanson Chalmers, MS, RD, LDN, CDE, and Amy Peterson
16 Myths of a Diabetic Diet will tell you the truth about diabetes and how to eat when you have diabetes. Learn what the most common myths about diabetes meal plans are, where they came from, and how to overcome them. Diabetes doesn't have to be a life sentence of boring, dull meals. Let experts Karen Chalmers and Amy Campbell show you how to create and follow a healthy, enjoyable way of eating.

Order no. 4829-02; Price $14.95

To order these and other great American Diabetes Association titles, call **1-800-232-6733** or visit http://store.diabetes.org. American Diabetes Association titles are also available in bookstores nationwide.